HERBAL COSMETICS
AND
BEAUTY PRODUCTS

Useful Books on COSMETICS TECHNOLOGIES

HAND BOOK OF SYNTHETIC & HERBAL COSMETICS

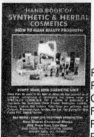

The Book covers Production Problems & Recommendations, Cosmetic and Drugs, Face Powder, Variations of Face Powder, Toilet Powder, Creams, Vanishing Creams, Foundation Creams, Hand Lotions, After Shaving Lotions, Deodorants, Mascara-eyebrow Pencils-Eye Shadows, Lipsticks, Shampoos, Depilatories, Shaving Cream, Cosmetics for Nails, Tooth Powder, Tooth Paste, Mouth Washes, Facial Masks, Cosmetics for Eyes, Cosmetic for Babies, Herbal Cosmetic for the Skin, Hair Shampoos, Anti Dandruff Preparations, Hair Straighteners, Hair Dyes, Bleaches, Colourings and Dye Removers, Oral Herbal Preparations, Govt.. Regulations & Acts on Drugs & Cosmetics, Bath Preparations, Baby Preparations, Home Made Cosmetics, Herbal Preparations for Body, Skin Cleansing, Herbal Preparations for Feet & Hands, Herbal Shampoo and Setting, How to Layout a Cosmetic Factory, Project Profiles on Various Cosmetics with Herbal etc.

HERBAL COSMETICS & BEAUTY PRODUCTS

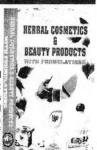

The major chapters and details of the book are : Useful Cosmetic Herbs : This chapter covers the detailed information on herbs used in herbal cosmetics, List of Common Cosmetics Herbs their active constituents and cosmetic applications, Plant and Equipments for Herbal Cosmetics Manufacture, Skin Cream and Lotions, Pomades and Beauty Masks, Hair Washes and Shampoo, Aromatic and Toilet Waters, Natural Perfumes, Herbal Extraction, Packaging of Herbal Cosmetics, Herbal Cosmetic Technology with various formulations, Herbal Cosmetics for beauty parlours with formulae i.e. Shampoo, Lotions, Cleansing creams, Moisturizer, Face scrubs, Egg Face pack, Cucumber face packs, Face packs for for patchy skin, Tomato face pack, Methi Shikakai Shampoo, Sandalwood shampoo, Neem Shampoo, Sunflower Hair Conditioner, Clove Hair Setting Preparation, Anti dandruff preparation etc. Details of setting up an establishment of a herbal beauty parlour, Herbal beauty products manufacture, List and their addresses of Herbs Suppliers, Apart from these details, the book also discloses the major other untold chapters which are quite important for those who wish to enter into herbal cosmetic trade. Frankly speaking- the book is also quite indispensable for those who have also setup their industry.

COSMETICS PROCESSES & FORMULATIONS HAND BOOK (WITH HERBAL COSMETICS TECHNOLOGY & FORMULAE)

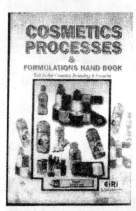

The Book covers Processes and Formulations of Cosmetics and Important chapters are Equipments and Raw Materials with Packaging of Cosmetics, Skin Cream, Skin Products, Bath Products, Deodorants and Antiperspirants Preparations, Depilatories, Foot Cosmetics, Shaving Preparations, Sunscreen, Suntan and Anti Sunburn Products, Face Powders and Makeup, Coloured Makeup, Oral Hygiene, Hair Colourants, Shampoo, Nail and Manicure Products, Hair Setting Lotions and Conditioners, Tooth Paste and Powder, Mouth Washes, Permanent Waving, Herbal Cosmetics, Skin Lighteners or Bleaches, Quality Control of Cosmetics, Testing of Cosmetics, Plant Economics of Herbal Cosmetics, Shampoo, Soap & Herbal Soap, Herbal Hair Oil, Nail Enamel, Talcum Powder, Modern Cosmetic Project, Antisep[tic Cream, Tooth Paste (Gel Type), Lipsticks, Baby Oil, Details of Plant Equipment and Machinery used to produce Cosmetic Products, Manufacturers/Suppliers of Plant and Machinery and Raw Materials, Packaging Materials etc.

ENGINEERS INDIA RESEARCH INSTITUTE   4449, Nai Sarak, Main Road, Delhi-6

HERBAL COSMETICS AND BEAUTY PRODUCTS

Written By
EIRI BOARD OF CONSULTANTS & ENGINEERS

ENGINEERS INDIA RESEARCH INSTITUTE

4449, Nai Sarak, Main Road, Delhi - 110 006 (India)
Ph:. 91-11- 3918117, 3916431, 3920361, 3960797
Fax: 91-11- 391 6431
* E-Mail : eirisidi@bol.net.in
* Website: www.startindustry.com

Sole Distributor :

INDIAN INSTITUTE OF CONSULTANTS, 4/27, ROOP NAGAR, DELHI - 110 007

PRINTED & PUBLISHED BY

ENGINEERS INDIA RESEARCH INSTITUTE

4449, Nai Sarak, Main Road, Delhi - 110 006 (India)
Ph:. 91-11- 3918117, 3916431, 3920361, 3960797
* Fax: 91-11- 3916431, 3918117
* E-Mail : eirisidi@bol.net.in
* Website: www.startindustry.com

DISTRIBUTED BY

SMALL INDUSTRY RESEARCH INSTITUTE
INDIAN INSTITUTE OF CONSULTANTS

© Copy Reserved by Sudhir Gupta, Delhi.

ISBN : 81- 86732-45-4
Printed in New Delhi (INDIA)

The book is sold subject to the condition that it shall not, by way or trade or otherwise, be lent, resold, hired out, or otherwise circulated without the publisher's prior written cinsent, in any form of binding or cover other than in which it is published/compiled and without a similar consent including this condition being imposed on the subsequent purchaser and without limiting the rights under copy rights reserved above, no part of this publication may be reproduced, stored in or introduced into a retrieval system, of transmitted in any form or by any means (electronic, mechanical, photocopying or otherwise), without the written prior permission of both the copyright owner and above mentioned publisher of this book. While the book has been prepared carefully, yet the publisher's, printer and compiler do not hold any responsibility on the subject of the book. All disputes regarding this book are Subject to Delhi Jurisdiction only

Rs. 750

Printed & Published by Sudhir Gupta for **"Engineers India Research Institute"** 4449 Nai Sarak, Main Road, New Delhi - 110 006 and Printed at Swastik Offset, Shahadra, Delhi - 32

NEW DETAILED PROJECT REPORTS AVAILABLE ON
COSMETICS WITH HERBAL INDUSTRIES @ Rs. 3675/- each

LIST OF READILY AVAILABLE DETAILED PROJECT REPORTS

- AFTER SHAVE LOTION
- ANTISEPTIC CREAM
- ALLETHRIN MOSQUITO REPELLENT OIL
- AGARBATTI SYNTHETIC PERFUMERY COMPOUND
- AGARBATTI BY MACHINE
- AYURVEDIC CREAM
- BABY OIL
- BOROPLUS TYPE ANTISEPTIC CREAM
- AYURVEDIC MEDICINE
- BINDIYA
- BLACK TOOTH POWDER (MONKEY BRAND TYPE)
- BLACK HAIR DYE IN FORM OF HAIR OIL
- CAR SHAMPOO
- COLD CREAM
- COLD WAVE FOR HAIR CURLING
- COSMETIC UNIT (HERBAL AND SYNTHETIC)
- COSMETIC (MODERN)
- COSMETIC INDUSTRY, SHAMPOO,
- SPRAY PERFUME, TALCUM POWDER
- EGG SHAMPOO
- FACE MASK (LIQUID FORM)
- FACE CREAM & BODY CREAM
- FISH OIL SOAP
- HAIR FIXER
- HAIR DYE POWDER
- HAIR DYE IN CREAM FORM
- HAIR REMOVING CREAM
- HAIR REMOVING WAX
- HAIR OILS
- HAIR FIXER & HAIR GEL
- HAIR STYLING GEL
- HENNA PASTE
- HERBAL COSMETICS
- HERBAL HAIR OIL
- HERBAL SHAMPOO & CREAM
- HERBAL TOOTH PASTE AND TOOTH POWDER
- HERBAL PRODUCTS COMPLEX
- KALI MEHANDI (HENNA)
- KAJAL
- KESH KALA TEL (HAIR DYE LOTION)
- LIQUID BINDI (KUMKUM TYPE)
- LIQUID BINDI AND SINDUR
- LIPSTICKS
- MEDICATED OIL
- MOSQUITO COIL & MATS
- NAIL POLISH & NAIL POLISH REMOVER
- NAIL ENAMEL
- NEUTRALIZER (FOR HAIR CURLING)
- SCENTS & PERFUMES
- SHAVING CREAM
- SINDUR
- SHAMPOO
- TALCUM POWDER
- TOOTH PASTE AND POWDER
- TOILET AND HERBAL SOAP
- TOILET SOAP
- TOOTH PASTE (GEL TYPE)
- TOOTH PASTE FROM TOBACCO DUST
- WASHING AND LAUNDRY SOAP
- TOILET CLEANER (HARPIK TYPE)
- DOG SOAP

Each 'EIRI' *Market Survey Cum Detailed Techno Economic Feasibility Report (Detailed Project Report)* covers Introduction, Uses & Applications, Properties, Market Survey, Present Manufacturers, Process of Manufacture, Formulations, Process Flow Sheet Diagram, Cost Economics with Profitability Analysis, B.E.P., Resources of Finance Suppliers of Plant & Machineries and Raw Materials, Cash Flow Statement, Repayment Schedule, Depreciation Chart, Projected Balance Sheet etc.

* Price **Rs. 3675/-** (Rs. Three Thousand Six Hundred Seventy Five Only) for Each Report OR US$ 250/- for overseas clients. Just Send Draft/M.O./Cash in favour of **"ENGINEERS INDIA RESEARCH INSTITUTE"**, DELHI. (Payable In India) (Delivery within Two Days)

Send your remittance through Draft/M.O. only at:

ENGINEERS INDIA RESEARCH INSTITUTE
4449, Nai Sarak, Main Road, Delhi - 110 006 (INDIA)
Ph./Fax : 91-11- 3918117, 3916431, 3920361, 3960797
E-Mail : eirisidf@bol.net.in Website: www.startindustry.com

ISBN : 81-86732-45-4

Preface

The book *'Herbal Cosmetics & Beauty Products'* covers almost all the basic and advanced details to setup own Herbals Cosmetic unit. Be it at home, beauty parlour or on industry level. The major chapters and details of the book are : Useful Cosmetic Herbs : This chapter covers the detailed information on herbs used in herbal cosmetics, List of Common Cosmetics Herbs their active constituents and cosmetic applications, Plant and Equipments for Herbal Cosmetics Manufacture, Skin Cream and Lotions, Pomades and Beauty Masks, Hair Washes and Shampoo, Aromatic and Toilet Waters, Natural Perfumes, Herbal Extraction, Packaging of Herbal Cosmetics, Herbal Cosmetic Technology with various formulations, Herbal Cosmetics for beauty parlours with formulae i.e. Shampoo, Lotions, Cleansing creams, Moisturizer, Face scrubs, Egg Face pack, Cucumber face packs, Face packs for for patchy skin, Tomato face pack, Methi Shikakai Shampoo, Sandalwood shampoo, Neem Shampoo, Sunflower Hair Conditioner, Clove Hair Setting Preparation, Anti dandruff preparation etc. Details of setting up an establishment of a herbal beauty parlour, Herbal beauty products manufacture, List and their addresses of Herbs Suppliers, Apart from these details, the book also discloses the major other untold chapters which are quite important for those who wish to enter into herbal cosmetic trade. Frankly speaking- the book is also quite indispensable for those who have also setup their industry.

The book has been written for the benefit and to prove an asset and a handy reference guide in the hands of new entrepreneurs & well established industrialists.

Director
ENGINEERS INDIA RESEARCH INSTITUTE
Nai Sarak, New Delhi (INDIA)
E-Mail : eirisidi@bol.net.in

Contents and Subject Index

Chapters	Page No.
Chapter 1	
USEFUL COSMETIC HERBS	**1-37**
- Aloe Vera Linn. (Ghrita Kumari/Kumari)	1
- Buchanania Lanzan Spreng (Chironji)	2
- Cucumis Sativa Linn. (Kheera)	2
- Datura Stramonium Linn. (Dhatura)	3
- Eclipta alba Hassk (Bhringraj)	4
- Foeniculum Vulgare Mill (Saunf)	4
- Glycyrrhiz Glabra Linn. (Mulatthi)	5
- Hibiscus ros-sinensis Linn. (Jasut/China Rose)	6
- Impatiens balsamina Linn. (Gul Mehandi)	7
- Impatiens Linn. (Gulmendi)	8
- Indigofera Linn.	8
- Inula Linn.	8
- Ipomea Linn.	8
- Ipomoea obscura (Linn.)	8
- Ipomea pescaprae Sw.	8
- Ipomoea pes-tigridis Linn.	9
- Iris Linn.	9
- Iris nepalensis D. Don	9
- Iris germanica Linn.	9
- Ixora Linn.	9
- Jasminum officinale Linn. (Chameli)	10
- Jasminum Linn.	11
- Jatropha curcas Linn.	11
- Jateorhiza palmata (Lam.)	11
- Juglans Linn.	11
- Juniperus oxycedrus Linn.	12
- Juniperus Virginiana Linn.	12
- Jussiaea tenella Burm.f.	12
- Lawsonia inermis Linn. (Henna)	13

Chapters	Page No.
- Lactuca Linn.	14
- Lactuca scariola Linn.	14
- Lagenandra Dalz.	14
- Lagenaria Ser.	14
- Lagerstroemia Linn.	14
- Mours alba Linn. (Shah-Tut)	15
- Nardostachys jatamansi DC. (Jatmansi)	15
- Nardostachys Dc.	17
- Neea Ruiz & Pav.	17
- Neocallitropsis Florin	17
- Nicandra Adans.	17
- Nelumbo (Tourn.) Adans	17
- Nepeta Linn.	17
- Nepeta cateria Linn.	18
- Nepeta hindostana(Roth) Haines	18
- Nerium Linn.	18
- Nyctanthes Linn.	18
- Nymphaea Linn.	18
- Ocimum sanctum Linn. (Tulsi)	19
- Ocimum Linn.	20
- Ocimum canum sims.	20
- Oenothera Linn.	20
- Oncnotis Benth.	20
- Ononis Linn.	20
- Olendra Cav.	20
- Ophioglossum Linn.	20
- Origanum Linn.	21
- Oxalis Linn.	21
- Oxystelma R.Br.	21
- Pennisetum glaucum R.Br.	22
- Quillaja saponaria Molina (Soap Bark)	22
- Quassia Linn.	23
- Quillaja Molina	23
- Rosa damascena Mill (Rose)	24
- Radermachera Zoll. & Moritzi	25
- Rafflesia R.Br.	25
- Randia Linn.	25
- Ranunculus Linn.	25
- Simmondsia Chinensis (Link)	

Chapters	Page No.
C.Schneid	26
- Saccharomyes Meyenx Hansen.	27
- Salacia Linn.	27
- Salmea DC.	27
- Salvia Linn.	27
- Trigonella foenum-graecum Linn.	28
- Tacca J.R. and G.Frost	29
- Tamarindus Tourn.ex.Linn.	29
- Tamarix Linn.	29
- Tanacetum Linn.	29
- Urtica dioca Linn. (Bichoo Booti/Stinging Nettle)	30
- Urginea Steinh	31
- Urtica Linn.	31
- Usnea Linn.	31
- Vetiveria zizanioides (Linn.) Nash. (Khus)	32
- Vallaris Burm.f.	33
- Valeriana Linn.	33
- Vanilla Mill.	33
- Vauque Correa.ex.Humb & Bonpl.	33
- Ventilago Gaertn	33
- Withania somenifera Dunal (Ashwagandha)	34
- Wahlenbergia schard.ex.Roth.	35
- Waltheria Linn.	35
- Weinmannia Linn.	35
- Widelia Jacq.	35
- Withania Paug.	35
- Xylopia Linn.	36
- Yucca Linn.	36
- Zamia Linn.	36
- Zanthoxylum Linn.	36
- Zizyphus Toum.ex Linn.	37

Chapter 2

A LIST OF COMMON COSMETIC HERBS THEIR ACTIVE CONSTITUENTS AND COSMETIC APPLICATIONS	**38-47**
- Acacia Concinna (PODS) (Shikakai)	38
- Achillea millefolium (WH) (Millefoil)	38
- Allium cepa (Bulbs) (Onion)	38
- Aloe vera (exudate) (Aloe)	38
- Althea officinals (W/H) (Marsh Mallow)	38
- Ammi magis (Seeds) (Creater Ammi)	38

Chapters	Page No.
- Agnelica archangelica (Roots) (Angelica)	38
- Angelica keiskei (Leaves) (Angelica)	38
- Apium graveolens (Fruits) (Celery)	39
- Arctium lappa (Roots) (Burdock)	39
- Arnica montana (W/H) (Arnica)	39
- Artemesia abrotanum (Southern wood)	39
- Azadirachta indica (leaf & bark) (Neem Tree)	39
- Betula alba (sap) (Beech)	39
- Betula alba (Bark) (Beech)	39
- Bidens cernua (W/H) (Burr marigold)	39
- Borago officinalis (W/H) (Borage)	39
- Camellia sinesis (Leaves) (Tea)	39
- Carum carvi (Caraway)	40
- Centella asiatica (whole herb) (Gotukola)	40
- Citrus limonum (Lemon)	40
- Cola nitida (seeds) (Cola)	40
- Convallaria majlis (Lily of the valley)	40
- Coptis teeta (Rhizome) (Mamira)	40
- Cucumis Sativa (Fruit) (Cucumber)	40
- Curcuma longa(Rhizome)(Turmeric)	40
- Daucus carota (Rhizome) (Carrot)	40
- Echinalea angustifolia (W/H) (Coneflower)	40
- Eclipta alba (whole herb) (Bhringraj)	40
- Emblica officinalis (fruits) (Amla)	41
- Equisetum arvense (whole herb) (Horse tail)	41
- Erythrea centaurium(W/H) (Centaury)	41
- Euphrasia officinalis (W/H) (Eyebright)	41
- Foeneculum vulgare (Fruit) (Fennel)	41
- Fumaria officinails (W/H) (Fumitory)	41
- Geum urbanum (Roots) (Avens)	41
- Glycyrrhiza glabra (Roots) (Liquorice)	41
- Goosypium species (Roots) (Cotton)	41
- Hamamelis virginicus(Bark) (Witch hazel)	41
- Hibiscus rosa sinensis (Flowers) (Chinarose)	41
- Humulus lupulus (Catkins) (Hops)	42
- Hypericum perforatum (W/H)	42

New Books Published from EIRI

HAND BOOK OF SYNTHETIC DETERGENTS WITH FORMULATIONS

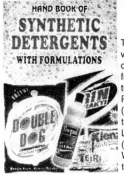

The unique and latest edition has just published. The book covers chapters viz. Group of Synthetic Detergents, Synthesis of Detergents, Manufacture of Finished Detergents, Formulations and Applications of Detergents, Perfuming of Soap and Detergents, Testing of Soaps and Detergents, Manufacturing of Herbal Synthetic Detergents, Detergents Bars, Herbal Liquid and Paste Detergents, Acid Slurry, Anionic Detergents, Detergent Washing Powder (Ariel Type- Enzyme Detergents), Synthetic Detergents (Blue Powder), Detergent Cake (Nirma Type), Cleaning Powder, Detergent Cake and Powder, Laundry and Dry Cleaners, Liquid Toilet Cleaner (Harpik Type), Acid Slurry (LAB), Nerol Laundry Soap, Liquid Detergents for Wool, Laundry for Clothes Washing, Nirma Type Detergent Powder, Non-Ionic Liquid Detergents, Detergent paste (Textile Grade), Spray Dried Detergent Powder, Washing & Laundry Soap, Zeolite -A Manufacturing (Detergent Grade), Detergent Washing Powder (Surf Excel Type), Detergent Powder Plants - Dry Mix Process, Laundry Soap Manufacturing Plant, Toilet (Bath) Soap Finishing Line, Detergent Cake Manufacturing Plants, Suppliers of Plant and Equipments and Raw materials etc.

HAND BOOK OF AGRO CHEMICAL INDUSTRIES (INSECTICIDES & PESTICIDES)

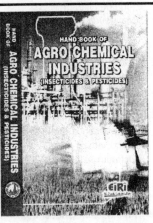

The Book covers Agro Chemical Industries with processes and Formulae including Organic Insecticides, BHC, Synthetic Insecticides, Fungicides, Nematicides, Rodenticides, Molluscicides, Fumigants, Acaricides, Herbicides, Plant Growth Regulators, Repellents, Attractants, Pheromones, Synergists, Synthetic Inhibitors & Proinsecticides, Toxicology and Safe Use of Pesticides, Insecticide Act, Pesticide Formulations, Pesticide Mixtures, Modern Equipments for a Pesticide Formulation Laboratory and Pilot Plant, Aerosol Formulations, Advances in Pesticides Formulations, Various different Project Profiles related with Insecticides and Pesticides including Neem Pesticides, Insecticides, Mosquito Agarbatti, Aerosol Insecticide Spray etc., Suppliers of Plant and Equipments and Raw Materials have also been provided for the new entrants in this line.

PAINT VARNISH SOLVENTS AND COATING TECHNOLOGY

The Book 'Paint Varnish Solvents and Coating Technology' covers Introduction, General Pigments Physical Properties, Pigments Processing, Plasticizers and Solvents, Synthetic Resins, Cellulose Ester and Ether Products, Varnishes, Pigmentation, Paints (Decorative & Building), Coatings (Water Borne), Methods of Applications, Industrial Paints and Coatings, Industrial Finishes, Miscellaneous Coatings and Ancillary Materials, Testing and Evaluation, Miscellaneous Formulae, Project Profiles of Aluminium Paints, Cement Paints, Acrylic Emulsion Paints, Insulating Varnish, Powder Coating, Primer Paints and many others. Suppliers of Raw Materials, Suppliers of Plant and Machinery, Present Manufacturers, Packaging Material Addresses and many other details.

Chapters	Page No.
- Inula helenium (Roots) (Elecampane)	42
- Jasminum officinale (flowers) (Jasmine)	42
- Juniperus spp. (leaves) (Juniper)	42
- Lactuca sativa (fruits) (Lettuce)	42
- Lavandula vera (Flowers) (Lavender)	42
- Lawsonia inermis (Leaves) (Henna)	
- Levisticum officinale (W/H) (Lovage)	42
- Lonicera perclymenum (W/H) (Honey suckle)	43
- Lycopersicum pimpinellifolium (F) (Currant tomato)	43
- Magnolia officinalis (Bark) (Magrolia Bark)	43
- Matricharia chamoilla (Flowers) (chamomille)	43
- Malaleuca alternifolia (Leaves) (Tea Tree Oil)	43
- Malalenca leucodendron (Leaves) (Cajupat)	43
- Mentha piperita(Leaves)(Peppermint)	43
- Morus alba (Bark) (Mulberry)	43
- Myrtus communis (leaves) (Vilayati Mehandi)	43
- Nardostachys jatamansi (Roots) (Jatamansi)	43
- Ocimum sanctum (W/H) (Holy Basil)	43
- Oenothera biennis (Seeds) (Evening primerose)	44
- Panax quinquefolia(Roots)(Ginseng)	44
- Pennesetum glaucum (Grain) (Pearl millet)	44
- Persea gratissma(Leaves)(Avocada)	44
- Petroselinum crispum (W/H) (Common Parsley)	44
- Phaseolus vulgaris (Peels) (Garden bean)	44
- Pilocarpus jaborandi (Leaves) (jaborandi)	44
- Pimpinella anisum (W/H)(Star Anise)	44
- Plantago major (W/H) (Plantain)	44
- Polygonum multiflorum (Roots)	44
- Pongamia Pinnata (Karanj Tree)	45

Chapters	Page No.
- Primula vulgaris(Flowers)(Primrose)	45
- Rose damascena (Petals) (Rose)	45
- Rosemarianus officinailis (Leaves) (Rosemary)	45
- Salix species (leaves) (Willow)	45
- Salvia officinails (W/H) (Sage)	45
- Salvia sclarea (W/H) (Clary sage)	45
- Sambucus nigra (Flower) (Elder)	45
- Sanguinaria canadensis (Roots) (Blood Root)	45
- Santalum album (Wood) (Sandal)	45
- Sapindus mukorassi (Fruits) (Soap nut)	46
- Saponaria officinalis(bark) (Soapwort)	46
- Simmondsia chinensis (Seeds) (Jojoba)	46
- Stellaria media (W/H) (Chickweed)	46
- Swertia species (whole herb) (Swertia)	46
- Syphytum officinale (Roots) (Comfrey)	46
- Taraxacum officinale (whole Herb) (Dandelion)	46
- Thuja occidentalis (Leaves) (White Cedar)	46
- Thymus serpyllum (W/H) (Wild Thyme)	46
- Thymus vulgaris (W/H) (Thyme)	46
- Trigonella foenum graecum (Seeds) (Fenugreek)	46
- Tropaeolum majus (W/H)	47
- Tussilago Farfara (leaves) (Colt's foot)	47
- Urtica urens (W/H) (Nettle)	47
- Veronica officinalis (W/H) (Spped well)	47
- Vetiveria zizaniodes (Roots) (Khus)	47
- Viola odorata (W/H) (Sweet violet)	47
- Viola tricolor (whole herb) (Heartease)	47
- Viscum album (Leaves & Fruits) (Mistletoe)	47
- Vitis vInifera (leaves/fruits) (Grapes)	
- Zingiber officinale (Rhizome)	47

Chapters	Page No.
Chapter 3	
EQUIPMENT USED IN THE MANUFACTURE OF COSMETICS	**48-75**
- Introduction	48
- Manufacture of Bulk Product	48
- Unit Manufacture	50
- Mixing	50
- Solid-Solid Mixing	51
- Manufacture of Pigmented Powder Products	51
- Hammer Mill	51
- Batch Colour Correction	53
- Vertical vortex mixer	54
- Plough-Shear	55
- Mixing Processes involving fluids	55
- General Principles of Fluid Mixing	55
- Mixing Equipment for Fluids	56
- Paddle Mixers	57
- Turbines	57
- Propeller Mixers	58
- Mixing in Non-Newtonian Liquids of Low or Medium Viscosity	59
- Impeller Types and Mixers for High Viscosity Fluids	59
- High Shear Mixers and Dispersion Equipment	61
- Solid-Liquid Mixing	64
- Suspension of Solids in agitated Tanks	68
- Complete Suspension	68
- Homogeneous Suspension	68
- Liquid-Liquid Mixing	69
- Miscible Liquids	69
- Immiscible Liquids	69
- The emulsification Process	69
- Orientation of Phases	70
- Addition of Surfactant	70
- Batch Processing Equipment	71
- Continuous Processing	72
- Emulsion Temperature	74
- Storage of Cosmetic powders	75

Chapters	Page No.
Chapter 4	
PLANT & EQUIPMENT FOR HERBAL COSMETICS MANUFACTURE	**76-85**
- Heating Equipment	77
- Grinders/Micro Pulverisers	77
- Sieving & Grading Equipment	78
- Dry-Mixing Equipment	78
- Wet Mixing Equipment	79
- Homogenizing Equipment	79
- Emulsification Equipment	79
- Preparation of cosmetic emulsion	80
- Ingredient	80
- Some oil phase ingredients	81
- Method of preparation	82
- Control of the thickness of emulsion	82
- Cause of failure of emulsion Preparations	83
- Emulsification process for preparation of herbal creams	83
- Straining, Filtering & Clarifying	84
- Filling liquids	84
- Filling Pastes - Creams	84
- Labelling Equipment	85
Chapter 5	
QUALITY CONTROL OF COSMETICS	**86-92**
- Introduction	86
- The Microbiological Laboratory Assurance of Purity and Hygiene	87
- Raw Material Inspection	87
- Inspection of the Finished Product	88
- Inspection of Containers and Packaging Materials	88
- Skip Lot Inspection	88
- Source Inspection	89
- Vendor Certification	89
- Computer-Assisted Delivery Testing	89
- In-Process Control	89
- Integrated Inspection Processes in the Manufacture of the Finished Product	90
- Finished Goods Control	90

Books on Paints, Plastic, Adhesive, Paints & Inks

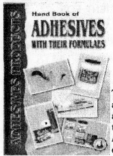

HAND BOOK OF ADHESIVES WITH THEIR FORMULAES

The book covers almost all the basic and advanced details to setup own unit of Adhesives & Gums etc., Manufacturers & suppliers of machinery & equipments and suppliers of raw materials & chemicals used in adhesive, glues & sealants industries. Apart from these, present manufacturers, dealers & suppliers of glue & adhesives have also been provided.

RUBBER CHEMICALS & PROCESSING INDUSTRIES

The Book covers Natural & Synthetic Rubber, Acrylic Rubber, ABR, Butyl Rubber, Nitrile Rubber, Silicone Rubber, Urethane Rubber, Rubber Powder, Rubber Reclamation, Pigments and Colours, Rubber Blowing Agents, Latex Dipped Goods, Latex Foam Products, Latex Based Adhesive and Rubber Solution, Rubber Moulded Articles, Rubber Beltings, Rubber Rollers, Rubber Footwears, Tyres & Tubes, Rubber Gaskets, Seals and Washers, Rubber Auto Parts, Various Other Important Formulaes, Polymers Related to Rubber, Compounding, Processing Methods, Testing, Trade Names & Chemical Compositions, Suppliers of Plant & Machinery, Suppliers of Raw Materials, Project Profiles, Details of Rubber Process Equipments & Machineries etc.

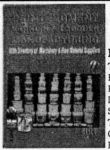

PAINT PIGMENT VARNISH & LACQUER MANUFACTURING

The book covers Paint & Enamels, Solvent & Plasticisers, More Other Important Details on Solvent and Plasticisers, Thinners, Powder Coating, Bituminous Paint, Synthetic Enamel Paints, Emulsion Paints, Distempers, N.C. Lacquers, Pigments & Extenders, Varnishes, Paints Formulaes, Varnish Formulaes, Important Formulations of Ready Mixed and Stiff Paints, Insulating Varnishes and Wire Enamels, Testing & Evaluation of Paints, Project Profiles, Suppliers of Plant, Equipments and Machineries, Suppliers of Raw Materials, Details of Plant Equipments and Machineries etc.

MODERN INKS FORMULAES & MANUFACTURING INDUSTRIES

The book contains Colour Matching, Raw Materials, Waxes & Additives, Typographic Inks, Formuations, Photogravure Inks for Three & Four Colour Re-production, Screen Process Inks, Ball Point Pen Inks, Testing of Finished Inks, Formulae, Toner Inks for Automatic Machine, Printing Inks, Screen Printing Inks, Offset Printing Inks, Stamp Pad Inks, Flexographic and Rotogravure Ink, Printing Inks (Flexographic Inks), Duplicating Ink, Ball Pen Refill Ink, Plastic Ink (Flexographic & Rotogravure Ink) and Golden Silver Paste, Suppliers of Plant & Machinery, Suppliers of Raw Materials etc.

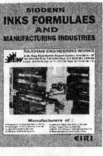

PLASTIC PROCESSING & PACKAGING INDUSTRIES

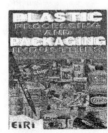

The book Introduction, Technical Specifications, Plastic Processing, Injection Moulding, Extrusion, Blow Moulding, Other Processes, Compounding of PVC, Processing of PVC, Applications of PVC, Improving Moulding Through Melt-Flow Oscillation, Polymides to Extend High Wear, Applications to Replace Metal, Polyurethanes, Project profiles and directory section. The book is covering with the 54 fully detailed and exhaustive chapters excluding a directory section which covers various addresses of Plant and Machineries suppliers and manufacturers of Plastics Processing and Packaging Industries.

ENGINEERS INDIA RESEARCH INSTITUTE 4449, Nai Sarak, Delhi-6

Chapters	Page No.
- Good Laboratory Practice (GLP) and Good Manufacturing Practice (GMP)	91
- Environmental Protection	91
- Quality Promotion	91
- Works Proposal System	92

Chapter 6

DETAILS OF PLANT, MACHINERY & EQUIPMENTS   93-108

- Mixer   93
- Multimill   93
- Herbs Grinder   93
- Hot Air Oven/Tray Dryer   93
- Portable Mechanical Shifter   94
- Oscillating Granulator   94
- Semi Automatic-2-Track Strip Packing Machine   94
- Automatic 4 Track Strip Packing Machine   94
- Packing Conveyor Belt   94
- Double Cone Blender   94
- Foil Sealer/Tagger Sealing Machine   94
- Batch Printing Machine (Motorised)   95
- Pulverizer S.S.   95
- Pulverizer M.S.   95
- Label Gumming Machine Motorised   95
- Dehumidifier   95
- Plate Form Balance   95
- S.S. Sieve   95
- S.S. Sieves, Mounted in Non Friable Wooden Frame   96
- Stainless Steel Scoops S.S. 304 Quality   96
- Bottle Washing Machine   96
- Bottle Drying Oven   96
- Automatic Volumetric Liquid Filling Machine   96
- Semi Automatic Volumetric Liquid Filling Machine   96
- Semi Automatic All-purpose filling Machine (Single Head)   97
- Foot/Hand Operated All purpose Filling Machine   97
- Bottle Inspection Table (Size 18"x36")   97
- High Speed Dissolver &

- Stirrer Machine   97
- Stainless Steel Mixing/Storage Tanks   97
- Primary Syrup Vessels   97
- P.P. Cap Sealing Machine (Floor Model)   97
- Stainless Steel Chain Conveyer Machine (10 Ft. Length)   98
- Packing Conveyer Belt Machine   98
- Emulsifier/Homogeniser with Lifting System   98
- Horizontal Plate Filter Press M/c   98
- Water Deioniser Plant   98
- H.D. Purified Water Storage Tank   99
- Double Cone Blender   99
- Portable Mechanical Shifter   99
- Dehumidifier   99
- Three Speed Planetary Mixer   99
- Double Speed Planetary Mixer (Special Type) Machine   99
- Double Speed Planetary Mixer   100
- Vacuum Planetary Mixer Machine   100
- Semi Automatic All-purpose Filling Machine (Single Head)   100
- Foot/Hand Operated All purpose Filling Machine   100
- Homogenizer   100
- Hot Air Oven   101
- Vacuum Oven   101
- Stainless steel Water Distillation Apparatus   101
- Autoclave Vertical   101
- Friability Test Apparatus   101
- Herbs Grinder   101
- Hot Air Oven/Tray Dryer   102
- Portable Mechanical Shifter   102
- Double Cone Blender   102
- Pulverizer S.S.   102
- Pulverizer M.S.   102

Chapter 7

SKIN CREAMS & LOTIONS   109-127

- Cleansing Creams   109
- Formulation for cleansing cream   110
- Formulation for Cucumber Cleasing Cream   110
- Manufacturing Procedure   110

Chapters	Page No.
- Formulation for rosewater Cleansing Cream	110
- Manufacturing Procedure	111
- Cold Creams	112
- Vanishing Creams	115
- Skin Tonics & Moisturizers	119
- Formulation for Skin Tonic	120
- Moisturizers & Nourishing Creams	120
- Moisturizers	120
- Sunflower Cream	121
- Avocado and Almond Cream	121
- Jasmine moisture cream	121
- Nourishing Creams	122
- Cocoa Butter Cream	122
- Elder Flower Cream	122
- Wheat Germ Cream	122
- Vitamin Cream	123
- Mixed Vegetable Cream	123
- Oily Nourishing Cream	123
- Orange Flower Skin Food	124
- Lime Juice Cream	124
- Lime Juice Glycerine	124
- Wrinkle Removing Cream	125
- Anti-Acne herbal preparation	125
- Face Lotions	126
- Shampoos for all hair types	127

Chapter 8

POMADES & BEAUTY MASKS 128-134

- The Mode of Preparation	128
- Pomade A La Rose	130
- Pomade A La Jasmine	130
- Beauty Masks	130
- High-Viscosity or Paste Masks	130
- Low Viscosity of liquid masks	130
- Manufacturing Procedure	131
- Efficay of masks	132
- Formulation for Gelatine Mask	132
- Aromatic Masks	132

Chapter 9

FACE POWDERS & TALCUM POWDERS 135-136

- Talcum Toilet Powder	136

Chapters	Page No.

Chapter 10

HAIR WASHES & SHAMPOOS 137-140

- Function of A Shampoo & hair wash	137
- Shampoo Types and Forms	137
- Lavender Shampoo	138
- Methi Shikakai Shampoo	138
- Coconut Oil Shampoo	138

Chapter 11

HAIR OILS & HAIR LOTIONS 141-147

- Herbal Hair Oil	141
- Herbal Hair Oil Extract	141
- Efficacy of Herbal Hair Oils	142
- Typical Formulation & Procedure for Hair Oil	142
- Addition of scents	145
- Colouring Hair Oils	146
- Packaging	146
- Herbal Hair Dyes	146
- Henna Hair Dye	146
- Saffron Hair Dye	147
- Walnut Hair Dye	147

Chapter 12

AROMATIC & TOILER WATERS 148-151 WITH COSMETICS FOR MAKEUP

- Commercial Rose Water	148
- Toilet Water	148
- Lavender Water	148
- Violet Water	149
- Eau De Cologne	149
- Cosmetics for Make-up	150
- Finger-tip colouring	150
- Bindi Stick	150
- Taral Alta	150
- Formulation for rose based alta	151
- Packaging of Taral Alta	151

Chapter 13

HERBAL COSMETICS 152-178

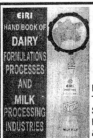

HAND BOOK OF DAIRY FORMULATIONS PROCESSES & MILK PROCESSING INDUSTRIES

The book is covering Introduction, Manufacturing, Technologies, Packaging, Statistical, Figures & Formulations of various Milk & Milk Based Products, Project Profiles on Dairy & Milk Products, Directory Section.

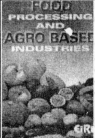

FOOD PROCESSING & AGRO BASED INDUSTRIES

The book is covering 31 detailed and exchaustive chapters including dairy, confectionery, fruit juice, chocolate, frozen desserts, honey, chewing gum, tomato products, jams and jellies, chutney, dehydration of fruit and vegetables, packing of food & alllied products, new development in technologies for food processing, aseptic packaging of food and beverages, packaging of dairy & milk products, breads, buns, pies, pasta products, cakes, biscuits and other allied bakery products. Among all the project profiles on different

AGRO BASED INDUSTRIES HANDBOOK (PLANTATION & FARMING)

The Book Covers almost all the lucrative Plantation Cultivation & Farming methods related with Piggery Farm, Aquaculture Shrimp Farming, Poultry & Broiler Farming, Dairy Farm & Dairy (Milk) Products (Pasteurised Milk, Butter Ghee & Paneer), Teak Tree Plantation, Suger Cane Plantation, Floriculture (Cut Flower-Rose) with Green House Technology, Silk Cocoon Cultivation (Growing of Silk Cocoon From Silk Worm), Mushroom Growing & Processing by Deep Freezing Method (Export Oriented), Papaya Cultivation and Papain Manufacture.

World Importers Directory of Agro Based & Food Processing Industries

The Directory provides Importers addresses of food & Agro Based industries with their Phone and Fax number alongwith complete addresses. This will help to find global overseas customers to the traders/exporters/ manufacturers.

START YOUR OWN COLD STORAGE UNIT

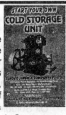

The major chapters in the book are Special features of Cold Storage Project, Selection of the location for the Cold Storage production details and process of manufacture, Operating Conditions, Selection of the Refrigeration Plant Capacity & Machinery, Main Features of Ammonia Compressors

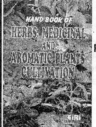

HAND BOOK OF HERBS, MEDICINAL & AROMATIC PLANTS CULTIVATION

The book is covering allmost all the Herbs, Medicinal & Aromatic Plants cultivation details.

Manufacture of Snacks Food, Namkeen, Pappad & Potato Products

The book covers Manufacturing of Potato Chips, Pappad, Snacks Food, Namkeen, Ready to Eat Food Products, Project Profiles, Manufacturers of Machinery & Raw Materials.

Hand Book of Essential Oils Manufacturing & Aromatic Plants

The book covers trade of essential oils, rose oil distillation method, cultivation of matricaria chamomilla, extraction of essential oils, essential chemical constituents profile in tree spice, folk medicinal, essential oil bearing plants status, promising aromatic plants of industrial value, essential oil industry waste utilization, fractionation of essential oil in perfumery & turpentine industry, citronella oil, ginger oil, jasmine rose & lily oil, jasmine flower oil etc.

Books Available at:
ENGINEERS INDIA RESEARCH INSTITUTE
4449, Nai Sarak, Main Road, Delhi-6
Ph:. 3918117, 3916431, 3920361,
3960797 * Fax: 91-11- 3916431
*E-Mail : eirisidi@bol.net.in

Chapters	Page No.
- Healing with Herbs	152
- Herbal or Plant Materials	152
- How to use herbs	157
- Infusions	157
- Decoctions	157
- Extracts and Tinctures	157
- Flower Waters	158
- Oil Soluble Extracts	158
- Herbal Cosmetics for the skin	160
- Equipment Used for Herbal Preparations	160
- Cleansing Creams	160
- Process of Manufacture	161
- Rose Water Cleansing Cream	161
- Cucumber Cleansing Cream	161
- Violet Cleansing Cream	162
- Masks	162
- Milk Mask	162
- Cleansing Mask	162
- Procedure	162
- Butter Milk Mask	162
- Meal Mask	163
- Carrot and Turnip Mask	163
- Oatmeal Mask	163
- Potato Mask	163
- Paw Paw Mask	163
- Luxurious Cleansing Mask	164
- Bath Salts	164
- Bath Oils	164
- Bath Oil - Formulation	164
- Procedure	164
- Massage Preparation	165
- Massage Paste	165
- Massage Oil	165
- Body Lotions	165
- Blue Ratin Body Lotion	166
- Lavender Body Lotion	166
- Almond Body Lotion	166
- Almond Oil Moisturising Creams	167
- Herb Cream(Comfrey Cream)	167
- Avocado Almond Cream	167
- Sun Flower Cream	167
- Jasmine Moisturising Cream	167
- Nourishing Creams	168
- Elderflower Cream	168
- Wheat Germ Cream	168
- Honey Cream	169
- Vitamin Cream	169
- Mixed Vegetable Cream	169

Chapters	Page No.
- Water-in-Oil Emulsions	169
- Formulations (Emulsified Hair Grooming Preparations	170
- Herbal Cosmetics for the Hair	170
- Herbal Hair Conditioners	171
- Herbal Hair Oil	171
- Herbal Henna	171
- Herbal Hair Tonic	171
- Herbal Henna Shampoo (for normal to oily hair)	171
- Herbal Amla Shampoo (for normal to dry hair)	171
- Hair Treatment Cream	171
- Herbal Mint/Hair Gloss conditioner	171
- Herbal Hair Rinse	172
- Herbal Hair Oils (Medicated)	172
- Base Formulation For Herbal hair oil	172
- Herbal Shampoos	173
- Hair Dye	173
- Henna	174
- Applications of Henna	174
- Henna Rinse	174
- Henna Pack	174
- Henna Mixtures	175
- Camomile	175
- Camomile Pack	175
- Camomile Shampoo	175
- Camomile-Henna Mixtures	175
- Henna Reng Dye	176
- Camomile Herbal Dye	176
- Fresh Soap-Wort Shampoo	176
- Procedure	177
- Dried Soap-Wort	177
- Nettle Rinse and Conditioner	178
- Lotion for Unruly Hair	178
- Horsetail Hair Rinse and Tonic	178
- Tonic Shampoo	178
- Herb Shampoo	178

Chapter 14

TESTING OF COSMETICS   179-243

- Introduction   179
- Spectroscopy in Cosmetic Analysis 179
- Ultraviolet and Visible Spectroscopy 180
- Constituents that Absorb in the Ultra-Violet   180

Chapters	Page No.
- Infrared Spectroscopy	180
- Sample Preparation	181
- Characteristic Absorbances	181
- Structural Elucidation	181
- Fluorometry	182
- Mass Spectrometry	182
- Nuclear Magnetic Resonance	183
- Adsorption Column chromatography	183
- Column Preparation, Sample Application and Elution	184
- Qualitative and Quantitative Analysis	184
- Variables and Efficiency	184
- Application to Cosmetic Analysis	185
- Partition Column Chromatography	185
- Solid Support	185
- Selection of the Liquid Phase	186
- Preparation of Column	186
- Application to Cosmetic Analysis	187
- Ion Exchange Chromatography	187
- Column Preparation, Sample Addition and Elution	188
- Applications to Cosmetic Analysis	189
- Thin Layer Chromatography	190
- General Techniques	190
- Variables	191
- Application to Cometic Analysis	191
- High Pressure Liquid Chromatography	192
- Gas Chromatography in Cosmetic Analysis	192
- Gas Liquid Chromatography	193
- Preparation of Packed Columns	194
- Preparatin of Solid Support	194
- Packing the Column	195
- Column Conditioning	195
- Sample Preparation	196
- Detectors	198
- Identification	200
- Determination	201
- Analysis of Creams and Lotions	202
- General Analysis	203
- Description of Product	203
- Type of Emulsion	203
- pH of Emulsion	204
- Ashing at 600°C	204
- Examination of Ash	204
- Non-volatile Matter at 105°C	205
- Infrared Examinations of Non-volatile Matter	205
- Chloroform-Extractable Matter	205
- Material Not Extractable by Chloroform from Acid Aqueous Solution	206
- Saponification of Chloroform-Extractable Matter	207
- Examination of the Saponifiable Matter	207
- Hydrocarbons and Alcohols in Unsaponifiable Matter	207
- Examination of Alcohols in Unsaponifiable Matter	208
- Composition of Chloroform-Extractable Matter	209
- Other Solvent Extraction Procedures	211
- Adsorption Chromatography on Silica Gel in Analysis of Isolated Fatty Materials	212
- Determination of Water by Toluene Distillation	213
- Examination of Aqueous Fraction from Toluene Distillation	213
- Silicons in Creams	214
- Determination of Esters of p-Hydroxybenzoic Acid	214
- Emulsifiers	214
- Aerosol Products	215
- Analysis of Lipsticks	215
- General Analysis	216
- Lakes and Fillers	216
- Trichloroethylene-Acetone Solubles	216
- Chromatographic Analysis of Tricholoroethylene-Acetone Solubles	217
- Gas-Liquid Chromatographic (GLC) Determination of Castor Oil	217
- Analysis of Shampoos	219
- General Analysis	220
- Description of Shampoo	220
- Infrared Examination of Non-volatile Matter	220
- Test for Ammonia	220
- Test for Basic Nitrogen Compounds Including Ammonia	220
- Lanolin and/or Sterols	221
- Water-soluble Gums	221
- Analysis of Nail Lacquers	221

Useful Books on Cosmetics, Perfumes & Essential Oils

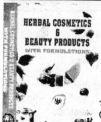

HERBAL COSMETICS & BEAUTY PRODUCTS
RS. 750/-

The book covers Useful Cosmetic Herbs, List of Common Cosmetics Herbs their active constituents and cosmetic applications, Plant and Equipments for Herbal Cosmetics, Skin Cream & Lotions, Pomades & Beauty Masks, Hair Washes & Shampoo, Aromatic & Toilet Waters, Natural Perfumes, Herbal Extraction, Packaging of Herbal Cosmetics, Herbal Cosmetic Technology with formulations, Herbal Cosmetics for beauty parlours with formulae i.e. Shampoo, Lotions, Cleansing creams, Moisturizer, Face scrubs, Egg Face pack, Cucumber face packs, Face packs for for patchy skin, Tomato face pack, Methi Shikakai Shampoo, Sandalwood shampoo, Neem Shampoo, Sunflower Hair Conditioner, Clove Hair Setting Preparation, Anti dandruff preparation etc. Details of setting up an establishment of a herbal beauty parlour, Herbal beauty products manufacture, List & addresses of Herbs Suppliers.

HAND BOOK OF ESSENTIAL OILS MANUFACTURING & AROMATIC PLANTS

With Directory of Plant & Machinery Suppliers, International Importers & Exporters and Manufacturers & Exporters of Essential Oils & Aromatic Chemicals

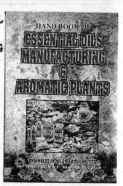

The book covers latest methods and formulaes to produce various type of Essential Oils and Aromatic Plants. The major chapters of the book are Trends in trade of essential oils, damask rose cultivation and processing, rose oil distillation method, chemistry of rose oil, cultivation of matricaria chamomilla, cultivation of davana for essential oil, cultivation and improvement of sweet marjoram, extraction of essential oils, essential chemical constituents profile in tree spice, folk medicinal uses of indigenous aromatic plants, essential oil bearing plants status, promising aromatic plants of industrial value, essential oil industry waste utilization, fractionation of essential oil in perfumery & turpentine industry, tagetes minuta, essential oil of hyptis suaveolens poit, super critical fluid extraction technology for spice extraction, citronella oil, clove oil, eucalyptus oil, ginger oil, jasmine rose & lily oil, jasmine flower oil etc.

HAND BOOK OF PERFUMES & FLAVOURS

(With Directory of Plant & Equipment, Raw Material & Manufacturer/ Exporters/ Suppliers of Perfumes)

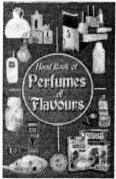

The book covers new formulaes of various kinds of perfumes & flavours. The major chapters of the book are Perfume, Formulary of Perfume, Formulary of Flavour, Chemicals Specifications for Perfume & Flavour Components, Natural Odours Simulated with Aromatic Chemicals, Simulated Flower Scents, Simulated Marine Scents (Algae), Plant & Equipment Suppliers, Suppliers of Raw Materials, Manufacturer/ Exporters/Suppliers of Perfumes. Project profiles has also included for the benefits of the new entrepreneurs.

HAND BOOK OF PERFUMES WITH FORMULATIONS
RS. 750/- OR US $ 125/-

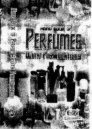

This book has just published and covering chapters viz; Creating a Perfume, Flower Perfumes and their Formulation, Sophisticated/ Fantasy Perfumes and their Formulation, Colognes : Perfumes for Men, Olfaction and Gustation : The Sense of Smell and Taste, Raw Materials of Perfumes (Natural Origin), Raw Materials of Perfumes (Synthetic Origin), Classification of Odours and Odourants, Applications of Perfumes, Packaging of Perfumes, Testing of Perfumes, Aerosol Spray, Aromatic Perfumery Compounds, Scents and Perfumes, Spray Perfumes, Perfumes for Soap, Detergent and Agarbatti etc. (Yara Yara), Suppliers of Raw Materials and Present Manufacturers etc.

Books Available at :
ENGINEERS INDIA RESEARCH INSTITUTE
4449, Nai Sarak, Main Road, Delhi-6
Ph:. 3918117, 3916431, 3920361, 3960797
* Fax: 91-11- 3916431
*E-Mail : eirisidi@bol.net.in

Chapters	Page No.	Chapters	Page No.
- General Analysis	222	- Testing of hair & bath preparations for eye irritation properties	240
- Net Contents	222	- Efficacy Testing	241
- Description of Nail Lacquer	222	- Cell Turnover Testing	241
- Infrared Film Spectrum of the Nail Lacquer	222	- Instrumental Tests	241
- Non-volatile Matter at 105°C	222	- Testing For Moisturises	242
- Determination of Non-volatile Constituents	222	- Test for Sebum	242
		- Test for Cleanser Mildness	242
- Separation of Nitrocellulose from Pigments	225	- Stability Testing	243
- Tricreasyl Phosphate in Nail Lacquers	226	**Chapter 15**	
- Acrylonitrile-Butadiene Polymer	226	**NATURAL PERFUMES**	**244-248**
- Base Coats	226		
- Infrared Spectrophotometric Analysis	226	- Vegetable Origin Perfumes	244
		- Animal Origin Perfumes	245
- Description and Interpretation of Spectra	226	- Musk	245
		- Amergris	245
- Infrared Spectra of Guanine and Tricresyl Phosphate	228	- Civet	245
		- Castor	246
- Gas-Liquid Chromatography	228	- Essences from natural herbal sources	246
- Gas-Liquid Chromatographic Determination of Acetone, Xylene, and Methyl Ethyl Ketone	229	- Sandalwood Oil	246
		- Rosemary Oil	246
		- Lavender Oil	246
- Analysis of Sunscren Products	229	- Bakul	246
- Infrared Examination of Non-Volatile Matter	230	- Henna	246
- Determination of Sunscreen	230	- Bela	247
- Analysis of Sunscreen Vehicle	230	- Champaka	247
- Skin Sensitisation and sensitivity Testing	231	- Rose	247
		- Chameli	247
- Sensitivity Testing	231	- Jasmine	247
- Patch Test	233	- Khus	247
- Open Patch Test	234	- Orange	247
- Prophetic Patch Test	234	- Lavender	248
- Repeated Insult Test	234	- Bergamot	248
- Photopatch Test	236	- Sandalwood	248
- Test for Sensitising Potential	236		
- Provocative Patch Test	236	**Chapter 16**	
- Use Test	237		
- Skin Testing with some Specific Cosmetics	237	**HERBAL EXTRACTION**	**249-252**
		- Extraction of Perfumes & Essences	250
- Creams	237		
- Deodorants and Antiperspirants	237	- Expression	250
- Depilatories	237	- Maceration	250
- Hair Dyes	238	- Digestion	251
- Cold Wave Lotion	239	- Infusion	251
- Lipsticks	239	- Absorption of Enflourage	251
- Nail Polish	239		

Chapters	Page No.
- Distillation	252
- Solvent extraction	252
- Solvent extraction of perfume	252
- Repening of perfumes	252

Chapter 17

PRESERVATION OF COSMETICS   253-259

- Antioxidants   253
- Factors for Deterioration of Cosmetics   254
- Presence of Molds   254
- Factors Influencing the Growth of Microorganisms   255
- Growth Factors   256
- Moisture Content   256
- PH   256
- Temperature   256
- Oxygen   257
- Other Ingrdients   257

Chapter 18

PACKAGING OF COSMETICS PRODUCTS   273-263

- Introduction   260
- Principles of Packaging   260
- Marketing and Packaging   260
- Technology and Components   261
- Plastics   261
- Metals   261
- Laminates   261
- Glass   261
- Paper and Board   262
- Printing and Decoration   262
- Package Development and Design   262
- Technical Aspects of Design   262
- Closures   262
- Package Testing and Compatibility   263
- Testing   263

Chapter 19

PACKAGING OF HERBAL COSMETICS   264-269

Chapters	Page No.
- Determining Factors for Packaging	265
- Technical Factors	265
- Aesthetic Factors	265
- Cost Factors	265
- Technical Factors	265
- Chemical Compatibility	265
- Physical Compatibility	265
- Retention of volatiles	265
- Leak Proof Caps	266
- Tamper-proof Seal	266
- Transport Hazards	266
- Aesthetic Factors	266
- Presentability/Appearance	266
- Packaging Design Technicalities	267
- Packaging Design-Practicability	268
- Packaging Design-Standard Weights and Measures for Packaged Commodities Act and Rules (SWAMPA RULES)	268
- Cost Factors	268
- Packaging Materials commonly Used for Cosmetics	269

Chapter 20

HERBAL COSMETICS FOR BEAUTY PARLOURS   270-299

- Skin Lotions   270
- Complexion lotions/sunscreen lotions for all skin types   270
- Lime Complexion Lotion   270
- Lavender Complexion Lotion   271
- Almond Complexion Lotion   271
- Sesame Complexion Lotion   271
- Brook Lime Complexion Lotion   271
- Witch Hazel Complexion Lotion   272
- Pimple Removing Lotions   272
- Pimple removing garlic lotion   272
- Pimple removing camphor lotion   272
- Astringent Lotions for All Skin Types   273
- Lemon Astringent Lotion   273
- Cornflowr Astringent Lotion   273
- Rose Astringent Lotion   273
- Lilly Astringent Lotion   273
- Nutmeg Astringent Lotion   274
- Peppermint Astringent Lotion   274
- Sandalwood Astringent Lotion   274
- Rosemary Astringent Lotion   274

Useful Books on Cosmetics, Perfumes, Essential

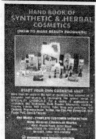

HAND BOOK OF SYNTHETIC & HERBAL COSMETICS

The Book covers Production Problems & Recommendations, Cosmetic and Drugs, Face Powder, Variations of Face Powder, Toilet Powder, Creams, Vanishing Creams, Foundation Creams, Hand Lotions, After Shaving Lotions, Deodorants, Mascara-eyebrow Pencils-Eye Shadows, Lipsticks, Shampoos, Depilatories, Shaving Cream, Cosmetics for Nails, Tooth Powder, Tooth Paste, Mouth Washes, Facial Masks, Cosmetics for Eyes, Cosmetic for Babies, Herbal Cosmetic for the Skin, Hair Shampoos, Anti Dandruff Preparations, Hair Straighteners, Hair Dyes, Bleaches, Colourings and Dye Removers, Oral Herbal Preparations, Govt. Regulations & Acts on Drugs & Cosmetics, Bath Preparations, Baby Preparations, Home Made Cosmetics, Herbal Preparations for Body, Skin Cleansing, Herbal Preparations for Feet & Hands, Herbal Shampoo and Setting, How to Layout a Cosmetic Factory, Project Profiles on Various Cosmetics with Herbal etc.

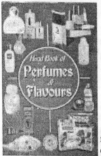

HAND BOOK OF PERFUMES & FLAVOURS

(With Directory of Plant & Equipment, Raw Material & Manufacturer/Exporters/Suppliers of Perfumes)

The book covers new formulae of various kinds of perfumes & flavours. The major chapters of the book are Perfume, Formulary of Perfume, Formulary of Flavour, Chemicals Specifications for Perfume & Flavour Components, Natural Odours Simulated with Aromatic Chemicals, Simulated Flower Scents, Simulated Marine Scents (Algae), Plant & Equipment Suppliers, Suppliers of Raw Materials, Manufacturer/Exporters/Suppliers of Perfumes. At the end of the book the last but not the least chapter project profiles has also included for the benefits of the new entrepreneurs.

HAND BOOK OF ESSENTIAL OILS MANUFACTURING & AROMATIC PLANTS

With Directory of Plant & Machinery Suppliers, International Importers & Exporters and Manufacturers & Exporters of Essential Oils & Aromatic Chemicals

The book covers latest methods and formulaes to produce various type of Essential Oils and Aromatic Plants. The major chapters of the book are Trends in trade of essential oils, damask rose cultivation and processing, rose oil distillation method, chemistry of rose oil, cultivation of matricaria chamomilla, cultivation of davana for essential oil, cultivation and improvement of sweet marjoram, extraction of essential oils, essential chemical constituents profile in tree spice, folk medicinal uses of indigenous aromatic plants, essential oil bearing plants status, promising aromatic plants of industrial value, essential oil industry waste utilization, fractionation of essential oil in perfumery & turpentine industry, tagetes minuta, essential oil of hyptis suaveolens poit, super critical fluid extraction technology for spice extraction, citronella oil, clove oil, eucalyptus oil, ginger oil, jasmine rose & lily oil, jasmine flower oil etc.

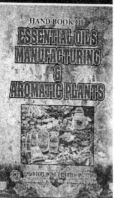

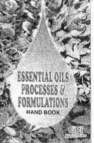

ESSENTIAL OILS PROCESSES & FORMULATIONS HAND BOOK

Essential Oils by Steam Distillation, Essential Oil Lemon Basil, Processing of Fresh Ginger (Zingiber Officinale Roscoe), Essential Oil from Cinnamomum glanduliferum (wal.) Nees, Kewda (Pandannus odoritissimus L.) flower distillation, Composition of essential oil from bottle brush (Callistemone lanceolatus) by capillary gas chromatography, Essentioal Oil of Ocimum basilicum L., Composition of essential oil from flowers of Keora (Pandanus odoratissimus Linn)., Manufacturers/Exporters/Importers & Traders of Essential oils and Aromatic Chemicals with Machinery Suppliers.

Books Available at :
ENGINEERS INDIA RESEARCH INSTITUTE
4449, Nai Sarak, Main Road, Delhi-6
Ph:. 3918117, 3916431, 3920361, 3960797
* Fax: 91-11- 3916431
*E-Mail : eirisidi@bol.net.in

Chapters	Page No.	Chapters	Page No.
- Witch Hazel Astringent Lotion	275	- Carrot Face Scrub	285
- Skin Toning Lotions	275	- Shaljam Face Scrub	285
- Sunflower Skin Toning Lotion	275	- Pea Face Scrub	285
- Skin Soothing Preparations	276	- Face scrubs for Combination Skin	286
- Yoghurt Skin Soothing Preparation	276	- Face Scrubs for Patchy Skin	286
- Witch Hazel Skin Soothing Preparation	276	- Oatmeal Face Scrub	286
		- Banana Face Scrub	286
- Cleansing Creams/Cold Creams	276	- Peach Face Scrub	286
- Almond Cleansing Cream (1)	276	- Sunflower Face Scrub	286
- Almond Cleansing Cream (2)	277	- Almond Face Scrub	287
- Almond Cleansing Cream (3)	277	- Strawberry Face Scrub	287
- Cucumber Cleansing Cream	277	- Face Scrubs for All Skin Types	287
- Oatmeal Cleansing Cream	278	- Oatmeal Face Scrub	287
- Chamomile Cleansing Cream	278	- Egg Face Scrub	287
- Night Creams	278	- Face Packs or Face Masks	288
- Garlic Night Cream	278	- Face Packs for Normal Skin	288
- Apple Night Cream	278	- Milk Face Pack	288
- Avocado Night Cream	279	- Apricot Face Pack	288
- Nourishing Creams/		- Bail Fruit Face Pack	288
Daytime creams	279	- Face Packs for Dry Skin	289
- Cucumber Nourishing Cream	279	- Egg Face Pack	289
- Oatmeal Nourishing Cream	279	- Face Packs for Oily Skin	289
- Almond Nourishing Cream	280	- Potato Face Pack	289
- Almond Nourishing Cream	280	- Cucumber Face Pack	289
- Marigold Nourishing Cream	280	- Papaya Face Pack	289
- Olive Nourishing Cream	280	- Face Pack for Combination Skin	290
- Red Elm Nourishing Cream	281	- Face Packs for Patchy Skin	290
- Anti-Wrinkle Creams	281	- Mint Face Pack	290
- Anti-Wrinkle Carrot Cream	281	- Coconut Face Pack	290
- Anti-Wrinkle Cucumber Cream	281	- Peppermint Face Pack	291
- Anti-Wrinkle Egg Cream	281	- Red Elm Face Pack	291
- Anti-Wrinkle Apricot(Khubani)		- Face Packs for All Skin Types	291
Cream	282	- Milk Face Pack	291
- Hand Creams	282	- Honey Face Pack	291
- Almond Hand Cream	282	- Egg Face Pack	292
- Vanilla Hand Cream	282	- Water Based Face Packs	292
- Witch Hazel hand Cream	283	- Tomato Face Pack	292
- Moisturizers for All Skin Types	283	- Orange Face Pack	292
- Lemon Moisturizer	283	- Honey Face Pack	292
- Watermelon Moisturizer	283	- Olive Face Pack	293
- Avocado Moisturizer	283	- Strawberry Face Pack	293
- Face Scrub	284	- Shampoos for All Hair Types	293
- Face Scrubs for Normal Skin	284	- Lime Shampoo	293
- Barley Face Scrub	284	- Lavender Shampoo	294
- Oatmeal Face Scrub	284	- Methi-Shikakai Shampoo	294
- Face Scrubs for dry skin	284	- Sandalwood Shampoo	294
- Oatmeal Face Scrub	284	- Neem Shampoo	295
- Almond Face Scrub	285	- Lime Hair Setting Preparation	295
- Face Scrubs for Oily Skin	285	- Hair Conditioners for All Hair Types	295

Chapters	Page No.
- Avocado Hair Conditioner	295
- Sunflower Hair Conditioner	295
- Wheat Hair Conditioner	296
- Hair Rinses	296
- Apple Hair Rinse	296
- Barley Hair Rinse	296
- Chamomile Hair Rinse	296
- Rosemary-Chamomile Hair Rinse	297
- Rosemary Hair Rinse	297
- Hair Setting Preparations for All Hair Types	297
- Bay-Rum Hair Setting Preparation	297
- Clove Hair Setting Preparation	297
- Gum Tragacanth Hair Setting Preparation	298
- Anti-Dandruff Preparation	298
- Anti-Dandruff Rosemary Preparation	298
- Anti-Dandruff Lemon Preparation	298
- Anti-Dandruff Lemon Preparation	298
- Anti-Dandruff Egg Preparation	299
- Anti-Dandruff Vinegar Preparation	299
- Anti-Dandruff Sesame Preparation	299

Chapter 21

	Page No.
PLANT ECONOMICS ON HERBAL COSMETICS	**300-302**
- Land & Building	300
- Plant & Machinery	300
- Fixed Capital	300
- Raw Materials	301
- Total Working Capital/Month	302
- Total Capital Investment	302
- Turn Over/Annum	302

Chapter 22

	Page No.
PLANT ECONOMICS ON HERBAL SHAMPOO AND CREAMS	**303-305**
- Land & Building	303
- Plant & Machinery	303
- Fixed Capital	304
- Raw Materials	304
- Total Working Capital/Month	305
- Total Capital Investment	305
- Turn Over/Annum	305

Chapter 23

	Page No.
PLANT ECONOMICS OF TOILET SOAP AND HERBAL SOAP	**306-307**
- Land & Building	306
- Plant & Machinery	306
- Fixed Capital	306
- Raw Materials	306
- Total Working Capital/Month	307
- Total Capital Investment	307
- Turn Over/Annum	307

Chapter 24

	Page No.
PLANT ECONOMICS OF HERBAL HAIR OIL (AYURVEDIC)	**308-309**
- Land & Building	308
- Plant & Machinery	308
- Fixed Capital	308
- Raw Materials	308
- Total Working Capital/Month	309
- Total Capital Investment	309
- Turn Over/Annum	309

Chapter 25

	Page No.
PLANT ECONOMICS OF ANTISEPTIC CREAM	**310-311**
- Land & Building	310
- Plant & Machinery	310
- Fixed Capital	310
- Raw Materials	310
- Total Working Capital/Month	311
- Total Capital Investment	311
- Turn Over/Annum	311

Chapter 26

	Page No.
PLANT ECONOMICS OF KESH KALA TEL	**312-313**
- Land & Building	312
- Plant & Machinery	312
- Fixed Capital	312
- Raw Materials	312
- Total Working Capital/Month	313

New Detailed Project Reports available on SPICES, FOOD ETC. INDUSTRIES @ Rs. 3675/- each

LIST OF READILY AVAILABLE DETAILED PROJECT REPORTS

- ASAFOETIDA (HING)
- ASAFOETIDA (SYNTHETIC)
- AJOWAN EXTRACTION FROM AJOWAN
- AMLA PLANTATION & PROCESSING (E.O.U)
- AMCHUR
- BLACK PEPPER
- BEE KEEPING
- BIO-FERTILIZER
- BREWERY & DISTILLERY
- CASHEW NUT SHELL LIQUID & KERNEL
- CHILLI OIL
- CORE OIL FROM CASHEW NUT OIL
- COCONUT PRODUCT & BY PRODUCTS
- CHILLI POWDER
- CARDANEL FROM CNSL
- CLOVE OIL
- COLD STORAGE & ICE
- DRYING OF RED CHILLI, HALDI, DHANIIA, PEAS ETC.
- DAIRY FARM & PRODUCTS
- DRY GINGER POWDER & OLEORESIN
- DRY GIBGER FROM GREEN
- GINGER
- EXTRACTION OF LARGE CARDAMOM
- FISH FARMING
- FLORICULTURE (CUT FLOWER)
- HERBS CULTIVATION
- HERBS DRYING
- GINGER PROCESSING
- GOAT & SHEEP FARMING
- GOAT FARMING
- GUAR GUM
- GARLIC OIL
- GARLIC POWDER
- GARLIC ACID
- GARLIC FLAKE & POWDER DEHYDRATION
- GINGER OIL
- GINGER OIL & GINGER DUST
- GINGER STORAGE
- MAIZE & ITS BY PRODUCTS
- MUSHROOM
- MINERAL WATER
- MUSTARD POWDE.
- PAPAYA
- OLEORESIN FROM CHILLI & GINGER
- OLEORESIN FROM CHILLI
- ONION FLAKES
- SPICES WITH PACKAGING & FORMULAES
- STARCH
- STRAWBERRY CULTIVATION
- THYMOL FROM AJOWAN OIL
- TOMATO CHILLI & SOYABEAN SAUCE
- TARMARIND JUICE CONCENTRATE
- TARMARIND SEED
- TURMERIC POWDER
- TURMERIC PLANTATION
- TURMERIC OIL OLEORESIN
- WATER COCONUT SWEET

*Each 'EIRI' **Market Survey Cum Detailed Techno Economic Feasibility Report (Detailed Project Report)** covers Introduction, Properties, Market Survey, Process of Manufacture, Cost Economics with Profitability Analysis, Suppliers of Plant & Machineries and Raw Materials, Cash Flow Statement, Repayment Schedule, Depreciation Chart, Projected Balance Sheet etc.

*Price **Rs. 3675/-** (Rs. Three Thousand Six Hundred Seventy Five Only) for Each Report. Send Draft/M.O./Cash in favour of **"ENGINEERS INDIA RESEARCH INSTITUTE"**, DELHI. (Payable In India) (Delivery within Two Days)

ENGINEERS INDIA RESEARCH INSTITUTE
4449, Nai Sarak (D), Main Road, Delhi - 110 006 (India)
Ph:. 3918117, 3916431, 3920361, 3960797 Fax: 91-11- 3916431
E-Mail : eirisidi@bol.net.in * Website:www.startindustry.com

Chapters	Page No.
- Total Capital Investment	313
- Turn Over/Annum	313

Chapter 27

PLANT ECONOMICS OF KALI MEHANDI — 314-315

- Land & Building — 314
- Plant & Machinery — 314
- Fixed Capital — 314
- Raw Materials — 315
- Total Working Capital/Month — 315
- Total Capital Investment — 315
- Turn Over/Annum — 315

Chapter 28

PLANT ECONOMICS ON HAIR OIL AND FORMULATION — 316-317

- Land & Building — 316
- Plant & Machinery — 316
- Fixed Capital — 316
- Raw Materials — 316
- Total Working Capital/Month — 317
- Total Capital Investment — 317
- Turn Over/Annum — 317

Chapter 29

PLANT ECONOMICS OF BABY OIL — 318-319

- Land & Building — 318
- Plant & Machinery — 318
- Fixed Capital — 318
- Raw Materials — 318
- Total Working Capital/Month — 319
- Total Capital Investment — 319
- Turn Over/Annum — 319

Chapter 30

ESTABLISHMENT OF A HERBAL BEAUTY PARLOUR — 320-324

- Present Status and viability of beauty parlours — 320
- Training for beauticians, consultancy and franchise assistance for beauty parlours — 320
- Requirement of Funds and the sources of Financial Assistance — 321
- Project Economics — 321
- Fixed Costs — 321
- Land and Building — 321
- Running Costs (Monthly) — 322
- Total Cost of Project — 322
- Means of Finance — 323
- Annual cost of production — 323
- Monthly Revenue — 323
- Profitablity — 324

Chapter 31

HERBAL BEAUTY PRODUCTS MANUFACTURERS — 325-329

- Product Mix — 325
- Formulation & Process of Manufacturers — 325
- Project Economics — 326
- Fixed Costs — 326
- Raw Materials — 326
- Salaries of Staff (monthly) — 327
- Total cost of project — 328
- Means of Finance — 328
- Annual cost of production — 328
- Monthly Sales Revenue — 328
- Profitability — 329

Chapter 32

LIST OF HERBS SUPPLIERS — 330-346

Chapter 33

SUPPLIERS OF PLANT, MACHINERY AND EQUIPMENTS — 347-355

- Consultants — 347
- Complete Plant Suppliers for Cosmetic Unit — 347
- Agitator — 347
- Weighing Balances — 348
- Blister Packing Machine — 348
- Bottle Filling Machine — 348
- Bottle Washing & Drying Machines — 349

Chapters	Page No.	Chapters	Page No.
- Cap Screwing Machine	349	- Film Plastic	358
- Collapsible Tube Sealing and		- Foils	358
Crimping Machines	350	- Lables	358
- Crushing & Grinding Machines		- Paper Waxed	359
(Disintegrators)	350	- Strip Packing Material	359
- Dryers & Drying Ovens	351	- Tubes Collapsible	359
- Experimental Cosmetic Testing		- Vials	359
Equipments	351	- Washers	360
- Labelling and Gumming Machine	351	- Wrappers	360
- Laboratory Equipments	352	- Pet Bottles/Containers	360
- Ball Mill	352		
- Mixers / Blenders	352	**Chapter 35**	
- Over-Printing Machine	353		
- Paste Filling Machines	353	**SUPPLIERS OF RAW**	**361-364**
- Powder Filling Machine	353	**MATERIALS**	
- Reaction Vessels / Storage Tanks	354		
- Sterilising Plants	354	- Herbs and Herbs Extract	361
- Strip Packing Machine	354	- Menthol	362
- Tanks (storage etc.)	355	- Balsum Peru	362
		- Coconut Oil	362
Chapter 34		- Cinnamon Leaf Oil	363
		- Herbal Extracts	363
PACKING MATERIALS	**356-360**	- Olive Oil	363
		- Detergents	363
- Bottles	356	- Essentials Oils	363
- Caps (Aluminium etc.)	356	- Perfumes, Fragrances and	
- Closures & Seals	357	Aromatic Chemicals	364
- Containers	357	- Perfumery Compound	364
- Corks	358	- Perfumery Chemicals	364
- Film Blister	358	❖	

OTHER USEFUL PUBLICATIONS

★ HANDBOOK OF SYNTHETIC & HERBAL COSMETICS
★ COSMETICS PROCESSES & FORMULATIONS HANDBOOK
★ HAND BOOK OF PERFUEMS WITH FORMULATIONS
★ ESSENTIAL OILS PROCESSES & FORMULATIONS HAND BOOK
★ HAND BOOK OF ESSENTIAL OILS MFG. & AROMATIC PLANTS
★ HANDBOOK OF PERFUMES & FLAVOURS
★ HAND BOOK OF HERBS, MEDICINAL & AROMATIC PLANTS CULTIVATION

AVAILABLE AT :

ENGINEERS INDIA RESEARCH INSTITUTE

Regd. Off. : 4449, Nai Sarak (S1), Main Road, Delhi-6 (India)
Ph. : 3918117, 3916431, 3960797, 3920361 Fax : 91-11-3916431
E-mail : eirisidi@bol.net.in Website : startindustry.com

New Detailed Project Reports available on FOOD & ALLIED INDUSTRIES @ Rs. 3675/-

LIST OF READILY AVAILABLE DETAILED PROJECT REPORTS

- ACTIVATED CARBON FROM COCONUT SHELL & RICE HUSK
- AGRICULTURE IMPLIMENTS
- AMALA PLANTATION & PROCESSING (E.O.U)
- AYURVEDIC MADICINES
- BAKERY (BREAD/BISCUIT)
- BEER PLANT (EOU)
- BANANA POWDER (EOU)
- BONE CRUSHING PLANT
- BEE KEEPING
- BIO-FERTILIZER
- BREWERY & DISTILLERY
- CASHEW NUT SHELL LIQUID & KERNEL
- CATTLE & POULTRY FEED
- COCONUT PRODUCT & BY PRODUCTS
- CURRY PASTE
- CONFECTIONERY
- CUSTARD POWDER
- COLD STORAGE & ICE
- DALL MILL
- DAIRY FARM & PRODUCTS
- DAIRY FARM (MILK)
- DEHYDRATION OF FRUITS & VEGETABLE BY FREEZE DRYING METHOD
- EGG POWDER (E.O.U)
- FISH FARMING
- FLORICULTURE (CUT FLOWER)
- FLOUR MILL
- FOOD PROCESSING UNIT
- FOOD DEHYDRATION
- FROZEN MEAT
- HERBS CULTIVATION
- HERBS DRYING
- GINGER PROCESSING
- GOAT & SHEEP FARMING
- GOAT FARMING
- GUAR GUM
- GRANULATED MIXED FERTILIZER
- HONEY PROCESSING
- HYBRID SEEDS
- ICE CREAM (FOR ALL TYPE)
- INSECTICIDES FROM NEEM SEEDS, NEEM OIL & LEAVE
- INSTANT FOOD
- INSTANT NOODLES
- INVERT SUGAR
- IODIZED SALT
- KATTHA & CUTCH
- MANGO JUICE BOTTLING
- MANGO PRODUCTS
- MANGO PULP
- MAIZE & ITS BY PRODUCTS
- MENTHOL FLAKES & BOLD
- MUSHROOM
- MINERAL WATER
- OLEORESINS FROM CHILLI
- PAPAYA
- PEANUT BUTTER
- PIGGERY FARM
- PORK FARMING
- POTATO CHIPS
- ONION FLAKES
- POPLAR TREE
- RICE MILL
- SOYA BEAN OIL
- SOFT DRINK
- SPICES
- STARCH FROM MAIZE
- STRAWBERRY CULTIVATION
- TEA & COFFEE
- TEAK PLANT

Each 'EIRI' *Market Survey Cum Detailed Techno Economic Feasibility Report (Detailed Project Report)* covers Introduction, Properties, Market Survey, Process of Manufacture, Cost Economics with Profitability Analysis, Suppliers of Plant & Machineries and Raw Materials, Cash Flow Statement, Repayment Schedule, Depreciation Chart, Projected Balance Sheet etc.

Price **Rs. 3675/-** (Rs. Three Thousand Six Hundred Seventy Five Only) for Each. Send Draft/M.O. in favour of "ENGINEERS INDIA RESEARCH INSTITUTE", DELHI.

ENGINEERS INDIA RESEARCH INSTITUTE
4449, Nai Sarak (D), Main Road, Delhi - 110 006 (India)
Ph:. 3918117, 3916431, 3920361, 3960797 Fax: 91-11- 3916431
E-Mail : eirisidi@bol.net.in Website:www.startindustry.com

New Publications from EIRI

1. HAND BOOK OF EXPORT ORIENTED INDUSTRIES
2. HAND BOOK OF PLASTIC PROJECTS (HI-TECH PLASTIC PROJECTS)
3. AGRO BASED & FOOD PROCESSING WITH EXPORT ORIENTED INDUSTRIES
4. HAND BOOK OF PACKAGING INDUSTRIES
5. ALL CHEMICALS AND ALLIED INDUSTRIES
6. HAND BOOK OF HOSIERY READYMADE GARMENTS & TEXTILE PROJECTS
7. AGRO BASED INDUSTRIES HAND BOOK (PLANTATION & FARMING)
8. REAL ESTATE PLAZAS, HOTEL, MOTEL, HOSPITAL & COMMERCIAL COMPLEXES
9. WORLD IMPORTERS DIRECTORY OF AGRO BASED & FOOD PROCESSING
10. WORLD IMPORTERS YELLOW PAGES (ALL TRADE BUYERS DIRECTORY)
11. HAND BOOK OF PRINTING PROCESSES TECHNOLOGIES & INDUSTRIES
12. SMALL MEDIUM & LARGE SCALE CHEMICAL INDUSTRES
13. DAIRY FORMAULATIONS, PROCESSES & MILK PACKAGING INDUSTRIES
14. PLASTIC PROCESSING AND PACKAGING INDUSTRIES
15. STATIONERY, PAPER CONVERTING & PACKAGING INDUSTRIES
16. INDUSTRIAL DIRECTORY (ALL INDIA TRADE DIRECTORY)
17. FOOD PROCESSING AND AGRO BASED INDUSTRIES
18. AGRO BASED PLANTATION CULTIVATION AND FARMING HAND-BOOK
19. RUBBER CHEMICALS AND PROCESSING INDUSTRIES
20. PAINT PIGMENT VARNISH AND LACQUER MANUFACTURING
21. MODERN INKS FORMULAES AND MANUFACTURING INDUSTRIES
22. HAND BOOK OF BAKERY INDUSTRIES
23. INDUSTRIAL DIRECTORY OF DELHI AND SURROUNDING AREAS ON CD-ROM
24. START YOUR OWN COLD STORAGE UNIT
25. GARMENTS EXPORT DIRECTORY OF DELHI AND AROUND
26. MOULDS DESIGN AND PROCESSING HAND BOOK
27. PROFITABLE SMALL SCALE MANUFACTURE OF SOAPS & DETERGENTS
28. PET PRE-FORM AND ITS PRODUCTS (BOTTLES ETC.) MFG.
29. INDIAN INDUSTRIAL AND BUSINESS DIRECTORY
30. ESSENTIAL OILS MANUFACTURING & AROMATIC PLANTS
31. MODERN PACKAGING TECHNOLOGY FOR PROCESSED FOOD, BAKERY, SPICE & ALLIED FOOD
32. AGRO BASED HAND BOOK ON CULTIVATION, PLANTATION & FARMING
33. HAND BOOK OF PERFUMES & FLAVOURS
34. HAND BOOK OF SPICES & PACKAGING WITH FORMULAES
35. HAND BOOK OF HERBAL & SYNTHETIC COSMETICS
36. HAND BOOK OF ADHESIVES WITH THEIR FORMULAES
37. ELECTROPLATING ANODIZING & SURFACE TREATMENT TECHNOLOGY
38. HAND BOOK OF AYURVEDIC & HERBAL MEDICINES WITH FORMULAES
39. FRUITS & VEGETABLES PROCESSING HAND BOOK
40. HAND BOOK OF HERBS, MEDICINAL & AROMATIC PLANTS CULTIVATION
41. HAND BOOK OF CONFECTIONERY WITH & FORMULATIONS
42. MANUFACTURE OF SNACKS FOOD, NAMKEEN, PAPPAD & POTATO PRODUCTS
43. ESSENTIAL OIL PROCESSES AND FORMULATIONS HAND BOOK
44. SYNTHETIC RESINS TECHNOLOGY WITH FORMULATIONS
45. PAINT VARNISH SOLVENTS AND COATING TECHNOLOGY
46. COSMETICS PROCESSES AND FORMULATIONS HAND BOOK
47. HAND BOOK OF SYNTHETIC DETERGENTS WITH FORMULATIONS
48. AGRO CHEMICAL INDUSTRIES (INSECTICIDES AND PESTICIDES)
49. HERBAL COSMETICS AND BEAUTY PRODUCTS

Above all books available at :

ENGINEERS INDIA RESEARCH INSTITUTE

Regd. Off. :4449, Nai Sarak (B), Main Road, Delhi-110 006.(India)
Ph: 3916431, 3918117, 3920361, 3960797 * Fax: 91-11- 3916431
E-mail : eirisidi@bol.net.in, Website : www.startindustry.com

Chapter - 1

USEFUL COSMETIC HERBS

Aloe Vera Linn.

"GHRITA KUMARI/KUMARI"

Hey Woman, Stay Girl

Aloe commonly known as Kumari or Kanya which means Virgrin Girl" perhaps has been named so as it gives tenderness, softness & juvenility of a young girl and makes you look younger than your age.

Aloe has been used in medicines & cosmetics since the time of Greeks & Egyptians, and believed to have used by Cleopatra to keep her complextion clear and soft.

The Aloe, Aloe vera Linn. (family:Liliaceae) is a very tall, strikingly attractive perennial plant which grows wild in the tropics, mainly in Africa & South Africa. Now it has been cultivated widely for medicinal and cosmetic purposes. The plant is xerophytic and bears a rosette of leaves which are thick, fleshy, sessile and spiny. Flowers are red or yellow.

The Aloe contains anthraglycosides as its active principles. The other constituents are polysaccharides steroids, organic acid, enzymes, antibiotic principles, amino acids, biogenic stimulators, wound healing hormones, saponins and minerals.

Aloe is reported to have various pharmacological activities like catahartic, purgative, anticancer & antiviral, immunomodulator, analgesic, anti-inflammatory, wound healing and antiaging. Fresh aloe vera gel is well known as a domestic medicine and the fresh gel has the property of relieving thermal burns and sunburn as well as promotring wound healing. It also has moisturising & emollient properties. One of the most valuable cosmetic property of aloe is its ability to stimulate the circulation of the skin and remove dead skin so giving freshness and younger appearance to skin. It also clear away blemishes, protects, the skin against infection and reduces wrinkles.

Aloe Vera shampoo help to combat dry brittle hair and used in shampoo for dry & damaged hair. Aloe Vera gel is soothing healing & astringent and when used externally it helps to keep the skin healthy.

Aloe Vera has been shown to have antiaging properties. Oil in water extracts of aloe when used externally claimed to significantly increase the soluble collagen level suggesting to topical antiaging effects.

BUCHANANIA LANZAN SPRENG.

"CHIRONJI"

FOR CLEAR & SPOTLESS FACE

Buchanania lanzan spreng., one of the common ingredients of pickles and a flavouring agent in India, is a secret of clear & spotless skin of the traditional Indian women.

Buchanania lanzan spreng commonly known as "CHIRONJI" or Piyala is used in skin care since antiquity. The plant belongs to family Anacardiaceae, is a small evergreen tree found through out the greater parts of India in dry deciduous forests up to an altitude of 1200 meters. The tree flowers during Jan-March and the fruits ripen during April-June.

The Chironji seeds has a great reputation as Body, Brain & Cardiotonic. The kernels are highly nutritious and contain good amount of proteins. The kernels are rich in proteins, fats, minerals and vitamins (thiamine, riboflavin, niacin & vitamin C). The kernels yield a light yellow sweet oil with a mild pleasant aroma. The oils is used as a substitute for olive and almond oils in indegenous medicine.

The kernels are worked up in to an ointment and used in skin diseases. The Chironji has a great reputation of clearing the face from all the spots and blemishes and traditionally been employed by Indian women. It is believed to cure pimples, prickly heat and itch.

The leaves are reported to be used for curing wounds and the healing properties of the leaf believed be due to presence of tannins (gallotannis), triterpenoids and flavonoids.

Cucumis sativa Linn.

"KHEERA"

The Secret of a Beautiful Skin

Out of the innumerable plants used in medicine and cosmetology, Cucumber or Kheera is one of the most common plant frequently used in cosmetic preparations. Application of fresh cucumber slices has for a long time been known to be effective in cases of rough skin, pigmented skin and freckled skin.

Cucumis sativa Linn. commonly known as Cucumber or kheera belongs to family cucurbitaceae. The plant is probably indegenous to north India. It is widely cultivated throughout India and in the tropical and subtropical parts of the world as a popular vegetable/salad crop.

Earlier it was believed that beneficial effect of Cucumber & Cucumber Juice are due to some growth promotring substances called auxins and also due to certain vitamins like biotin, niacin and pantothenic acid. Recently, however a mucoiytic enzyme known as Lysozym has been found to be the principle active susbstance reponsible for all the beneficial effect of Cucumber on skin. Lysozym has a considerable antibiotic effect which affect bacteriae lyticly. Other enzymes present in cucumbers are ascorbases and ascorbinases which have great effect on the stability of ascorbigen bound in the form of ascorbic acid.

The bleaching effect of this juice on pigmented skin is of a great historical and cosmetic value. Sufficient waters in the Cucumber fruit has a favourable effect on the rehydration of skin (humectant), particularly in dry skin.

Crude Cucumber juice or its biocomplexes can be easily incorporated with cosmetic preparations like skin water, lotions and tonics, jellies, lotions and creams for hands, cleansing lotions, shaving lotions, humectant creams, astringent lotions, antiperspirants and face packs. In recent years the so called streching masks containing cucumber juice and polyvinyl alcohol are extensively in use.

Datura Stramonium Linn.
"DHATURA"
A Poison that gives life to Hair & Skin

Dhatura once used for sucidal and homicidal purposes traditionally being used in skin and hair care in India.

Datura stramonium Linn. belongs to family solanaceae and commonly known as Datura or Dhatura. The herbs is glabrous or farinose, annual, usually 3 meter high, stem erect with spreading branches; leaves; ovate or triangular, irregularly toothed; flowers; white or violet; fruit; a spiny capsule. The plant is distributed from Kashmir to Sikkim up to 8000ft, & in hilly districts of central and South India.

The herb contains alkaloids, chlrogenic acid, a dark essential oil and others. The herb is a narcotic, antispasmodic and anodyne and is used chiefly to relieve spasm of the bronchioles in asthma. The leaves are applied to boils, sores fish bites, bruises and wounds, carcinomatous ulcers, & running sores. The powdered root is used to relieve pain from the gums in toothache.

The seeds are useful in leucoderma, skin diseases, ulcers itching and boils; applied topically it removes the pain of tumors and piles. The roots and seeds are claimed to have anti-inflammatory properties. The green fruits are use to treat carbuncles. The fruit juice is applied to the scalp for falling hair and dandruff.

Eclipta alba Hassk

"BHRINGRAJ"

No Grey Hair as long as Bhringraj is available

Eclipta Hassk is a small genus of herbs distributed in the tropical and subtropical regions of the world.

The Eclipta alba Hassk is a member of Asteraceae family, common in China, Taiwan, India Indochina, Japan and in the Philippines. The herb is commonly known as Bhringraj, Maka, Bhangra and Mochkand. The herb is erect or prostrate, much branched often rooting at the nodes; leaves sessile, oblong lanceolate; flowers born in head, white and few cms in diameter.

Eclipta alba Hassk commonly known as safed Bhangra (white Bhringraj) when in flowers and as Kala Bhangra (Black Bhringraj) when in fruit. Bhringraj is medicinally used in eye and ear troubles, headache hepatic and spleen enlargement, liver cirrhosis, skin diseases, toothache and wind trouble in the cosmetics it is used as a hair darkner. It is traditionally used in hair care to check hair loss and stimulate hair growth. The herb is prescribed as an astringent and haemostatic. The extracted juice of the fresh herb is applied to the scalp to promote hair growth and taken internally it blackens the hair & beard. The plant possess a bluish blackdye and use as a staining herb in tattoing. The herb has skin toning properties, stimulate & invigorate peripheral blood circulation of the skin.

Eclipta alba is made into a hair oil in Ayurveda. In Hair Oil it may be used along with Centella Asiatica and Phyllanthus emblica. A paste is prepared by mincing the plants has an antiinflammatory effect. The shoot extract shows antibacterial activity.

Foeniculum Vulgare Mill.

"SAUNF"

Herbal care for most sensitive skins

"Saunf" or "Fennel" has increasingly being used in baby products and toiletries because of its irritation alleveiating and mild antiseptic properties and now a days frequently been used for the care of sensitive skins like that of babies.

"Saunf" botanically known as foeniculum vulgare Mill. belongs to family Umbelliferae. Fennel is a tall graceful, aromatic herb with tall stout stem which bears soft leathery bright green leaves. The yellow flowers are born in flate topped umbels in winters in India.

Fruits contain a volatile oil and fatty oils with relatively high concentratic.. of tocopherols. The fruits also contains flavonoids, vitamins and minerals (relatively high in calcium and potassium).

Fenel and it volatile oil have carminative and stimulplant properties and well known for its calming effect on the digestion. Fennel is a diuretic herb and can be helpful in a slimming programme. Fennel lotion in mildly antiseptic it helps to close the pores and smooth out small wrinkles as well as to protect the skin from infection, fennel extract are also incorporated in to face pack to smooth out wrinkles and to improve dull looking skin.

Hair preparations contaning extracts of fennel are belived to stimulate scalp and strengthen the hair.

Current use of fennel however is in bath preparation and baby toiletries because of its property to alleviate irritation and also due to its mild bactericidal properties.

Fennel is also a good source of minerals (paricularly calcium & potassium) which have been claimed to supply the skin with nutrients. They are said to regulatc the dermal water balance and to protect the skin against dehydration and therfore could be incorporated into facial and bath preparations.

Glycyrrhiz Glabra Linn.

"MULATTHI"

No Sweat, No Body Odour

Recently Glycyrrhiz glabra Linn. has been evaluated for its potential use in cosmetic preparations in a number of studies. The herb has been evaluated for its antiinflammatory and antioxidant properties and the herb is shown to have fair amount of these properties The traditional use of liquorice as antiperspirant in India has also been justified in some of the reports.

Glycyrrhiza glabra Linn. (Family, Leguminosae) commonly known as mulatthi or liquorice is a perennial herb distributed in the subtropical and warm temperate regions of the world, chiefly in mediterranean countries and China.

The principle constitutent of liquorice to which it owes it characteristic sweet taste is glycyrrhizin which is present in a conc. of 2-17%,. other constituents are glucose, sucrose, starch, a volatile oil, as paragine, and a colouring matter (Anthoxanthine glycoside).

The root is refrierant, tonic, aphrodisiac, alexetric, diuretic, alternative, galactagogue and expectorant. The roots have healing and antinflammatory properties and lycyrrhizin appears to be active component. Glycyrrhiza roots have also been evaluated for its anti oxidant (free radical scavanging) properties and reported to have fair amount of this property (148 mg/ml and SOD like activity of 17.8% of an extraction yield of 20.3%) In India leaves of Glycyrrhiza have been used in foul perspration of the armpits and also used for scalds of the head. The root is healing and used for wounds & ulcers. Roots are also reported to help control sebum production and could be used as antiperspirant in talc and other cosmetic products.

Hibiscus ros-sinensis Linn.

"JASUT/CHINA ROSE"

Keeps your Hair Black & Shining

Once used to blacken the shoes, China rose or Shoe flower is one of the most commonly used skin and hair care herb in India.

Hibiscus rosa-sinensis is a native of china. It is grown as an ornamental plant in gardens thorughout India. The herb belongs to family Malvaceae and locally known as jasum or jasut. The plant thrives in all type of soil. It can be propogated by cutting. It blossoms almost throughout the year and seldom sets seeds under cultivation.

Flowers are refrigerant, emollient, demulscent and aphrodisiac. Petals are demulscent; leaves are amollient, anodyne, aperient and laxative. Hibiscus is useful in menorrhagia, strangury, cystitis and other irritable condition of the genitouinary tract. The flowers are made in to a paste and applied to swellings and boils.

Crushed flowers yield a dark purpulish dye which was formerly employed for blackening shoes and hair, eyebrows, food & liquours. Hibiscus is useful as antidandruff, antinfectie, prophylactic against skin diseases and allergic conditions, cheks hair loss & stimulates hair growth. The herb is claimed to darken the colour of hair. Hibiscus is a useful ingredient of skin and hair care products for its skin & hair conditioning activity. It has ability to strike exact balance for skin moisture and normalize a skin which otherwise has an erratic behaviour.

Impatiens balsamina LinN.

"GUL MEHANDI"

Henna from the Flowers

Impatiens balsamina Lihn. commonly known as Gul Mehandi or Garden balsam belongs to family Balsaminaceae. Impatiens are chiefly native to the mountainous regions of tropical Asia and Africa but are also found in the north temperate zone and in South Africa Impatiens balsamina is found throughout India upto 5000 feets and extensively grown in gardens for beautiful flowers.

Th herb is an erect, branched, succulent, annual with shortly stalked, alternate, lanceolate, serrate leaves, flowers; solitary; or fasicled, purpule pink or nearly white with long incurved spur. The plant is of medicinal improtance and the acrid juice of plant is considered emetic cathartic and diuretic. The flowers are mucilaginous and cooling; they are reported to improve circulation and relieve stasis. Alcoholic extracts of the flowers posses marked antibiotic activity.

The flowers are a source of natural dye used as a substitute for henna for dyeing the finger nails. Flowers are considered cooling and emollient and applied to burns and scalds.

OTHER USEFUL PUBLICATIONS

★ HANDBOOK OF SYNTHETIC & HERBAL COSMETICS
★ COSMETICS PROCESSES & FORMULATIONS HANDBOOK
★ HAND BOOK OF PERFUEMS WITH FORMULATIONS
★ ESSENTIAL OILS PROCESSES & FORMULATIONS HAND BOOK
★ HAND BOOK OF ESSENTIAL OILS MFG. & AROMATIC PLANTS
★ HANDBOOK OF PERFUMES & FLAVOURS
★ HAND BOOK OF HERBS, MEDICINAL & AROMATIC PLANTS CULTIVATION

AVAILABLE AT :

ENGINEERS INDIA RESEARCH INSTITUTE

Regd. Off. : 4449, Nai Sarak (S1), Main Road, Delhi-6 (India)
Ph. : 3918117, 3916431, 3960797, 3920361 Fax : 91-11-3916431
E-mail : eirisidi@bol.net.in Website : startindustry.com

IMPATIENS Linn.
FAMILY-BALSAMINACEAE
Impatience balsamina Linn.
Common Names :-
English : Garden Balsam, Zangibar balsam, Yellow Balsam
Hindi : Gulmendi
Distribution : china, Cochin-china, Japan. In India found throughout up to 5,000ft.
Applications : The juice of the garden Balsam is used by women to dye their nails. The plant is used to treat wounds.
Category: Colour Cosmetics, Skin Care.

INDIGOFERA Linn.
FAMILY-LEGUMINOSAE
Indigofera aspalathoides Vahl. ex. DC.
Common Names :
Punjab : mil
Sanskrit : Sivanimbu
Distribution : Plains of Carnatic
Applications : The leaves are applied to abcesses. The roots are chewed in toothache and apthae. The whole plant is used is oedamatous tumours and the ashes of the plant is used in antidandruff preparations.
Category : Skin & Hair Care
Action : Antidandruff, reduce inflammation

INULA Linn.
FAMILY-ASTERACEAE
Inula helenium Linn.
Common Names : Elecampane
English : Alant, Elecampane, Horse heal
Distribution : South and central Europe, Balkan and central Asia.
Applications : A decoction of root is a good cleansing lotion for spots and pimples.
Category : Skin Care, Acne & Pimples
Action : Antiacne

IPOMEA Linn.
FAMILY - CONVOLVULACEAE
Ipomea murucoides Roem. & Schult.
Common Names : Arbol del muerto, Arbol del venado, Cazazuate, palo del muerto
Distribution : S.Mexico, Guatemala
Application : The ash is used as a soap in Guatemala.
Category : Soaps & Detergents
Action : Detergent

Ipomoea obscura (Linn.) Ker-Gawl.
Common Names :
Tamil : Chiruedali
Sanskrit : Vachagandha
Distribution : Throughout tropical India in moist regions.
Applications : The leaves of herb are mucilaginous. They are used as an application to apthous affections after toasting powdering and boiling in ghee. In admixture with the leaves of Argyreia mollis, they are used for sores.
Category : Skin Care
Action : Emollient

Ipomea pescaprae Sw.
Common Names :
Hindi : Dopatilata
Bengali : Chhagalkuri
Tamil : Adambu
Distribution : Throughout India, abundant near the sea.

Useful Cosmetic Herbs

Applications _: The plant is mucilaginous and is said to be useful for skin affections. In Malasia, leaf poultices are applied to boils, wounds, ulcers and carbuncles.
Category : Skin Care
Action : Emollient, Soothing

Ipomoea pes-tigridis Linn.
Common Names :
Bengali : Langulilata
Tamil : Puli chovadi
Delhi : Ghiabati
Distribution : More or less throughout India.
Applications : The herb is used in the treatment of boils and carbuncles. In Philippines and Indonesia leaves are applied as poultices to boils pimples and sores.
Category : Skin Care, Acne & Pimples
Action : Antiacne

IRIS Linn.
FAMILY - IRIDACEAE

Iris germanica Linn.
Common Names :
English : German Iris, Flag Iris
Distribution : Mediterranean
Applications : Cultivated extensively. The rhizome (Radix Iridis, Rhizoma Iridis, Verona Orris Root) is used to make tooth-powders and sachets. Small pieces of the rhizome are given to children to chew during teething. It is used in some parts of Italy to make rosary beads.
Category : Dental & Oral Care

Iris nepalensis D. Don
Common Names :
Himalayas : Chalnundar, Chiluchi, Shoti, Sosan
Distribution : Temperate Himalayas from the Punjab and western Tibet, east wards 5000-10,000 ft and Khasia Hills, 5000-8000ft.
Applications to sores and pimples.
Category : Skin Care, Acne & Pimples
Action : Antiacne

Iris germanica Linn.
Common Names :
Hindi : Keore ka mul
Sanskrit : Padma-Pushkara
Distribution : Cultivated in Kashmir
Applications : The leaves are rich source of Vitamin C and have been applied for the treatment of frozen feets.
Category : Foot, Hand & Lip Care
Action ; Antiscorbutic

IXORA Linn.
FAMILY- RUBIACEAE

Ixora coccinea Linn.
Common Names :
English : Jungle Flame Ixora
Hindi : Rangan, Rookmani
Sanskrit : Raktaka, Bandhuka
Distribution : Indegenous in Western peninsula. Cultivated throughout India.
Applications : The roots possess astringent and antiseptic properties and are applied to sores and chronic ulcers. A decoction of the bark & flowers is also applied as a lotion for sores and ulcers.
Category : Skin Care
Action : Astringent, & Antiseptic

Jasminum officinale Linn.
"CHAMELI"
For a Smooth and Babysoft Skin

The jasmine oil is used in high grade perfumes. It blends with any floral scent imparting smoothness and elegance to perfume composition. Jasmine oil is used for perfumery, expensive soaps, cosmetics, mouth washes, dentrifices, bath salts and tobacco. Recently the jasmine oil has been recomended in skin care product because of its skin stimulant properties.

Jasminum officinale Linn. (family oleaceae) commonly known as Royal Jasmine or Chameli is an evergreen or decidous shrub with very fragrant flowers distributed in subtropical N.W.Himalayas, 2000-5000 feets, salt range, trans-indus, eastward to kumaon, hills of Rajputana and Central India, often cultivated in Indian gardens.

In Indian system of medicine the flower is considered good for diseases of skin, ear, eye and mouth. The flowers are good for tooth-ache, dental caries, inflammations, scabies, ulcers, etc. The oil is good for old people, lesson the inflammation and soften the skin. The oil is considered cooling and jasmine attars (oil) from the flowers are valued for their cooling effect in skin diseases.

The leaves contain salicylic acid, an alkaloid, an astringent principle resin etc. and considered good for skin diseases. The fresh juice of the leaves is applied to the soft corn between the toes & to mouth ulcers. Jasmine oil is claimed to have skin stimulating properties and it has been observed that oil of jasmine stimulate fibroblast growth which translate into an increase in epidermal cell turnover and belivered to have skin regenerative properties.

Jasmine sambac (Linn.) Ait. commonly known as chamba or mogra is a closely related species of Royal Jasmine is used in the same way as Jasmimum officinale Linn. The flower are made into face and eye lotion to wash the face, flowers are also used in scentring coconut oil. Leaves are applied to skin complaints and ulcers.

JASMINUM Linn.
FAMILY-OLEACEAE

Jasminium sambac (Linn.) Ait.
Common Names :
English : Arabian Jasmine, Tuscan Jasmine
Hindi : Banmallika, moghra, Chamba
Sanskrit : Mallika
Distribution : Cultivated throughout India.
Applications : The leaves are applied as a poultice for skin complaints and ulcers. A lotion made from flowers is used for washing face and eyes. In Malaya flowers are used in scenting coconut hair oil.
Category : Skin & Hair Care

JATROPHA Linn.
FAMILY-EUPHORBIACEAE

Jatropha curcas Linn.
English : Physic Nut, Purgingnut
Hindi : Jangli-Arand, safed Arand.
Sanskrit : Kanan aeranda, parvata randa.
Distribution : Grown in various parts of India as a field barrier especially on the coromandal coast and in Travancore, common hedge plant in konkan, a native of tropical America.
Applications : The oil from the seeds is used as an external application for skin diseases. In Java the oil is applied to hair as growth stimulator. It is also used as an application for sores on domestic stock. Tender twigs of the plant are used for cleaning teeth; the juice is reported to relieve toothache and strengthen gums. The juice of the plant is used as haemostatic in Java. The twing sap is considered styptic and used for dressing wounds and ulcers; an emulsion of the sap with benzyl benzoate is said to be effective against scabies, eczema and dermatitis. The root bark is used as an external aplication for sores.
Category : Skin, Hair, Dental & Oral Care
Action ; Cleaning, Heamostatic, Promote Hair growth, Antiseptic

JATEORHIZA Miers.
FAMILY-MENISPERMACE

Jateorhiza palmata (Lam.) Miers.Syn.
J. Calumba Miers.
Common Names :
Hindi : Kalamb
Tamil : Kalamba
Distribution : Cultivated in some parts of India
Applications : Powdered roots are used in dressring sores.
Category : Skin Care
Action : Healing

JUGLANS Linn.
FAMILY-JUGLANDACEAE

Juglans insularis Griseb
Common Names : Nogal, Palo del Nuez
Distribution : Cuba
Applications : The leaves are used locally in astringent baths to treat skin diseases of the heads of children.
Category : Skin Care, Aromatic & Medicated Baths.

Actin : Astringent

Juglans regia Linn.
Common Names :
English : Common Walnut, Persian walnut, European walnut
Hindi : Akhrot
Sanskirt : Akschota
Distribution : Temperate Himalayas 3,000-10,000ft., wild and cultivated in Khasia Hills and Baluchistan.
Applications : The bark is used for cleaning teeth or for chewing to redden the lips. Green walnut shells have be used as hairdye in the form of an oily or alchoholic extracts mordanted with alum, used as a dentrificealso.
Category : Skin, Hair, Dental & Oral Care
Action : Astringent, Source of brown Dye

JUNIPERUS Linn.
FAMILY-CUPRESSACEAE

Juniperus oxycedrus Linn.
Common Names :
English : Pricky Juniper
Distribution : Mediterranean region
Applications : Distillation of the heartwood yields an oil (Oil of Cade) used as an antiseptic and to kill external parasites.
Category : Skin & Hair Care
Action : Antiseptic, Disinfectant

Juniperus Virginiana Linn.
Common Names :
English : Red cedar, Pencil cedar
Distribution : N.Hemisphere
Applications : Cedar wood oil is used as an insecticide, in perfumery, soaps, liniments, cleansing and polishing preparations. The leaves were formerly used as an ingredient of a counter-irritant liniment.
Category : Perfumery, Skin Care
Action : Insecticidal, Counter irritant

Jussiaea Linn.
FAMILY-ONAGRACEAE

Jussiaea tenella Burm. f.
Applications : In Celebes, the plant is employed in poultices for pimples.
Category : Acne & Pimples

Lawsonia inermis Linn.

"HENNA"

A Cure for almost all Hair Problems

Henna has been used as a hair dye since the dawn of history. The earliest use of henna as a hair dye dates back to 3300 year. Famous beauties like Nefertiti & Cleopatra used henna to enhance their hair colouring. Natural Henna is leaves of a small shrub Lawsonia inermis Linn. (family Lythraceaes) commonly known as Henna. Lawsone, 2-hydroxyl-1-4-napthaquinone is the principle active constituent as a dye.

Today the use of henna has increased considerably not only for hair colouring but also for hair conditioning, as a hair growth promoter, hair brighther, antidandruff, astringent and sunscreen. The oil from the flower is used in perfumery.

Henna has long been used in India and Middle East countries for colouring palms, soles and finger nails. It is also used for dyeing hair, beard and eyebrows for personel adornment. For use as a colouring matter henna leaves are pulverised into a paste with water and applied to the part to be dye. For dyeing hair it is applied as a pack & it acts as a substantive dye for keratin and imparts and orange red colour. It is harmless and causes no irritation of skin.

Henna leaves are reported to have properties like antifungal, antibacterial, antitumor, antispasmodic, anti-inflammatory and analgesic. The leaves are used to cure leucoderma, insanity, headache, lumbago bronchitis etc. The leaves are used to allay burning sensation. The leaves are believed to favour the growth of hair and used to treat skin problem like scabies, sores, boil, ulcers, burns and scalds.

LACTUCA Linn.
FAMILY-ASTERACEAE

Lactuca sativa Linn.
Common Names :
English : Garden Lettuce
Hindi : Kahu, Salad
Distribution : The garden lettuce is cultivated throughout India.
Applications : Concentrates of Vitamine-E and Antioxidants have been prepared from lettuce. Lettuce is used in poultices for burns and painful ulcers.
Category : Skin & Hair Care
Action : Antioxidant, source of Vit. E

Lactuca scariola Linn.
Common Names :
Hindi : Kahu
Tamil : Salattu
Distribution : Western Himalayas, 6000-12000ft.
Applications : The seed oil is considered as a cure for falling hairs.
Category : Hair Care
Action : Prevent Hair loss

LAGENANDRA Dalz.
FAMILY-ARACEAE

Lagenandra ovata (Linn.) Thw.
Common Names :
Bombay: Rukhalu
Malayalam : Andavazha
Distribution : From Konkan to N. Kanara, Mysore, Curg, Cochin & Travancore.
Applications : The plant contains an acrid juice and used in ointments for itch.
Category : Skin Care
Action : Antiitch

LAGENARIA Ser.
FAMILY-CUCURBITACEAE

Lagenaria siceraria (Mol.) Standl.
Common Names :
English : Bottle gourd
Hindi : Kaddu
Sanskrit : Alabu
Distribution : Cultivated throughout India.
Applications : The juice of the fruit extract mixed with lime juice as an application for pimples. The leaf juice is used for baldness. The fruit is a good source of B vitamins and a fair source of ascorbic acid.
Category : Skin Care, Hair Care, Acne & Pimples
Action : vitamin B & C, Prevent Hair loss, Anti-pimples

LAGERSTROEMIA Linn.
FAMILY-LYTHRACEAE

Lagerstroemia indica Linn.
Common Names :
English : Common crape myrtle
Hindi : Pharash
Bombay : Chinai-mendhi
Distribution : Throughout India, common in gardens.
Applications : The roots are astringent and used as gargle.
Category : Dental & Oral Care
Action : Astringent

Useful Cosmetic Herbs 15

Mours alba Linn.
"SHAH-TUT"
A Fairness Herb

Mours alba Linn. commanly known as tut or shahtut or mulberry is one of the popular unani medicine for throat troubles. Fruits and leaves are used medicinally to enrich and cool the blood, better the apetite and improve complexion.

Mours alba Linn. a member of family Moraceae is native to china and extensively cultivated throughout the plains of India and in the hilly areas of Himalayas upto an elevation of 3,300m. The Leaves are rich in proteins, free amino acids, calcium, phosphorus and potassium. Leaves are a good source of vitamin C (200mg-300mg/100gr). The leaf contains carotene, vitamin B, folic acid, folinic acid and vitamin D. The leaves also contain organic acids, glucoside, essential oil, tanins etc. The fruit contain organic acids, glucoside, essential oil, tanins etc. The fruit contains sugars, clacium, phosphorous, iron, carotenes (Vitamin A), thiamine, nicotinic acid, riboflavin, vitamin C, flavonoids and others. The bark contain isoprenyl flavonoids and coumarins as active principles.

Mulberry leaves are considerd diaphoretic and emollient. A decotion of leaves is used as a gargle in inflammations of the throat, dyspepsia and melancholia. The root is reported to posses anthelmintic and astringent properties & the leaf extracts possess antibacterical activity. In yunani system of medicine the fruits and leaves are recommended to improve the complexton and dose of 25 ml of leaf juice is sufficient. The root bark contains isoprenyl flavonoids and coumarins as its major components and responsible for the skin whitening and protective (antimicrobial) action. The seeds are a used to heal cracked sole of the foot.

Nardostachys jatamansi DC.
"JATAMANSI"
The Secret of Long & Black Hair of Your Granny

Jatamansi also known as Balchir of Balchhadi (Ka Tel) is still a popular preparation among traditional Indian and older women, particularly in North India The roots are extracted in vegetable oil and used on hair to make hair long and black.

Nardostachys jatamansi DC. (family; Valerianaceac) is an erect perennial herb, 2 feet high with stout woody rootstock found in the alpine Himalayas from Punjab to Sikkim and Bhutan. It is valued for its rhizome used in India as a drug, cosmetic and also in perfumery. Jatamansi has an agreeable odour with a bitter aromatic taste and is used as a substitute for valerian. It yields an essential Oil (Jatamansi Oil, Balchir Ka Tel) with a pleasant odour. The oil contains a saturated bicyclic sesquiterpene Ketone Jatamansone, an alcohol and its isovaleric ester and Jatamanshic acid. The Oil possesses antiarrthymic, anticonvulsant and hypotensive activity. In Ayurveda, the rhizome is considerd as tonic, cooling, antipyretic, alexipharmic and fattening, cure burning sensation erysipelas, skin diseases, ulcers and improve complexion.

In Yunani system the herb is considerd good for eye and hair besides other uses. It is believed that the herb increases the luminosity of the eyes and promote the growth and blackness of the hair.

OTHER USEFUL PUBLICATIONS

★ HANDBOOK OF SYNTHETIC & HERBAL COSMETICS
★ COSMETICS PROCESSES & FORMULATIONS HANDBOOK
★ HAND BOOK OF PERFUEMS WITH FORMULATIONS
★ ESSENTIAL OILS PROCESSES & FORMULATIONS HAND BOOK
★ HAND BOOK OF ESSENTIAL OILS MFG. & AROMATIC PLANTS
★ HANDBOOK OF PERFUMES & FLAVOURS
★ HAND BOOK OF HERBS, MEDICINAL & AROMATIC PLANTS CULTIVATION

AVAILABLE AT :

ENGINEERS INDIA RESEARCH INSTITUTE

Regd. Off. : 4449, Nai Sarak (S1), Main Road, Delhi-6 (India)
Ph. : 3918117, 3916431, 3960797, 3920361 Fax : 91-11-3916431
E-mail : eirisidi@bol.net.in Website : startindustry.com

NARDOSTACHYS DC.
FAMILY-VALERIANACEAE

Nardostachys jatamanasi DC.
Common Names :
English : Spikenard, Indian Nard
Hindi : Balchir, Jatamansi
Distribution : Alpine Himalayas, 11,000-15,000 ft. extending eastwards from Kumaon to Sikkim, 17,000 ft. and Bhutan.
Applications : The rhizome is reported to promote the growth of hair and also impart blackness.
Category : Hair Care
Action : Promote hair growth, darkens hair

NEEA Ruiz & Pav.
FAMILY-NYCTAGINACINACE

Neena parviflora Poepp. and Endl.
Distribution : Tropical S. America
Applications : The leaves (Yana muco) are chewed by the Peruvian Indians to preserve and blacken the teeth.
Category : Dental & Oral Care
Action : Strengthen gums

NEOCALLITROPSIS Florin.
FAMILY-CUPRESSACEAE

Neocallitropsis araucariodes Compton
Applications : A viscid rosescented oil (Oil of Araucaria) is distilled from the wood. It is used as a fixative in scenting cosmetics, soaps, creams etc.
Category : Perfumery

NICANDRA Adans.
FAMILY-SOLANACEAE

Nicandra physaloides (Linn.) Gaertn.
Common Names :
English : Apple of Peru
Bombay : Ran-popati
Distribution : Subtempemperate Himalayas, 3,000-6,000 ft. from Kashmir to Sikkim, Mts. of W. Deccan Peninsula, introduced.
Applications : In malagasy (madagascar) a decoction of the leaves is used for killing head lice.
Category : Hair Care
Action : Antilice

NELUMBO (Tourn.) Adans
FAMILY-NYMPHAEACEAE

Nelumbo nucifera Gaertn.
Common Names :
English : Indian lotus
Hindi : Kamal, Ambuj
Sanskrit : Ambhoja, padama
Distribution : Throughout the warmer parts of India
Applications : In Ayurveda anthers are used to cure ulcers and sores of mouth. In china & malaya dried red petals are used as a cosmetic application to the face to improve the complexion. The dried yellow fragrant stamens are also used as a cosmetic.
Category : Skin Care
Action : Improve complexion

NEPETA Linn.
FAMILY-LABIATAE

Nepeta cateria Linn.
Common Names :
English : Catnip, Catmint Catnep
Distribution : Kashmir, N.W. Frontier provinces, Kumaun valley and Baluchistan.
Applications : A decoction of the catnep flowering tops is effective in cleaning dandruff & catnep leaves are chewed to relieve toothache.
Category : Hair, Dental & Oral Care
Action : Antidandruff, Antiseptic

Nepeta hindostana (Roth) Haines
Common Names :
Punjab : Badrang
Nepal : Niasbo
Distribution : Hilly parts of Punjab, Bengal Bihar, Kumaon, N.W. Frontier Province, Rajputana, Madhya Bharat, Deccan and Konkan.
Applications : A decoction of the plant is used as a gargle for sore throat.
Category : Dental & Oral Care
Action : Antiseptic

NERIUM Linn.
FAMILY-APOCYNACEAE

Nerium indicum Mill.
Common Names :
English : Indian Oleandera
Hindi : Kaner
Distribution : Mediterranean region cultivated in Indian gardens.
Applications : An oil extracted from the root bark is used in skin diseases of scaly nature.
Category : Skin Care

NYCTANTHES Linn.
FAMILY-OLEACEAE

Nyctanthes arbor-tristis Linn.
Common Names :
English : Night Jasmine
Hindi : Har Singhar
Sanskrit : Parijata
Distribution : Outer Himalayan ranges from the Chenab to Nepal, Assam, Bengal, Madhya Bharat, Southwards to the Godavari. Cultivated in many parts of India.
Applications : Powered seeds are used as an application for scurfy affections of the scalp (dandruff).
Category : Hair Care
Action : Anti dandruff

NYMPHAEA Linn.
FAMILY-NYMPHAEACEAE

Nymphaea lotus Linn.
Distribution : Tropical Africa and Asia
Applications : The seeds are used in the Sudan to treat skin diseases.
Category : Skin Care

Nymphaea stellata Wild.
Common Names :
English : Blue water lily
Hindi : lilophal, Nilkamal
Sanskrit : Asitopala, Indiwar.
Distribution : Warmer parts of India.
Applications : Flowers are said to promote the growth of hair.
Category : Hair Care
Action : Promote Hair growth

Useful Cosmetic Herbs

Ocimum sanctum Linn.
"TULSI"
A Cure for Acne

Octimum sanctum Linn. (family Umbelliferae) is one of the most sacred herb in India and found in almost every hindoo house. The herb has been used since antiquity for its medicinal properties. The plant is an erect glabrous herb few feet tall native of Central Asia and North-West Asia, cultivated throughout the greater parts of India.

The leaves yield an essential oil possessing a pleasant odour characteristic of plant. The oil contains eugenol, eugenol methyl ether and carvacrol, other constitutents include methyl chaivcol, ciniole and linalool. The herb is of great medicinal vlaue and has pharmacological action like anti- catarrah, demulcent, diphoretic, digestive, diuretic, ex-pectorant and febrifuge Tulsi is indicated in bronchitis catarrhal fever, cold cought, hepatic affections, genitourinary troubles, ringworm, skin diseases etc.

In cosmetics. Tusli is used for skin care, indicated for skin diseases, ringworm, as skin softner, prophylactic, anti-inflammatory and removes skin blemishes. The oil possess antibacterial and insecticidal properties. The basil oil has been tested in India as an antibacterial treatment for acne and the oil shown very good result in curing acne even at very low dilutions. That is why the ocimum increasingly find use in a number of antiseptic/antimicrobial preparations particularly for acne.

OCIMUM LINN.
FAMILY-LABIATAE
Ocimum americanum Linn.
Common Names :
English : Hoary basil
Hindi : kalatulsi
Sanskrit : Ajaka
Distribution : Plains and lower hills of India.
Applications : Used as a mouth wash for relieving toothache. A paste of leaf is used as an external application for parasitical skin affections. Plant is antibacterial.
Category : Skin, Dental & Oral Care
Action : Antibacterial, Antilice

Ocimum canum sims.
Common Names :
English : Hoary Basil
Distribution : Old World Tropics
Applications : In the Sudan a paste of the leaves is used as a poultice for skin diseases.
Category : Skin Care
Action : Antibacterial

OENOTHERA Linn.
FAMIOLY-ONAGRACEAE

Oenothera biennis Linn.
Common Names :
English : Evening prime rose
Distribution : Europe & North America.
Applications : The oils is externally used to moisturise hair and skin. The oil is rich source of Gamma linoleic acid(GLA).
Category : Skin & Hair Care
Action : Emollient, Source of GLA

ONCNOTIS Benth.
FAMILY-APOCYNACEAE

Oncnotis echinata Oliv.
Distribution : Tropical W. Africa
Applications : Cultivated in Central America for the seeds which yield an oil (Gorli Oil, Gorli Seeds Oil) used in the treatment of leprosy and other skin diseases.
Category : Skin Care

ONONIS Linn.
FAMILY-LEGUMINOSAE

Ononis spinosa Linn.
Common Names :
English : Restharrow
Distribution : Europe to Turkestan
Applications : A decoction of the stem and leaves is used in Central Europe to treat skin diseases. An infusion of the flowers is used to clean the blood.
Category : Skin Care

OLENDRA Cav.
FAMILY-POLYPODIACEAE

Oleandra Wallichii Presl.
Distribution : Tropics
Applications : The rhizome is reported to posses rejuvenating properties and beneficial to the aged.
Category : Skin, Care
Action : Rejuvenating

OPHIOGLOSSUM Linn.
FAMILY-OPHIOGLOSSACEAE

Ophioglossum pendulum Linn.
Distribution : Hawaii

Useful Cosmetic Herbs

Applications : The fronds of fern are shreded into coconut oil which is applied as an ointment in the scalp to improve the hair.
Categoy : Hair Care

ORIGANUM Linn.
FAMILY-LABIATAE

Origanum vulgare Linn.
Common Names :
English : Origano, Pot Marjoram
Distribution : Europe
Applications : A decoction of the leaves is used in home remedies for dental problems. The origanum oil is used as an external application for toothache. It is also used externaly as lotion for healing wounds usually in conjection with other herbs. The oil is used in gargles & baths. It is claimed to stimulates the growth of hair.
Category : Dental & Oral Care

OXALIS Linn.
FAMILY-OXALIDACEAE

Oxalis corniculata Linn.
Common Names :
English : Indian sorrel
Hindi : Amrul Sak
Sanskrit : Amlika
Distribution : Nearly all regions throughout the warmer parts of India, in the Himalayas up to 8,000 ft.
Applications : Good source of vitamine C (125 mg/100 g). The plant posses antiseptic and astringent properties. They are used for removing corns, warts and other excrescences of skin. A decoction of the leaves used as a gargle.
Category : Skin Care
Action : Astringent, Antiseptic

OXYSTELMA R.Br.
FAMILY-ASCLEPEDIACEAE

Oxystelma esculentum R.Br.
Common Names :
Hindi : Dudhilata
Tamil : Uippala
Distribution : Throughout the plains and lower hills of India, usually near water Ceylon & Java.
Applications : A decoction of the plant is used as a gargle in aphthous ulcers of the mouth and in sore throat. The milky sap forms a wash for ulcers in Sind. In combination with turpentine it is prescribed for itch.
Category : Skin, Dental & Oral Care
Action : Healing

Pennisetum glaucum R.Br.

"BAJRA"

Ceramides not from Bovine or Swine

Cerebrosides are produced in basal epidermal cells and secreted externally where they form protective coating around the viable cells. As the stratum corneum keratinizes, the cerebrosides in part, are hydrolyzed to yield ceramides. The ceramides are an integral part of skin intercellular memberance network. These membranes are ultimately responsible for skin hydration and suppleness.

Though crude extracts and purified extracts of Bovine brain are used in cosmetic preparations, the main obstacles in using them in cosmetic preparations are their animal like odour, colour, solubility and high cost. Pennisetum glaucum R.Br. commonly known as "BAJRA" or Pearl Millet is one of the major food crop in India and extensively cultivated for their seeds which are highly nutritive. The plant is considered tonic and useful in diseases of heart. The seeds contains glycolipids and an extract prepared from the seeds contains nearly 5% cerebrosides along with cholesterol, hydrocarbons, fatty acids and triglycerides.

While the extract contains less cerebroside then the animal extracts but the extract is excellent.as far as odour, colour & solubility is concerned Also, they add aesthetic and marketing benefits by being of plant origin. Ceramides are used in a variety of cosmetic preparations and are claimed to make skin soft, luminous and well hydrated. By using ceramides of plant origin we could also help in stopping the butchering animals for ceramide extraction which is the ugly face of beauty business.

Quillaja saponaria Molina

"SOAP BARK"

Say no to Synthetic Shampoos

Quillaja saponaria Molina commonly known as Soap Bark is an evergreen tree, native of the western slopes of Andes in Chile and Peru, and has been introduced in to India and grown in Botanic Garden of Ootacammund, Nilgiris. The bark consists almost entirely of the saponaceous innerbark (Phloem) and is marketed in the form of odourless flat pieces.

The Bark powder yield copious later in water and is used for washing delicate fabrics. It is employed as a detergent emulsifying and foaming agent in shampoos, hair tonics and other cosmetics. Medicinally the bark is reported to be an expectorant and diuretic and a dermal stimultant. Its liquid extract is employed in lotions used as a wash for the scalp in certain troubles.

Because of its copious foaming and external stimulant properties it has great potential to be used in a variety of cosmetic products like shampoos, face washes, tonics, lotions, facial scrubs etc.

QUASSIA Linn.
FAMILY-SIMAROUBACEAE

Quassia indica Nootiboom
Common Names :
Marathi : Lokhandi
Malayalam : Karinjotta
Distribution : Tropics, found in India.
Applications : In Solomon Islands, the macerated leaves mixed with coconut oil are used for cleansing hair. An infusion of the leaves is used to kill lice and for itch.
Category : Hair Care
Action : Cleaning, Antilice

QUILLAJA Molina
FAMILY-ROSACEAE

Quillaja brasiliensis (St.Hil.) Mart.
Distribution : S. Brazil, E. Argentine, Uruguay, Chile
Applications : The bark is used as a soap for washing fine textiles.
Category : Soaps & Detergents
Action : Detergent (Cleaning)

Quillaja saponaria Molina.
Common Names :
English : Soapbark Tree, Quillaja
Distribution : Peru, Chile
Applications : The dried inner bark (Soap Bark, Soap Tree Bark, Panama Bark) is used for washing clothes and as an emulsifying agent in tars. It is also used for washing hair. The Quillaja powder is used in laundering delicate fabrics, detergent shampoo hair tonics, and other cosmetics, cutaneous stimulants. Its liquid extracts is employed in lotions used as a wash for the scalp.
Category : Skin, Hair Care
Action : Detergent

Rosa damascena Mill.

"ROSE"

The Symbol of Beauty

The rose has been treasured for its lovely fragrance over many centuries. The poet sappho called it the Queen of flowers.

The damask rose, Rosa damascena Mill. (family; Rosaceae) is a sweatly scented flowering shrub cultivated on a large scale for its lovely perfume. In India it is made in to a number of rose products such as Rosewater, Gulkand, Rose Attar, Otto of rose, Gul roghan (Hair Oil), Rose hips and rose petals.

The rose petals/flowers contains geraniol glycosides, flavonoids & tannins as major components which have antiseptic, stimulatory and astringent action respectively. In medicine, rose petals are used as mild laxative, useful for sour throat or enlarged tonsils, cooling, astringent and used to relive uterine haemorrhage, brain trouble, headache, heart trouble impotency, skin diseases and burning sensation of the body due to high fever.

Rose petal is widely accepted herbal skin toner and conditioning agent, the chief uses of rose are in perfumery, skin care & hair care. It is used as skin antiseptic, skin softner, coolant, antiflammatory, astringent haemostatic & styptic. In India, a hair oil is produced from rose petals by enfleurage with wet sesamum seeds, chiefly produced in U.P. and known as Gul-Roghan.

RADERMACHERA Zoll. & Moritzi
FAMILY-BIGNONIACEAE
Radermachera xylocarpa (Roxb.) K. Schum.
Common Names :
English : Padri tree
Marathi : Kharsing
Malayalam : Vedangkonna
Distribution : Khandesh, Konkan, Deccan, S. Mahrata Country. W. Ghats of Madras State and N. Circars.
Applications : The plant is acredited with antiseptic properties and a resin extracted from the wood is used for the treatment of skin troubles.
Category : Skin Care
Action : Antiseptic

RAFFLESIA R.Br.
FAMILY-RAFLESIACEAE

Rafflesia patma Blume.
Distribution : Java
Applications : The flowers are used locally as an astringent.
Categoy : Skin, Dental & Oral Care
Action : Astringent

RANDIA LINN.
FAMILY-RUBIACEAE

Randia maculata DC.
Distribution : Tropical Africa
Applications : The fruits yield a dye, used locally for tattooing.
Category : Tatooing, Body Colouring & Skin Painting

Randia malleifera Benth and Hook
Distribution : Tropical Africa
Applications : The juice from the fruit is used as ink in the regions of white Nite. The dark sap is used locally to stain the skin.
Category : Tatooing, Body Colouring & Skin Painting

Randia spinosa Poir.
Common Names :
English ; Common Emetic tree
Hindi : Mainphal
Sanskrit : Madana
Distribution : Sub Himalayan tract from the Rawalpindi district eastwards, ascending in Sikkim up to 4000 ft. Southwards extends to Chittagong and Peninsular India.
Applications : The unripe fruits are used as a soap in some areas (saponin 2-3% in fresh fruits & 10% in dried fruits).
Category : Soaps & Detergents
Action : Cleaning, Detergent

RANUNCULUS Linn.
FAMILY-RANUNCULACEAE

Ranunculus scelaratus Linn.
Common Names :
English : Blister butter cup
Hindi : Jal Dhania
Distribution : Warm valleys of Himalayas, Northern India. Mt. Abu, Bengal, Sind and Waziristan.
Applications : Rubifacient. Used against skin disorders in homeopathy & popular medicine, seeds used to destroy foul breath.
Category : Skin, Hair, Dental Care
Action : Rubifacient, Breath Freshner

SIMMONDSIA CHINENSIS (LINK) C.SCHNEID
"JOJOBA"
A NATURAL MOISTURIZER AND SKIN & HAIR CONDITIONER

Traditionally a hair restorer, jojoba oil is one of the most popular natural emollient and skin & hair conditioning agent of the modern days cosmetics and it has replaced the petroleum waxes from modern cosmetic products to a great extent.

"JOJOBA" botanically known as Simmondsia chinensis (Link) C.Schneid belongs to family Simmondsiaceae, commanly known as pignut, goatnut and deernut is an attractive shrub, 1-2 meter high bearing opposite, entire, oblong-ovate beautiful leaves. The shrub bears unisexual flowers and nut like ovoid leathery fruits.

"JOJOBA" mostly found in arid and drier regions of the world and cheifly distributed in tropical America particularly in Southern Arizona, Sourthern California, Sonora and Baza California & also in Argentina. Jojoba has also been introduced in India in the arid regions.

The plant part of cosmetic importance of the herb is its seeds which contains a waxy liquid, popularly known as "JOJOBA OIL" which is obtained by solvent extraction. The "JOJOBA OIL" composed of high molecular Weight C_{20} and C_{22} esters of straight long chain monounsaturated fatty acids and alcohols including monoethylenic acids (eicosenoic acid and docosenoic acid); alcohols (eicosenol and docosenol) traces of oleic and palmitoleic acids and a glucoside (Simmondsin).

The "JOJOBA OIL" is highly stable and does not oxidize volatize or become rancid after standing for long periods of time. The "JOJOBA OIL" is considered as an excellent emollient and skin & hair conditioning agent. The Oil is included in a variety of cosmetic products such as shampoos, lipsticks, makeup products, cleansing products, face, body/hand creams & lotions. JOJOBA wax beads (Hydrogenated JOJOBA OIL) are used as an exfoliating agent in facial scrub, body polishing preparations, soaps and shower gels.

Hydrogenated JOJOBA wax is used in Lipsticks, Lotions, Creams Ointments, hair styling gels and other products because it provides lubricity and emolliency in creams and lotions, forms matrix with other waxes for nolding pigments and oils in lipsticks. Increases viscosity of the products and itself is an excellent skin and hair conditioner & moisturizer.

Useful Cosmetic Herbs

SACCHAROMYES Meyenx Hansen.
FAMILY-SACCHAROMYCETACEAE
Saccharomyes cerevisiae Hansen
Common Names :
English : Brewers' Yeast, Bakers' Yeast
Applications : The compressed yeast is sold dried (Cerevisiae Fermentum Compressum) as a source of Vitamin B complex.
Category : Skin & Hair Care
Action : Source of Natural Vitamins

SALACIA Linn.
FAMILY-CELASTRACEAE

Salacia macrophylla Blume.
Common Names : Katji pot
Distribution : Malaya
Applications : A paste of the leaves is used to treat skin diseases.
Category : Skin Care

SALMEA DC.
FAMILY-COMPOSITAE

Salmea eupatoria DC.
Distribution : Mexico
Applications : When root is chewed it has a local anaesthetic effect on the tongue and gums and is used locally to treat tooth-ache.
Category : Dental & Oral Care
Action : Local Anaesthetic

SALVIA Linn.
FAMILY-LABIATAE

Salvia lyrata Linn.
Common Names :
English : Lyre-leaved Sage

Distribution : E.N. America
Applications : The local Indians use an ointment made from the roots to treat sores.
Category : Skin Care

Salvia moorcroftiana Wall
Common Names :
Punjab : Kaligarri, Shobri, that
Distribution : W.Himalayas from Kashmir to kumaon; 6,000-9000ft.
Applications : Leaves applied as poultice to boils, wounds and ulcers.
Category : Skin Care
Action : Healing, Antiseptic

Salvia officinalis Linn.
Common Names :
English : Sage, Garden sage
Hindi : Sefakuss
Distribution : Introduced into some Indian gardens.
Application : Leaves are used as dentrifice. The herb has been used in tooth and mouth washes, gargles, poultices, powders, hair tonics and hair dressings.
Category : Hair, Dental & Oral Care
Action : Tonic, Dentrifice

Salvia plebeia R.Br.
Common Names :
Bengali : bhu-tulasi
Bombay : Kamarkass Seeds
Distribution : Throuhout India
Applications : Seeds mucilaginous. Mucilage is employed to give gloss to the hair.
Category : Tatooing Body Colouring & Skin Painting.

Trigonella foenum-graecum Linn.
"METHI OR FENUGREEK"
Youthfullness forever

"Methi" of Fenugreek Elixir is an ancient reciepe for youthfullness forever and fenugreek was highly esteemed for its rejuvenating properties and it was believed that the fenugreek elixir would turn an old man into a youngman.

"METHI" botanically known as Trigonella foenum-graecum Linn. belongs to family Fabaceae is an annual herb and grown as a rabi crop in India. It has been used for millenia as a drug, food and spice in Egypt, India & Middle East.

The methi seeds are important from cosmetic and medicinal point of view. The seeds contains simple alkaloids, saponins, flavonoids, proteins and mucilage. The seeds are aromatic carminative, tonic and galactagogue. They are used externally in poultices for boils, abcesses and ulcers and internally as emollient for inflammation of intestinal tracts. The seeds are also used for chapped lips and as a hair tonic to cure baldness.

Ayurveda recommends seeds as tonic, antipyretic, anthelmintic, increase the appetite, astringent to the bowels; remove bad taste from mouth & useful in heart diseases.

Fenugreek (Methi) is a traditional component of hair care products mainly for its cleansing & softening activity through stimultory and protective behaviours to bring back normal health for dull hair. In Indian system of medicine fenugreek (Methi) is claimed to have properties like cleansing, skin toning and stimulation, checks hairloss, stimulates hair growth and darkness them. In Egypt, the herb is a reciepe for youthfullness and spotless skin.

TACCA J. R. and G. Frost
FAMILY-TACACACEAE

Tacca fatsiifolia Warb.
Common Names : Kanalong, Nonno, Rayung-payungar
Distribution : Indonesia, Philippines
Applications : The plant is used locally as a poultice for wounds.
Category : Skin Care

Tacca palmata Blume=T.monaena
Common Names : Gadoong ti koos, Koom is ootjing, Temoo giling
Distribution : Malaysia, Philippines
Applications : The tubers are used as a poultice for boils.
Category : Skin Care

TAMARINDUS Tourn. ex. Linn.
FAMILY-CAESALPINIACEAE, LEGUMINOSAE

Tamarindus indica Linn.
Common Names :
English : Tamarind Hindi : Imli
Sanskrit : Abdika, panktipatra
Distribution : Grown for fruits & tannins.
Applications : The leaves are applied to reduce lings, ringworms and tumors. Bark has astringent & tonic properties & heal ulcers. The seeds are astringent, they are boiled and used as a poultice to the boils.
Category : Skin Care.
Action : Astringent, Reduce inflammation

TAMARIX Linn.
FAMILY-TAMARICACEAE.

Tamarix chinensis Lour.
Common Names : Tcheng lieou
Distribution : China, Japan, Indonesia, Indochina.
Applications : The Chinese use the leaves as a poultice on wounds.
Category : Skin Care, Aromatic & Medicated Baths

TANACETUM Linn.
FAMILY-ASTERACEAE

Tanacetum balsamina Linn.
Common Names :
English : Balsamic Tansy
Distribution : N.Temperate
Applications : The leaves, flowers or oils is used in mild cases of burns, bruises and mild irritation of the skin.
Category : Skin Care, Anti-irritant
Action : Antiitch

Urtica dioca Linn.
"BICHOO BOOTI / STINGING NETTLE"
The Secret of Healthy Hair

Stringing Nettle, botanically known as Urtica dioca Linn. is a member of family Urticaceae has been named so because this species is armed with stinging hair on the leaves and stems, which on contact with the skin cause irritation and symptoms of urticaria or nettle rash.

The herb found in the Himalayas from Kashmir to Kumaun at altitudes of 2100-3200m. The herb is few meter high with grooved stems abundantly armed with stringing hair; leaves are cordate, serrate; flowers greenish.

Herb contains amines including histamine, serotonin, acetylcholine, flavonoids, lecithin, carotenoids, vitamin C, triterpenes, organic acids and relatively high amount of calcium, potassium and silicic acid.

The herb is diuretic, antiallergenic, haemostatic, and antispasmodic. The extracts of nettle also possess marked antibacterial activity against a wide range of bacteria. The leaves have been used as an expectorant and blood purifier. Urtica is used as a hair stimulant, stimulating the circulation of the capillary vessels of the skin (scalp) and increasing the supply of nutrient materials to the epidermis thereby improving the hair growth. The aerial parts are claimed to have anti-dandruff properties are also cleanse the hair of waxes. Ethanolic extracts of Urtica dioca, along with those of Arctium lappa, Thymus serpyllum and Matricaria chamomilla forms an ingredient of the preparation for hair & scalp. The nettle also contains tannins, silicic acid and calcium in fair amount which have astringent, firming and re-mineralising effects respectively on the skin. A massage preparation is made from the roots and leaves for relaxation of the muscles after sports.

Because of the above claimed virtues nettle extracts are used as a biological additive in a number of cosmetic preparations such as shampoos, conditioners, skin freshners and miscellaneous skin care products.

Useful Cosmetic Herbs

URGINEA Steinh.
FAMILY-LILIACEAE
Urginea indica Kunt.
Common Names :
English : Indian Squill, timesqull sea onion
Hindi : Jangli Piyaz
Sanskrit : Vana pandan
Distribution : W. Himalayas, Bihar, Chota Nagpur, Konkan and coromandel coast.
Applications : The bulbs are used to remove warts and corns. To relieve burning sensation of the soles the bulbs are heated bruised and applied to the feet.
Category : Skin Care
Action : Antitumour

URTICA Linn.
FAMILY-URTICACEAE

Urtica dioca Linn.
Common Names :
English : Stinging Nettle
Hindi : Bichoo Booti
Distribution : N.W. Himalayas from Kashmir and the salt range to Simla, 8000-10700 ft.
Applications : It enters into compresses for wounds and sores and is used as a hair stimulant and for cleaning hair wax and dandruff. Ethanolic extract of Urtica dioca along with those of Arctium lappa. Thymus serpyllum and Matricaria chamomilla forms an ingredient of the preparation of hair & scalp. They (Folia et Herba Urticae) are also used in home remedies for skin troubles and rashes, burns and to wash the hair. A decoction of the roots (Nettle Root, Radix Urticae, Rhizoma urticae) is used as an astringent and as a hair-wash.
Category : Skin & Hair Care
Action : Astringent, Antidandruff, Stimulant

USNEA Linn.
FAMILY-USNEACEAE

Usnea barbata Hoffin
Common Names :
English : Bearded Usnea, Old Man's Beard
Distribution : Temperate regions
Applications : Yields a red-brown dye, used for dyeing wool. The powdered plant (Cyprus Powder) was used in the 17th century as a toilet powder and for powdering wigs.
Category : Hair Care
Action : Hair Dye

Vetiveria zizanioides (Linn.) Nash.

"KHUS"

Keeps You Cool

Since ancient times khus has a great reputation as coolant or refrigerant. In earlier times the roots have been used for making screns (Khus Chicks) mats, hand fans and baskets. The screens were hung like curtains in the house and when sprinkled with water impart a fragrant coolness to air. In indegenous medicine system, the khus had a great reputation as cooling medicine useful in burning sensation, excessive sweating, foul breath, thirst, headache and cooling to the brain; A paste of pulverised roots is used as a cooling external application in fevers.

Vetiveria zizaniodes (Linn.) Nash is a member of grass family (graminae) found throughout the plains and lower hills of India, particularly on the river banks and in rich marshy soil ascending to an altitude of 1,200 meter. The grass is chiefly cultivated in Kerala.

The roots contains an essential oil known as vetiver oil containing cadinane and eucadesmane, sesqueterpenes, khusilal and others. The khus root posses cooling, tonic, alexteric, stomachic and astringent properties useful to ally thirst in fever and inflammatory affections. The root is cooling to the brain relieves oppressive heat or burning sensation of the body.

Khus is used as a paste to relieve oppressive heat, to cure skin diseases, allergic condition, sweat and ulcers. The roots possess styptic and haemostatic properties remove skin blemishes, useful for facial skin and hair care.

Khus is a useful ingredient in traditional Indian cosmetic preparations. It has mostly protective activity to promote skin & scalp conditions as well as it could offer a soothing benefit to dry and bruised skin and scalp.

VALLARIS Burm. f.
FAMILY-APOCYNACEAE

Vallaris solanacea Kuntze.
Common Names :
Hindi : Ramsar
Sanskrit : Bhadravalli
Kumaon : Dudhi
Distribution : More or less throughout India commonly cultivated.
Applications : The milky sap or latex produced by plant is applied to wounds and old sores. It is said to has ten healing. It is popular remedy for toothache and inflamed gums. The bark is astringent and is used by the kols tribals for fixing loose teeth. It is one of ingredients of vishagarbha taila.
Category : Skin, Dental & Oral Care
Action : Antiinflammatory, Astringent

VALERIANA Linn.
FAMILY-VALERIANACEAE

Valeriana officinalis Linn.
Common Names :
English : Valerian
Hindi : Billilotan
Distribution : Europe, India (Kashmir)
Applications : The valeriana is one of the plant which contains good amount of various mineral salts such as calcium magnesium, potassium, phosphorous and iron & have been claimed to supply the skin with trace elements which are often absent in normal human diet. The are said to regulate the dermal water balance and protect the skin from dehydration.
Category : Skin & Hair Care
Action : Stimulant, Source of natural minerals

VANILLA Mill.
FAMILY-ORCHIDACEAE

Vanilla griffithii Reichb.
Common Names :
English : Telinga kerbaoo
Distribution : India, Malaysia
Applications : The juice from the leaves is used as a hair tonic.
Category : Hair Care
Action : Stimulant

VAUQUE Correa. ex. Humb & Bonpl.
FAMILY-BOSACEAE

Vauque linia correa.
Distribution : Mexico
Applications : A yellow dye from the bark is used locally to stain goat skins.
Category : Natural Colour

VENTILAGO Gaertn
FAMILY-RHAMACEAE

Ventilago madraspatana Gaertn.
Common Names :
English : Red Creeper
Hindi : Pitli
Sanskrit : Raktavall;
Distribution : Mumbai Presidency, Konkan, W.Ghats. S.M. Country, Madras State, Deccan Forests from Kistna to Mysore and Coimbatore.

Withania somenifera Dunal.

"ASHWAGANDHA"

The Indian Answer to Ginseng

Withania somenifera Dunal, is a member of family Solanaceae commonly known as "Ashwagandha" or Hair flower tree. The plant is an erect evergreen tomentose shrub found throughout the drier parts of India. Afganistan and as farwest as Israel.

It has always had a prominent place in Ayurvedic, Unani and Ancient Indian systems of medicines, where it is used to restore the balance of life forces much in the same way as Ginseng and Elutherococus are used. It is often referred to as Indian ginseng, the Ashwagandha roots contains alkaloids, glycosides, starch, free amino acids and reducing sugars.

Ashwagandha root is useful in the treatment of inflammatory conditions, ulcers and scabies when applied locally. The leaves are bruised and applied to lesions, painful swellings and sore eyes. Among the glycosides (withaniolides) withaferin A is extremely potent and shows marked antibacterial and antifungal action. The withaferin A exhibit fairly potent anti-arthritic and anti-inflammatory activities and could effectively supress the inflammation. The green berries of the herb is used to treat ringworm externally. The herb is used to kill lice in Afganistan.

A Leaf paste is used to cure erisepelas, eye sores, bed sores, boils and to kill lice. The flowers of Withania are exclusively hair-care remedy in India. Other parts of the shrub are considered for diverse applications including use as an aphrodisiac & immunostimulant. The plant is good for circulation of scalp improving the structure of the hair, used in preparations against greasy hair and dandruff. The herb is considered rejuvenatring in Ayurveda.

Useful Cosmetic Herbs

WAHLENBERGIA Schard.ex.Roth.
FAMILY-COMPANULACEAE

Wahlenbergia marginata (Thunb.) A. DC
Common Names :
Mundari : Tosad Kesari
Oraon : Dudma arka
Distribution : North & North East India
Application : The herb is crushed and used for strengthening the loose teeth and also for skin troubles.
Category : Skin, Dental & Oral Care
Action : Strenthen Gums

WALTHERIA Linn.
FAMILY-STERCULIACEAE

Waltheria indica Linn.
Common Names :
Bengali : Khardudhi
Telugu : Nallabenda
Mundari : Khain
Distribution : All the hotter parts of India
Applications : The plant is used as a resinous powder for drying and healing wounds. A decoction of the aerial parts is used in skin eruptions and for cleaning wounds.
Category : Skin Care
Action : Protective

WEINMANNIA Linn.
FAMILY-CUNONIACEAE

Weinmannia selloi Engl.
Distribution : S.America
Applications : The astringent bark is used locally in Brazil as a poultice for wounds.
Category : Skin Care
Action : Astringent

WIDELIA Jacq.
FAMILY-ASTERACEAE

Widelia chinensis Merill.
Common Names :
Hindi : Bhanra, Bhangra
Sanskrit : Bhringaraja, kesaraja
Distribution : Bengal, Assam, Konkan, Plain districts of the Madras state.
Applications : The herb is said to possesses properties similar to the Eclipta alba. The leaves are used for dyeing grey hair and for promoting the growth of hair, their juice is used for tattoing, the colour produced is deep bluish back and indelible. The root is bluish black. The root is pounded as a black dye with salts of Iron. The leaves are used for skin disorderers and alopecia.
Category : Hair Care
Action : Promote Hair Growth & Darkens Hair Colour

WITHANIA Paug.
FAMILY-SOLANCEAE

Withania somenifera Dunal.
Common Names :
Hindi : Asgandh
Sanskrit : Ashwagandha
Distribution : In the drier parts of India ascending to 5,500 ft. in the Himalayas.
Applications : It is useful for inflammatory conditions. ulcers, and scabies in the form of external applications. Leaves used as a

febrifuge and applied to lesions. painful swelling and sore eyes. The roots are used to kill lice.
Category : Hair & Skin Care
Action : Antiinflammatory, Antilice

XYLOPIA Linn.
FAMILY-ANNONACEAE

Xylopia caroliniana Walt
Distribution : E.N. America
Applications : The leaves and roots are used locally as a poultice for skin diseases.
Category : Skin Care

Xylopia communis Kunth.
Distribution : Tropical America.
Applications : The roots are used in Brazil to treat skin diseases, including leprosy.
Category : Skin Care

YUCCA Linn.
FAMILY-AGAVACEAE

Yucca filamentosa Linn.
Common Names :
English : Soap Tree Yucca
Distribution : S.U.S.A. to Mexico
Applications : The roots are used locally as a soap substitute.
Category : Soaps & Detergents
Action : Detergent

Yucca glauca Nutt.
Common Names :
English : Small Soapwort
Distribution :S.W.U.S.A. to Mexico
Applications : Local Indian use the roots as a soap substitute
Category : Soaps & Detergents

Action : Detergent

ZAMIA Linn.
FAMILY-ZAMIACEA

Zamia clalva-herculis Linn.
Common Names :
English : Hercules Club Prickly Ash, Toothache Tree.
Distribution :S.U.S.A
Applications : A decoction of the bark is used medicinally to treat toothache and rheumatism. The berries are used as a tonic and stimulant.
Categoy : Skin, Dental & Oral Care
Action : Astringent, Stimulant

ZANTHOXYLUM Linn.
FAMILY-RUTACEAE

Zanthoxylum alatum Roxb.
Common Names :
Hindi : Darmar. Tezmal Timur
Sanskrit : Andhaka, Driha. Sanuja
Distribution : Trans-Indus. Punjab along the foot of the Himalayas from the indus eastward upto 5,000 ft. Kumaon 5,000-7000ft. eastwards to Bhutan. Khasia Hills 2,000-3000ft.
Applications : The fruits are used for the diseases of the lips & leucodema.

The seeds are used to remove foul smell from the mouth. The fruits and branches are used as a remedy for toothache.
Category : Skin, Dental & Oral Care
Action : Healing, Breathfreshner, Astringent

Useful Cosmetic Herbs

ZIZYPHUS Toum.ex Linn.
FAMILY-RHAMNACEAE

Zizyphus endlichii Loes.
Distribution : Mexico
Applications : The bark is chewed to relieve toothache.
Category : Dental & Oral Care
Action : Local Anaesthetic

Zizyphus mummularia wight & Am. Prodr.
Common Names :

English : Wild jujube
Hindi : Jarberi, Jharberi
Sanskrit : Ajapriya
Distribution : Dry and arid regions W.Rajputana, Cutch Kathiarwar Gujrat & Khandesh.
Applications : The leaves are applied to scabies and to boils; the decoction of leaves used as gargle for bleeding gums.
Category : Dental, Oral & Sking Care
Action : Astringent, Styptic

OTHER USEFUL PUBLICATIONS

★ HANDBOOK OF SYNTHETIC & HERBAL COSMETICS
★ COSMETICS PROCESSES & FORMULATIONS HANDBOOK
★ HAND BOOK OF PERFUEMS WITH FORMULATIONS
★ ESSENTIAL OILS PROCESSES & FORMULATIONS HAND BOOK
★ HAND BOOK OF ESSENTIAL OILS MFG. & AROMATIC PLANTS
★ HANDBOOK OF PERFUMES & FLAVOURS
★ HAND BOOK OF HERBS, MEDICINAL & AROMATIC PLANTS CULTIVATION

AVAILABLE AT :

ENGINEERS INDIA RESEARCH INSTITUTE
Regd. Off. : 4449, Nai Sarak (S1), Main Road, Delhi-6 (India)
Ph. : 3918117, 3916431, 3960797, 3920361 Fax : 91-11-3916431
E-mail : eirisidi@bol.net.in Website : startindustry.com

Chapter - 2

A LIST OF COMMON COSMETIC HERBS THEIR ACTIVE CONSTITUENTS AND COSMETIC APPLICATIONS

Botanical Names : Acacia Concinna (PODS)
Common Name : Shikakai
Active Constituents : saponins, alkaloids, tannins
Applications : Foaming & cleaning agent, increase skin permeability, promotes hair growth & an astringent.

Botanical Names : Achillea millefolium (WH)
Common Name : Millefoil
Active Constituents : alkaloids, flavonoids, essential oils, salicylic acid, amino acids
Applications : Stimulate skin circulation, increase skin permeability, soften the hard epidermis, enhance nutrients absorption

Botanical Names : Allium cepa (Bulbs)
Common Name : Onion
Active constituents : Vitamin C, aminoacids & peptides, essential oils phenolic acids
Application : Antiacne, cure chilblains, blemished skin, boils, abcesses and blackheads; also effective in burns and scalds
Botanical Names : Aloe vera (exudate)

Common Name : Aloe
Active Constituents : poly saccharides
Applications : Glycosides anti-irritant, healing, antiaging, soothing

Botanical Names : Althea officinals (W/H)
Common Name : Marsh Mallow
Active Constituents : gums, sugars, pectins, starch
Applications : Emollient, humectant, enhances skin hydration and soothing

Botanical Names : Ammi magis (Seeds)
Common Name : Creater Ammi
Active Constituents : xanthotoxin
Increases kin pigmentation, used for treating leucoderma & an effective suntan promoting agent

Botanical Names : Agnelica archangelica (Roots)
Common Name : Angelica
Active Constituents : Essential Oil
Applications : Antiinflammatory, antiperspirant

Botanical Names : Angelica keiskei (Leaves)
Common Name : Angelica
Active Constituents : Chalkone, Coumarins

A List of Common Cosmetic Herbs their active constituents and cosmetic applications

Applications : U-V protection, stimulate blood circulation.

Botanical Names : Apium graveolens (Fruits)
Common Name : Celery
Active Constituents : Coumarins, Coumarin glycosides, essential oils, oleoresin
Applications : Suntanning of the skin, antioxidant & stem exhibit significant antiinflammatory activity

Botanical Name : Arctium lappa (Roots)
Common Name : Burdock
Active Constitutents : Inulin, arctin, polyacetylones
Application : Cure acne & psoriasis, healing in burns, hair restoring, bacteriostatic and fungistatic, antidandruff

Botanical Name : Arnica montana (W/H)
Common Name : Arnica
Active Constitutents : essential oils, arnicin
Application : Hyperaemic, stimulant (skin & scalp), prevent hair loss

Botanical Name : Artemesia abrotanum
Common Name : Southern wood

Botanical Name : Azadirachta indica (leaf & bark)
Common Name : Neem Tree
Active Constituents : Alkaloids, Terpenoids, essential oil sulphur compounds, tannins
Application : Astringent, antidandruff & stimulate hair growth.

Botanical Name : Betula alba (sap)
Common Name : Beech
Active Constitutents : fructose, dextrose, fruit acids, calcium & magnesium
Application : Improves hair texture, promotes hair growth.

Botanical Name : Betula alba (Bark)
Common Name : Beech
Active Constituents : betulin & methyl salicylate and others
Application : Antiseptic, antidandruff, skin stimulant

Botanical Name : Bidens cernua (W/H)
Common Name : Burr marigold
Active Constituents : Triyne
Application : Antibacterial, antifungal, antiinflammatory & antiparasitic in skin diseases.

Botanical Name : Borago officinalis (W/H)
Common Name : Borage
Active Constituents : alkaloids cholines silicic acid, calcium and potassium, mucilage
Application : Skin stimulant, strenhthen hair, provides elasticity & firmness to skin, enhances skin hydration and nutrition, oil is used for skin disease.

Botanical Name : Camellia sinesis (Leaves)
Common Name : Tea
Active Constituents : flavonoids, aminoacids, caffeine, vitamins
Application : Antioxidant, source of vitamins B & E of essential aminoacids

Botanical Name : Carum carvi
Common Name : Caraway
Active Constituents : essential oils, fatty oils
Application : Deodorant, disinfectant

Botanical Name : Centella asiatica (whole herb)
Common Name : Gotukola
Active Constituents : phytosterols, glycosides, tannins, essential oils
Application : Protective, promotes growth of hair, skin & nails, astringent, prevent hair loss

Botanical Name : Citrus limonum
Common Name : Lemon
Active Constituents : terpenoids, flavonoids, essential oils
Application : Antiseptic, antidandruff, skin stimulant

Botanical Name : Cola nitida (seeds)
Common Name : Cola
Active Constituents : Tannins
Application : Anti-irritant, enhances skin nutirition.

Botanical Name : Convallaria majlis
Common Name : Lily of the valley
Active Constituents : glycosides valeric acid, wax, tannins
Application : Stimulant, protective, astringent

Botanical Name : Coptis teeta (Rhizome)
Common Name : Mamira
Active Constituents : Berberine, palmitine
Application : U-V protection

Botanical Name : Cucumis Sativa (Fruit)
Common Name : Cucumber
Active Constituents : auxins, lysozym, vitamin C
Application : Antibacterial, antinflammatory, mild bleaching agent, enhances skin hydration

Botanical Name : Curcuma longa (Rhizome)
Common Name : Turmeric
Active Constituents : terpenoids, alkaoids carotenoids, essential oils
Application : Antiseptic, anti-inflammatory, improves complexion, soften hard skin

Botanical Name : Daucus carota (Rhizome)
Common Name : Carrot
Active Constituents : B-carotenses, tocopherols
Application : Source of vita. A and vita. E

Botanical Name : Echinalea angustifolia (W/H)
Common Name : Coneflower
Active Constituents : flavonoids, essential oil, cichoric acid, caffeic acid
Application : Antiseptic, healing, cure eczema, burns acne & boils.

Botanical Name : Eclipta alba (whole herb)
Common Name : Bhringraj
Active Constituents : alkaloids, free amonoacids, flavonoids
Application : Stimulate skin and scalp, tone and tighten the skin, stimulate skin circulation, promote hair growth and darkens them

A List of Common Cosmetic Herbs their active constituents and cosmetic applications

Botanical Name : Emblica officinalis (fruits)
Common Name : Amla
Active Constituents : glycosides, bioflavonoids, vitamin C, tannins
Application : Antioxidant, astringent, source of vitamin C, revitalize hair and skin

Botanical Name : Equisetum arvense (whole herb)
Common Name : Horse tail
Active Constituents : silicic acid, tannins etc.
Application : Make the connective tissues of the skin and hair firm, strengthen the hair, make skin firm & elastic

Botanical Name : Erythrea centaurium (W/H)
Common Name : Centaury
Acctive Constituents : glycosides, valeric acid, wax & tannin
Applications : Astringent, soothing, styptic

Botanical Name : Euphrasia officinalis (W/H)
Common Name : Eyebright
Active Constituents : Tannins
Applications : Astringent, styptic

Botanical Name : Foeneculum vulgare (Fruit)
Common Name : Fennel
Active Constituents : calcium compounds, essential oil
Applications : Strengthen hair, make skin firm & elastic, mild antiseptic, antiirritant close large skin pores

Botanical Name : Fumaria officinails (W/H)
Common Name : Fumitory
Active Constituents : alkaloids, tannins, pholobaphenes
Applications : Mild bleaching herb, effective in fading freckles and suntan

Botanical Name : Geum urbanum (Roots)
Common Name : Avens
Active Constituents : tannins
Applications : Astringent, haemostatic, antiseptic and antiinflammatory

Botanical Name : Glycyrrhiza glabra (Roots)
Common Name : Liquorice
Active Constituents : terephenoids
Applications : Antiinflammator, antiperspirant

Botanical Name : Goosypium species (Roots)
Common Name : Cotton
Active constituents : cerebrosides/ ceramides
Applications : Skin hydration, skin suppleness, integral part of skin intercellular memberane network.

Botanical Name : Hamamelis virginicus(Bark)
Common Name : Witch hazel
Active Constituents : tannins
Application : Astringent, retard inflammation, antiseptic, close large skin pores

Botanical Name : Hibiscus rosa

sinensis (Flowers)
Common Name : Chinarose
Active Constituents : flavonoids, tannins, albuminoids, soluble carbohydrates
Application : Stimulate circulation of scalp & skin, improves skin hydration, antiseptic, astringent, skin toning

Botanical Name : Humulus lupulus (Catkins)
Common Name : Hops
Active Constituents : Bacids, Phytohormones, essential oils
Application : Estrogenic activity, promote skin's blood circulation, antiacne, stimulates formation of new cells.

Botanical Name : Hypericum perforatum (W/H)
Common Name : St. Jhon's wort
Active Constituents : choline, stearine
Application : Astringent, retard inflammation, antiseptic, close large skin pores

Botanical Name : Inula helenium (Roots)
Common Name : Elecampane
Active Constituents : essential oils, sterols inulin, pectins
Application : Antibacterial and antifungal, prevent pimples, extract of herb make a good cleansing lotion for spots and pimples.

Botanical Name : Jasminum officinale (flowers)
Common Name : Jasmine
Active Constituents : essential oils

Application : Stimulate fibroblast growth

Botanical Name : Juniperus spp. (leaves)
Common Name : Juniper
Active Constituents : essential oils
Application : Stimulate fibroblast growth, skin stimulant

Botanical Name : Lactuca sativa (fruits)
Common Name : Lettuce
Active Constituents : Tocopherols, carotenes, folic acid, calcium pectate
Application : Rich source of vitamin E, concentrates of vitamin E and antioxidants have been prepared from the lettuce seeds used for burns and painful ulcers.

Botanical Name : Lavandula vera (Flowers)
Comon Name : Lavender
Active Constituents : essential oils, tannins, coumarins, flavanoids
Application : Skin toner, stimulate hair growth, improves complextion of the skin, astringent & styptic.

Botanical Name : Lawsonia inermis (Leaves)
Common Name : Henna
Active Constituents : napthoquinones, phytosterols, tannins, mucins
Application : Antiseptic, sunscreen agent, astringent, improves skin hydration, hair conditioners and a hair dye.

Botanical Name : Levisticum officinale (W/H)

A List of Common Cosmetic Herbs their active constituents and cosmetic applications

Common Name : Lovage
Active Constituents : essential oil, coumarins, terpenoids
Application : Deodorant, clear skin of spots and fade freckles.

Botanical Name : Lonicera perclymenum (W/H)
Common Name : Honey suckle
Active Constituents : caffeic acid tannins
Application : U-V protection

Botanical Name : Lycopersicum pimpinellifolium (F)
Common Name : Currant tomato
Active Constituents : Vitamin C tomatine
Application : Antiscorbutic, antifungal, especially against fungal affections of the skin

Botanical Name : Magnolia officinalis (Bark)
Common Name : Magrolia Bark
Active Constituents : phenolics
Application : Antiinflammatory, antioxidant

Botanical Name : Matricharia chamoilla (Flowers)
Common Name : chamomille
Active Constituents : chamazulens
Application : Healing, antiseptic

Botanical Name : Malaleuca alternifolia (Leaves)
Common Name : Tea Tree Oil
Active Constituents : essential oil
Application : Broadspectrum, antimicrobial

Botanical Name : Malalenca leucodendron (Leaves)
Common Name : Cajupat
Active Constituents : essential oil
Application : Antiacne, good for psoriasis, sores etc.

Botanical Name : Mentha piperita (Leaves)
Common Name : Peppermint
Active Constituents : essential oil
Application : Antiseptic, healing, antiirrtant

Botanical Name : Morus alba (Bark)
Common Name : Mulberry
Active Constituents : osoprenyl flavonoids coumarins, essential oil, tannins organic acid
Application : Antimicrobial, astringent used for eczema, wounds & ulcers promote skin whitening.

Botanical Name : Myrtus communis (leaves)
Common Name : Vilayati Mehandi
Active Constituents : essential oil
Application : Antimicrobial, skin whitening, darkens hair

Botanical Name : Nardostachys jatamansi (Roots)
Common Name : Jatamansi
Active Constituents : essential oil
Application : Promotes hair growth, imparts blackness to hair.

Botanical Name : Ocimum sanctum (W/H)
Common Name : Holy Basil
Active Constituents : terpenoids glycosides, essential oil
Applications : Antiseptic, antiirritant, effective against acne &

pimples, stimulate skin and scalp circulation

Botanical Name : Oenothera biennis (Seeds)
Common Name : Evening primrose
Active Constituents : Gamma linoliecacid
Applications : Emollient, good for treatment of eczema and other disorders of the skin, help cell proliferation, improves dull looking skin

Botanical Name : Panax quinquefolia (Roots)
Common Name : Ginseng
Active Constituents : glycosides
Applications : Enhanced skin nutrition, stimulates skin's blood circulation & cell proliferation, antiaging

Botanical Name : Pennesetum glaucum (Grain)
Common Name : Pearl millet
Active Constituents : cerebrosides/ceramides
Applications : Skin hydration, skin suppleness, integral part of intercellular membrance network

Botanical Name : Persea gratissma (Leaves)
Common Name : Avocado
Active Constituents : tannins
Applications : The leaves have antiseptic and astringent properties, close large skin pores, haemostatic, removes excess of oil from hair

Botanical Name : Petroselinum crispum (W/H)
Common Name : Common Parsley
Active Constituents : Essential oils, oleoresins coumarins xanthotoxins, flavonoids
Application : Stimulates skin and scalp circulation, increases skin pigmentation, antiinflammatory

Botanical Name : Phaseolus vulgaris (Peels)
Common Name : Garden bean
Active Constituents : silicic acid, tannins
Applications : Strengthen hair, make skin firm & elastic

Botanical Name : Pilocarpus jaborandi (Leaves)
Common Name : jaborandi
Active Constituents : alkaloids
Applications : Stimulant, promote hair growth, prevent hair loss

Botanical Name : Pimpinella anisum (W/H)
Common Name : Star Anise
Active Constituents : essential oils, coumarins, terpenoids
Applications : Mild antiseptic, antifungal & used to kill head lice

Botanical Name : Plantago major (W/H)
Common Name : Plantain
Active Constituents : glycosides
Applications : Antiinflammatory, good for treating sunburns and minor skin disorders

Botanical Name : Polygonum multiflorum (Roots)
Common Name :
Active Constituents : silicic acid,

A List of Common Cosmetic Herbs their active constituents and cosmetic applications

tannins etc.
Applications : Anti perspirant, make skin firm, improves hair strength

Botanical Name : Pongamia Pinnata
Common Name : Karanj Tree
Active Constituents : napthoquinones
Applications : U-V protection, used to cure chronic skin diseases

Botanical Name : Primula vulgaris (Flowers)
Common Name : Primrose
Active Constituents : essential oil, Tannins
Application : Astringent and mild bleaching agent, clear the skin of spots and fade freckles

Botanical Name : Rose damascena (Petals)
Common Name : Rose
Active Constituents : geraniol glycosides, flavanoids tannins, essential oil
Application : Cooling and soothing effect on skin

Botanical Name : Rosemarianus officinailis (Leaves)
Common Name : Rosemary
Active Constituents : essential oil
Application : Stimulate fibroblast growth & skin stimulant

Botanical Name : Salix species (leaves)
Common Name : Willow
Active Constituents : salicylic acid
Application : Antimicrobial, antiseptic, antidandruff, antiinflammatory

Botanical Name : Salvia officinails (W/H)
Common Name : Sage
Active Constituents : essential oils
Application : Antioxidant, astringent, skin stiumlant, promotes hair growth and darkens them, antidandruff, antimicrobial, antiseptic, antiinflammatory.

Botanical Name : Salvia sclarea (W/H)
Common Name : Clary sage
Active Constituents : essential oils, tannins deterpene alcohols
Application : Reduce inflammation, cure diseases like boils & spots, used as a fragrance component in cosmetics.

Botanical Name : Sambucus nigra (Flower)
Common Name : Elder
Active Constituents : essential oils, glucoside, alkaloids, cholines
Application : Cleansing & soothing, antiinflammatory, beneficial for scaly skin, softens, tones and whitens the skin

Botanical Name : Sanguinaria canadensis (Roots)
Common Name : Blood Root
Active Constituents : tannins
Application : Astringent, styptic

Botanical Name : Santalum album (Wood)
Common Name : Sandal
Active Constituents : essential oils
Application : Stimulant of skin & scalp

Botanical Name : Sapindus mukorassi (Fruits)
Common Name : Soap nut
Active Constituents : Saponins
Application : Cleansing & foaming agent, used in hair rinses and washes

Botanical Name : Saponaria officinalis (bark)
Common Name : Soapwort
Active Constituents : saponins
Application : Antibacterial, cleanser & foaming agent

Botanical Name : simmondsia chinensis (Seeds)
Common Name : Jojoba
Active Constituents : liquid wax
Application : Hair & Skin conditioner & moisturiser

Botanical Name : Stellaria media (W/H)
Common Name : Chickweed
Active Constituents : coumarins, coumarin glycosides, essential
Application : Antibacterial, cleansing, antiacne, used in scrofula and skin diseases

Botanical Name : Swertia species (whole herb)
Common Name : Swertia
Active Constituents : oils, oleoresin glycosides, flavonoids
Application : Expand capillary vessels, raises skin temperature, enhance skin nutrition

Botanical Name : Syphytum officinale (Roots)
Common Name : Comfrey
Active Constituents : allantion, alkaloid, mucopolysaccharides, tannins
Application : Antiinflammatory, astringent, emollient, haemostatic

Botanical Name : Taraxacum officinale (whole Herb)
Common Name : Dandelion
Active Constituents : sulphur, Silicic acid
Application : Antiinflammatory, antimicrobial, promotes hair growth (prevent alopecia)

Botanical Name : Thuja occidentalis (Leaves)
Common Name : White Cedar
Active Constituents : Pinene (terpenes)
Applications : Stimulate fibroblast growth

Botanical Name : Thymus serpyllum (W/H)
Common Name : Wild Thyme
Active Constituents : Essential oils
Applications : Stimulate skin & scalp, antiseptic and antidandruff

Botanical Name : Thymus vulgaris (W/H)
Common Name : Thyme
Active Constituents : Essential oils
Applications : Stimulate fibroblast growth, antiseptic and antidandruff

Botanical Name : Trigonella foenum graecum (Seeds)
Common name : Fenugreek
Active Constituents : alkaloids, essential oils Phytosterols, saponins
Applications : Protective and stimulant, soften and cleanses the skin, makes hair soft and shining,

A List of Common Cosmetic Herbs their active constituents and cosmetic applications

rejuvenating

Botanical Name : Tropaeolum majus (W/H)
Common Name : Nasturtium chloragenic acid, vitamin C, benzisothiocyanate, sulphur
Active Constituents : Glucosides,
Applications : Antimicrobial, antiscorbutic, good for hair and scalp

Botanical Name : Tussilago Farfara (leaves)
Common Name : Colt's foot
Active Constituents : Sulphur, silicic acid
Applications : Antidandruff, in minor skin disorders

Botanical Name : Urtica urens (W/H)
Common Name : Nettle
Active Constituents : Histamines, acetylcholine, flavonoids, vit. C
Application : Antiscorbutic, antifungal especially against fungal affections of the skin

Botanical Name : Veronica officinalis (W/H)
Common Name : Spped well
Active Constituents : tannins
Applications : Astringent, styptic

Botanical Name : Vetiveria zizaniodes (Roots)
Common Name : Khus
Active Constituents : tannins sesquiterpenoids, essential oils, refrigerant
Application : Promotes skin and scalp condition, soothing to skin and scalp, removes skin blemishes,

astringent

Botanical Name : Viola odorata (W/H)
Common Name : Sweet violet
Active Constituents : Alkaloids (Violin), essential oils, glycosides, saponins
Application : Antimicrobial & antifungal, antiinflammatory, improves dull complextion, emollient, keeps the skin soft & supple

Botanical Name : Viola tricolor (whole herb)
Common Name : Heartease
Active Constituents : salicylic acid
Application : Antidandruff, antimicrobial, antiseptic, antiinflammatory

Botanical Name : Viscum album (Leaves & Fruits)
Common Name : Mistletoe
Active Constituents : acetylcholines, histamines flavones, vitamin C, resin
Application : Antiseptic, relax nervous tension externally, sedative & nervine

Botanical Name : Vitis vInifera (leaves/fruits)
Common Name : Grapes
Active Constituents : essential oil
Application : Antiirritant

Botanical Name : Zingiber officinale (Rhizome)
Common Name : Zinger
Active Constituents : Shagoal
Application : Antiinflammatory, healing, antimicrobial, astringent, used for eczema, wounds & ulcers.

Chapter - 3

EQUIPMENT USED IN THE MANUFACTURE OF COSMETICS

INTRODUCTION

Cosmetics manufacture is concerned with a very broad range of processes, there are enough common elements to allow a relatively simple overall view of the subject; this helps considerably in a study of the basic principles of cosmetic production technology. The manufacture of cosmetics is conveniently divided into two parts: (i) Bulk manufacture; and (ii) Unit manufacture. The bulk manufacture is carried out in three steps. They are: (i) Mixing; (ii) Pumping; and (iii) Filtering. The most important step is mixing.

MANUFACTURE OF BULK PRODUCT

A convenient way of classifying the mixing processes is represented in table 1. Every single cosmetics manufacturing process contains minimum one mixing operation.

Table - 1
Scope of mixing operations within the cosmetics industry

	Type of mixing	Examples
1.	Solid/Solid	
	(a) Segregating	None
	(b) Cohesive	Face powders, eye shadows and all dry mixing
2.	Solid/Liquid	(i) Dissolution (of water–soluble dyes, preservatives, powder surfactants, etc.)
		(ii) Suspensions and dispersions (pigments in castor oil and in other liquids)
3.	Liquid/Liquid	
	(a) Miscible	(i) Chemical reactions (formation of soaps from acid and base)

(Cont'd)

Type of mixing	Examples
	(ii) pH control
	(iii) Blending (spirituous preparations, clear lip gloss products)
(b) Immiscible	(i) Extraction (none)
	(ii) Dispersion (emulsions)
4. Gas/Liquid	(i) Absorption (none)
	(ii) Dispersion (aeration and de-aeration)
5. Distributive	
(a) Fluid motion	Heat transfer (during emulsion and other manufacture)
(b) Limited flow	Pumping (pastes and other highly viscous products)

e.g. The manufacture of pigmented emulsion–based cream include four mixing steps. They are :

1. Preliminary dry blending of pigments and excipient (type Ib).

2. Dissolution of oil–soluble and water–soluble materials separately in their appropriate phase (type 2 example i and type 3a).

3. Dispersion or suspension of pigments in the oil or water phase (type 2, example ii).

4. Mixing of the two phases to form an emulsion, possibly with the formation *in situ* of a soap as part of the emulsifier (types 3a and 3b).

5. Adjustment of pH (type 3a).

6. De-aeration of the bulk (type 4).

7. Cooling to ambient temperature and pumping into a storage vessel (type 5a).

The subject of pumping is not clearly separated from that of mixing since pumping implies the forced flow of product. Any flow will naturally introduce an element of mixing if the product is not already homogeneous. Further, since flow is a common element of both processes, the same product characteristics (for example, rheological behaviour) must be taken into account.

Filtering is not usually a unit operation of major importance in cosmetics manufacture except in the production of spirituous preparations (colognes, aftershave and perfumes). It is possible to regard filtering as un-mixing and certainly the flow characteristics of the filtered product are again of prime importance.

Unit Manufacture

Most cosmetic products are filled from bulk in machines specifically designed to handle the units of a particular product type. While it is true that great care must be taken in the choice and the setting up of such machines, the main problems encountered are often concerned with the characteristics of the machines themselves rather than with the manufacture or processing of the product. There are at least two areas, however, where special understanding of the product units and their characteristics are essential for the achievement of efficient production: these are the moulding processes (lipsticks, wax–based sticks, alcohol–stearate gels) and compression processes (compressed eyeshadow, blushers and face powders). A description of unit manufacture could include all filling and packaging operations.

THE MANUFACTURE OF BULK COSMETIC PRODUCTS

Mixing

The object of a mixing operation is to reduce the inhomogeneities in the material being mixed. As Table - 1 shows, inhomogeneity may be of physical or chemical identity or of heat. Further, in the processes demanded by cosmetic manufacture, the mixing is designed to be permanent–or as permanent as it is possible to make it.

The reduction in inhomogeneity depends on the efficiency of the mixing apparatus used and also on the physical characteristics of the materials constituting the mixture. For miscible liquids, homogeneity can be produced at a molecular level whereas for mixture of powders homogeneity is limited to the sizes of the powder particles themselves. When examining a mixture for quality, therefore, the *scale of scrutiny*–the magnification at which the mixture is examined–must vary from product to product. At an acceptable scale of scrutiny, *perfect mixing* implies that all samples removed from the mixture will have exactly the same composition. This is rarely achievable. *Random mixing* is achieved if the probability of finding a particle of a given component in a sample is the same as the proportion of that component in the whole mixture. Random mixing is the aim of all industrial mixing operations and whereas samples removed from such a mixture will not be identical, the variations should be very small. If the scale of scrutiny is reduced sufficiently, however, this may no longer be true.

Mixing can only occur by relative movement between the particles of the constituent components of the mixture. Three basic mechanisms for achieving this relative movement have been identified: bulk flow, convective mixing and diffusive mixing. *Bulk flow* (which includes shear mixing, cutting, folding and tumbling) occurs in pastes and solids, when relatively large volumes of mixture are first separated and then redistributed to another part of the mixing vessel. *Convective mixing* involves the establishment of circulation patterns within the mixture. Finally, *diffusive mixing* occurs by particle collisions and deviation from a straight line. In miscible liquids of sufficiently low viscosity, the thermal energy which is possessed by the constituent molecules may be enough to achieve a good mixture quality by thermal diffusion without additional energy being applied, although this process is usually too slow for industrial purposes.

Many mixing problems arise from the tendency of mixture particles to segregate during attempts to mix them. *Segregation* is defined as the preference of the particles of one component to be in one or more places in a mixer rather than in other places. The size of the non–uniformities in an imperfect mixture is sometimes referred to as the 'scale of segregation' and the difference in composition between neighbouring lumps of volumes is the 'intensity of segregation'. Segregation is not, fortunately, a major problem in cosmetics manufacture although it does manifest itself occasionally (as, for example, in the flotation of pigments during lipstick processing).

SOLID–SOLID MIXING

Solid–solid mixing is of two types: (i) Segregating; and (ii) Cohesive. Free flowing powders exhibit many process advantages (such as easy storage, easy flow from hoppers, smooth flow of product), but have the disadvantage that they tend to segregate unless all the constituent particles are of very similar shape and size. Cohesive powder, on the other hand, lacks mobility, and individual particles are bonded together and move as clumps or aggregates. Although segregation does not appear to be a problem (except, as will be seen, at very small scales of scutiny), cohesive powders are difficult to store and do not easily flow from hoppers.

MANUFACTURE OF PIGMENTED POWDER PRODUCTS

Powder eyeshadows, face powders and powder blushers are commonly composed of the following types of material : Talc, Pigments, pearl agents, Liquid binder and preservative.

The order in which these ingredients are mixed and the process by which the mixing is carried out depend largely upon the type of equipment that is available.

Hammer Mill

The processing of bulk pigmented powder products is carried out using the hammer mill Fig. 18.1. The hammer mill was designed as a comminution machine. It consists of a fast rotating shaft fitted with freely swinging hammers mounted in a cage which is equipped with a breaker plate against which the feed is disintegrated, chiefly by impact from the hammer. The very high speed at which the hammers move (60–100 ms⁻¹) increases the chance of a hammer making contact with each particle and the dwell–time of particles within the chamber is increased by the placement of a variable size screen over the exit.

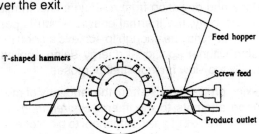

Fig. 18.1. Hammer mill.

Hammer mills are very efficient in the comminution of brittle particles in the range of 1500–50 μm but below this size their efficiency (the probability of direct impact) falls off rapidly. The very high rotational speed of the hammers and the air flow within the chamber ensure that there are enough weak secondary impacts (particle-wall and particle-particle) to break the much weaker pigment agglomerates–which may be up to 50 μm in diameter. The disintegrated agglomerate fractions then stabilise by becoming coated on a larger talc particles and should not be further changed by subsequent passes through the mill.

Hammer mill, has certain disadvantages. For example, from the viewpoint of energy consumption, a hammer mill used is very inefficient. The feed-rate and therefore, the processing time for all but the smallest batch sizes of powder is very slow. Increasing the residence time of powder within the grinding chamber by decreasing this mesh size can cause the screen to become blocked with compacted powder, resulting in overheating and damage to machine and product. The hammer mill is a continuous processing device being used for batch processing. For this reason, it must be fed with a powder mixture which has already been effectively mixed, otherwise the colour of the milled product changes as each section of unmixed bulk passes through. This preliminary mixing must be efficient although it is not necessary for any extension to be achieved at this stage.

The most widely used is the 'ribbon blender' which comprises a horizontal drum containing a rotating axial shaft which carried ribbon-like paddles. In such a device, the pre-mix can take anything between 20 and 60 minutes. Other mixers are now available which utilise higher energy input but are quicker. Table - 2 summarises the properties of some of the more conventional powder mixers. Since it is relatively easy to achieve good mixture quality (at a large scale of scrutiny) in cohesive powders, any mixing device will eventually produce a satisfactory even distribution of components provided that it contains no dead spots where mixing does not take place.

Table - 2
Conventional powder mixers

Type of mixer	Batch/ continuous	Main mixing mechanism	Speed of mixing	Ease of cleaning	Energy consumption	Quality of extension
Horizontal drum	B	Diffusive	Poor	Good	Low	Poor
Loedige-type	B	Convective	Good	Fair	Medium	Fair
Ribbon blender	B or C	Convective	poor	Fair	Low	Poor
Nauta mixer	B	Convective	Good	Poor	Low	poor
V-mixer (with cutters)	B	Diffusive	Poor	Good	Medium	Unknown
Airmix	B	Convective	Good	Fair	Low	Unknown

It is usual to add the liquid binder during this preliminary mixing stage. The binder may be poured into a suitable orifice in the mixer although many production chemists prefer to spray it into the mixer cavity as an aerosol through a venturi or similar device. This procedure helps to distribute the liquid more evenly and avoids the formation of wet, lumpy areas in the powder body. The separation of large agglomerates which takes place subsequently in the mill normally assures the completion of the wetting process provided only that the binder is correctly chosen. Should the binder still appear to be unevenly distributed after the passage of the powder through the mill, the product can often be rescued by passing it through as fine a mesh sieve as possible.

Batch Colour Correction

It is not unusual for the bulk powder product, even though it has been correctly processed, to require colour correction in order to obtain a satisfactory match to the standard. Since any addition of pigment or talc needs to be extended, a passage through the mill is necessary. A common procedure is as follows. After the preliminary coarse mix has been completed, a small amount of the bulk (usually about 5 kg), which is assumed to be representative of the whole, is passed through the mill. This is examined in the laboratory, and if necessary, a pigment addition specified. This correction is added to the 5 kg of milled product, mixing in roughly by hand and the 5 kg is re-milled. The twice-milled sample is returned to the remainder of the bulk and re-mixed in the original mixer. A further 5 kg is then removed and the process is repeated until a match is obtained. The use of pigments previously extended on talc and stored as such. This has the merit of speeding up the correction process.

When pearl agents are part of the formulation, unless an un-pearlised standard is provide, the pearl must be added in the correct proportion to the laboratory sample before colour can be assessed. Pearl is only added to the bulk in the last stage of the manufacturing procedure. The ideal equipment would probably have the following properties :

1. It would be capable of breaking up weak particles in the size range 50–0.5 µm without damaging talc or mica particles of similar diameter.

2. It would be a low energy device, consuming little power itself without heating the powder mixture excessively.

3. It would be a batch processing device capable of mixing and extending in one operation.

4. It would be rapid: processing times of less than 10 minutes would be acceptable.

5. It would not cause excessive aeration of the powder (since this causes further processing problems in later processing).

6. It would be easy to clean.

7. Its efficiency would not vary with the cohesiveness of the powder; it would not be affected by poor flow characteristics.

8. It would be quiet and clean in operation.

Other comminution devices have been shown to produce extension, particularly pin mills and fluid energy mills, yet none seems to work as efficiently as the hammer mill. Recently two types of mixers have been developed. They are : (i) Vertical vortex mixer; (ii) Plough-shear.

Vertical vortex mixer

The powder mixture is placed in a vertical, cylindrical chamber and is then accelerated outwards and upwards into a fluidised vortex motion. The motion may be produced by compressed air blasted sequentially from a series of nozzles contained in a lower cone-shaped section; alternatively, a propeller-shaped tool of 'poor aerodynamic' design may be used which rotates rapidly in the dished base of the mixing bowl. Mixing and dispersion occur at the point of conversion of the powder particles (in the upper point of the mixing bowl) by particle-particle collisions.

Plough-Shear

The high-speed mixer is often referred to as a 'plough-shear' device, because of the unusual shape of the mixing paddles which rotate on an axial shaft in a cylindrical horizontal mixing chamber. These paddles cause the powder from all parts of the chamber to be thrown about in such a way that it all passes rapidly through a zone occupied by a series of rapidly revolving blades on a separate shaft, referred to as a 'chopper'. The chopper is largely responsible for the powder extension and may be switched on or off independently of the main axial drive.

Both types of mixer have been used as partial or complete replacement for the traditional blender-hammer mill combination. The plough-shear type may also be used for wet-processing.

MIXING PROCESSES INVOLVING FLUIDS

Although there are similarities between the flow of powders and the flow of liquids it is obviously easier to set up and sustain flow patterns in the latter. On the whole this makes the mixing processes easier to perform and a much larger variety of equipment is consequently available to choose from.

General principles of Fluid Mixing

Some mixing operations can be thought of as simple blending – for example, the blending of colour solutions into miscible bulk liquids and the blending of oils, alcohol and water in perfumes and colognes. On the other hand, the formation of an emulsion, the suspending of a gelling agent and the distribution of pigment agglomerates in a viscous liquid all involve the breaking up of one of the constituents of the mixture into finer particles during the mixing process. For this reason, it is referred to as 'dispersive' mixing to distinguish it from simple blending.

On the industrial scale, mixing occurs as the result of forced bulk flow within the mixing vessel. Two types of flow can be distinguished, laminar and turbulent. Laminar flow occurs when the fluid particles move along streamlines parallel to the direction of flow. The only mode of mass transfer is by molecular diffusion between adjacent layers of fluid (Brownian motion). In turbulent flow, the fluid elements move not only in the parallel paths but also on erratic and random paths, thus producing eddies which transfer matter from one layer to another. For this reason, turbulent mixing is rapid compared with other mixing mechanisms.

When a quiescent liquid is slowly stirred the flow is laminar but as the velocity increases it may become turbulent; thus the velocity is a significant factor in determining the type of flow set up in the mixing vessel. A valuable aid in describing the critical point at which laminar flow becomes turbulent is due to Reynolds who, in 1883, first demonstrated turbulence. The dimensionless number which bears his name, Re, can be calculated for agitated vessels as follows :

$$Re = \frac{D^2 N \rho}{\eta} \qquad 18.1$$

Where D is the diameter of the impeller, N the impeller speed (rpm), ρ the density of the mixture and h its viscosity.

Although little is known about the mechanism of turbulence, experience has shown that in agitated tanks the onset of turbulence occurs at Reynolds numbers of about 2×10^3. For fully developed turbulence, Reynolds numbers greater than 10^4 are required and are found in many cosmetic mixing processes. The majority of products exhibit non-ideal (non-Newtonian) behaviour which can often be more appropriately described by the expression

$$F = (\eta_{app})^n A \times \text{velocity gradient} \qquad 18.2$$

In this case η_{app} is termed as the 'apparent viscosity' and n usually has a value between 0 and 1. The name given to this type of behaviour is 'pseudoplastic' and the basic difference between materials exhibiting this property and ideal or 'Newtonian' fluids is illustrated in Figure. 18.2. As can be seen, pseudoplasticity is manifested by a fall in viscosity with increasing shear rate at constant temperature. Many cosmetic liquids exhibit this behaviour – especially emulsions and suspensions of particles of the order of 1 mm or less in size.

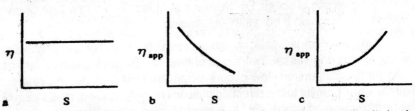

Fig. 18.2 Rate of shear (S) plotted against viscosity (η) or apparent viscosity (η_{app}).

Mixing Equipment for Fluids

In the mixing of fluids, all three mixing mechanisms – bulk flow, turbulent diffusion and molecular diffusion – are usually present. As viscosity increases, however, and turbulence becomes correspondingly more difficult to establish, the parts played by turbulent and molecular diffusion become less important.

Mixing equipment can therefore be divided into two categories, laminar shear and turbulent mixers.

Laminar shear/distributive mixers	Turbulent mixers
Helical screw/ribbon blenders	Turbine-agitated vessels
Two-blade mixers	Pipes
Kneaders	Jet mixers
Extrusion devices	Sparged systems
Calenders	High-speed shear mixers
Static mixers: low Re	Static mixers: high Re

Paddle mixers

Paddle mixers are simple and cheap but very inefficient for all but very low viscosity liquids. They produce mainly tangential flow and are usually mounted centrally because of their large diameter compared with that of the tank.

Turbines

Turbines are probably the most common impeller type used in cosmetic processing since they can cope with a wide range of viscosities and densities. For liquids of low viscosity, the flat-blade impeller is sometimes used Figs. 18.3 (a) and (b). For very viscous materials the blades may be curved backwards in the direction opposite to the rotation, since these require a lower starting torque and seem to give better energy transfer from impeller to liquid Fig 18.3 (c).

Fig. 18.3 (d) illustrates a fixed-pitch *axial flow* impeller. Used without baffles, however, the axial component generated by such turbines remains secondary to the radial flow component. Typically, impellers of this kind are used at rotational speeds of 100–2000 rpm as distinct from the low speed (15–50 rpm) of paddles.

Equipment used in the Manufacture of Cosmetics

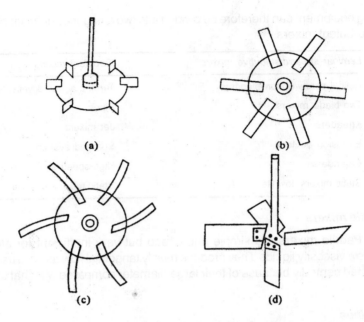

Fig. 18.3 Various designs of turbine impeller.

Propeller mixers

Propeller mixers are restricted to use with low viscosity fluids. They have pitched blades of which the blade angle varies along the length from centre to tip. Flow patterns developed by propeller mixers have a high axial component and the rate of circulation is high. They are usually of relatively small diameter, typically three-bladed, and are used at speeds between 450–2500 rpm. Such stirrers are used extensively in the cosmetics industry for simple blending operations but are not suitable for the suspension of particles which settle rapidly or for the dissolution of sparingly soluble heavier materials.

Many portable mixers are of the propeller type. If the mixer is mounted centrally in the mixing tank Fig. 18.4 (a), because of the entrainment of liquid above the impeller, the surface becomes depressed and a vortex is formed. Generally, vortices are to be avoided because of the low order of turbulence and the air-entrapment which they cause. When they are mounted eccentrically, however Fig. 18.4 (b) turbulence is increased and vortices avoided.

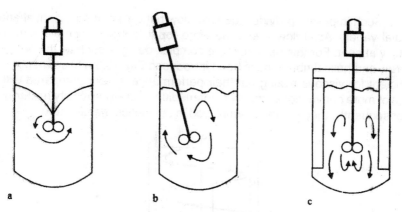

Fig. 18.4 Portable mixers

Mixing in Non-Newtonian Liquids of Low or Medium Viscosity

Many liquids – perhaps the majority – encountered in cosmetics processing are of the shear-thinning and/or elastic rheological type. Naturally, if the liquid is already of low viscosity, the effect of shear-thinning may not be noticeable. On the other hand, more viscous liquids showing these characteristics present considerable problems to the cosmetics processor. The fluid close to the rotating impeller of a mixer is sheared at a high rate and so becomes relatively mobile, but as this is pumped away from the impeller it encounters regions of less intense flow and hence of much higher viscosity. Turbulence is therefore rapidly damped out, decreasing the turnover in the vessel and slowing down the mixing process. Moreover any elasticity shown by the liquid results in the absorption of energy by deformation of a recoverable variety, thus damping out turbulence even further.

Impeller Types and Mixers for High Viscosity Fluids

Propellers and turbines, as already mentioned, work best under turbulent conditions at relatively high rotational speeds. In viscous products, given that such speeds are attainable at all, flow is confined to the regions very close to the impeller, and large stagnant regions in the mixer exist where no mixing can occur without the employment of some secondary mechanism. To eliminate these stagnant regions, large impellers such as paddles, gates, anchors and leaf impellers may be used; these sweep a much greater proportion of the vessel and produce more extensive flow. Usually such impellers are designed to have close clearances with walls, giving a degree of wall-scraping. This help to eliminate build-up of unmixed materials at walls provides a region of high shear for dispersing aggregates and lumps, and may improve the wall heat transfer to and from the bulk.

Such impellers provide extensive flow but only of the tangential and radial variety. Axial flow – and therefore top-to-bottom mixing–is almost totally absent. For this reason, more complex designs such as the helical screw and helical ribbon have been introduced Fig. 18.5. These are more efficient for viscous mixing but their performance is poor compared with that of more conventional impellers for medium and low viscosity mixtures. Consequently, they are rarely employed in cosmetics manufacture.

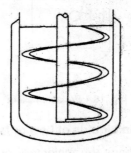

Fig. 18.5 Helical impeller

Axial flow cannot be achieved by the introduction of baffles as when mixing lower viscosity fluids, but some success has been achieved by the use of impeller-draught tube combinations. As the name implies a draught tube is a tubular, axially orientated enclosed space within the main mixing chamber containing an impeller or some other means of forcing the flow of mixture along it. Small impellers or helical screws designed to fill most of the cross-section of such a tube have been successfully used to promote axial flow in most liquids, even those of very high viscosity.

An alternative approach to the problem created by lack of flow in viscous media is the use of impellers which progressively sweep the whole contents of the vessel while the mixture remains stationary. Examples of this include the 'Nauta'-type mixer in which a helical screw sweeps the wall of a conical mixing chamber.

For even more viscous products such as mascara and very thick pastes, equipment which exhibits a greater degree of distributive mixing may be utilised. Such mixers are designed to produce bulk flow and laminar shear by spatial redistribution of elements of the mixture. Perhaps the most commonly encountered mixers of this type are of the single or double action planetary type or the two-blade 'dough' mixer. Their essential feature involves the cutting and folding of a volume of the mixture and the physical replacement of it into another part of the mixer where it is cut and folded again. An example of this distributive mechanism is illustrated in Fig. 18.6, in which for clarity a volume of a mixture has been isolated and divided into six equal segments, one of which consists of a black minor component. The cube is compressed to one quarter of its initial height, cut and reassembled as shown. Redistribution of the minor component has been achieved which, were the process to be repeated often enough, would eventually achieve the desired level of homogeneity.

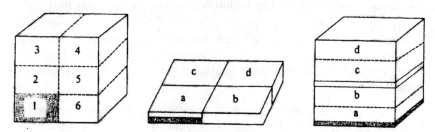

Fig. 18.6 Distributive mixing mechanism

A more recent innovation is the so-called static mixer, of which several designs are now commercially available. Static mixers are essentially in-line mixing devices in which mixtures flowing through a pipe are cut and folded by a series of helical elements in a circular tube Fig. 18.6. These elements (which do not move – hence the name 'static') turn the flowing mixture through an angle of 180°. since alternative elements have opposite pitch and are displaced 90° to each other, this causes the bulk flow to reverse direction at each junction, and thus the leading edge of each element becomes a cutting device, splitting ;and re-folding the mixture in on itself.

Finally, mention must be made of extruders, in which a helical screw forces the bulk mixture to flow down a tube. Here, the pressure generated can be enormous, as in soap-plodding, and such energy can cause materials with the viscosity of toilet soap to undergo laminar flow. The actual flow pattern produced is complex, being a combination of pressure and drag flow within the tube.

High Shear Mixers and Dispersion Equipment

Generally, a high shear rotor-stator mixer may be used either for batch processing all-enveloping chamber. Used as a batch mixer, it is capable of generating considerable turbulence because of the great velocity with which fluid is pumped out of the mixing head. As with other devices, however, this high energy is increasingly converted into heat with increasing viscosity of the mixture. A serious disadvantage for certain processes is the tendency of the mixer to cause aeration when used in the top-entry mode. For this reason such devices are often incorporated into the bottom of processing vessels.

Equipment used in the Manufacture of Cosmetics

Another high shear rotor-stator device in common use is the colloid or stone mill. Such equipment is commonly thought of as a comminution device; this serves to illustrate the fineness of the dividing line between mixing and comminution with high shear equipment. While it is true that colloid mills may be used for the comminution of very soft materials in a slurry, they find application in the cosmetics industry for the dispersion of pigments and the size reduction of internal phase droplets in emulsions. In principle, the colloid mill consists of a rapidly rotating conical member (which may be toothed or grooved) and a similarly coned stator into which the former fits. The fluid mixture is forced through the small clearance between rotor and stator (0.5 - 0.05 mm) as before. Fig. 18.7 illustrates the design of colloid mills in greater detail.

Colloid mills are used exclusively as an 'in-line' or continuous device. They may be water-cooled and can be adjusted as the moving parts wear down.

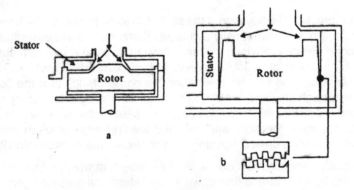

Fig. 18.7. Colloid mills (a) Stone (b) Toothed.

for more viscous products, an alternative device is the triple roll mill Fig. 18.8. The device consists of three steel rollers which rotate in the directions indicated in the diagram. Each roller is water-cooled and machined to great accuracy so that the gaps between each pair of rollers can be set very fine. The product is applied at the top of roller A, passes between A and B and round the underside of B between rollers B and C. As it traverses each gap, the product is subjected to enormous compression forces which are particularly effective in breaking down pigment agglomerates. Strictly speaking, therefore, the triple roll mill is not a high shear device but a compression device. It is included here, however, as a real alternative to the rotor-stator mixers in bringing about effective pigment dispersion in liquids - particularly in viscous liquids.

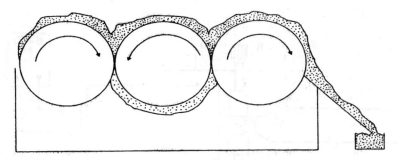

Fig. 18.8. Triple roller mill.

Perhaps the highest shear stress of all is generated by a valve homogeniser, which is still extensively used in the production of emulsions with very fine internal phase droplets.

An interesting alternative to the valve homogeniser, and one which is finding increasing use in cosmetics manufacture, is the ultrasonic homogeniser. When high intensity ultrasonic energy is applied to liquids, a phenomenon known as cavitation occurs. Cavitation is complex and not fully understood. As ultrasonic waves are propagated through the fluid, areas of compression and rarefaction are formed and cavities are produced in these rarefied areas. When the wave passes on, these cavities collapse and change to an area of compression and it has been demonstrated that the pressure in these cavities just before their collapse can be as much as several thousand atmospheres. Most of the effects of ultrasonic radiation in liquids are attributed to the powerful shock waves produced immediately following the collapse of such cavities. One design of ultrasonic homogeniser is illustrated in Fig. 18.9.

No description of dispersing equipment would be complete without mention of ball mills and sand mills. In both these devices the breakdown of agglomerates is achieved by attrition between rapidly moving grinding elements which take the form of pebbles, balls or (in the case of sandmills) finer sand-like particles < 1 mm diameter. The movement of these grinding particles may be achieved in a number of ways. In a tumbling mill, the elements tumble over each other as a horizontal drum is rotated on trunnions Fig. 18.10. Sand mills may be horizontal or vertical cylinders in which the grinding medium is stirred by a rotating agitator (Fig. 18.11), whereas in vibration mills movement of the whole chamber may be caused by eccentric cams, by out-of-balance weights on a drive shaft, or electrically.

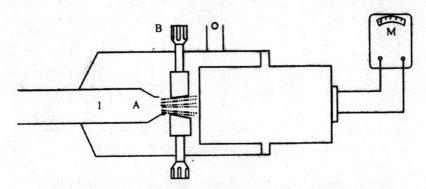

Fig. 18.9. Ultrasonic homogeniser.

The roughly premixed product enters at I and, on passing through orifice A, is subjected to intense ultrasonic energy by vibrating blade B. The treated product leaves via O. The meter, M, and 'tuning' devices at B combine to allow the operator to achieve maximum effect with each different product type.

Small ball mills and sand mills are used extensively in the dispersion of pigments into liquids (as, for example, in the production of castor oil lipstick pastes) and for the dispersion of bentone into nail varnish media. Although they are very effective, their chief disadvantage is the extremely protracted cleaning time required when changing from one colour to another. For this reason many users prefer to keep separate sets of grinding media for each different colour they wish to produce.

The basic mechanism by which mills of this kind produce their effect is attrition between grinding elements. Very little shear is developed.

SOLID-LIQUID MIXING

The production of a cosmetic product often involves the incorporation of a powdered solid material into a liquid. The objective may be to dissolve the powder completely (as with salt or preservatives in water), to effect a colloidal dispersion of water-swellable particles (as with bentones and other gelling agents) or simply the dispersion of insoluble materials such as pigments. To do this efficiently with a wide range of powder particle size and surface characteristics and with a range of different liquids of varying viscosity, quite a variety of mixing equipment is available.

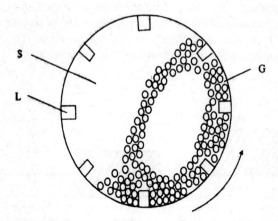

Fig. 18.10. Ball mill showing ball pattern in rotating drum. (G–Grinding medium; L–Lifter elements; S–Slurry).

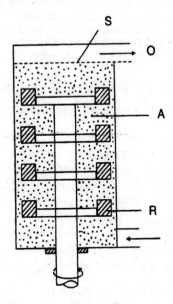

Fig. 18.11. Sand mill. (I-Slurry in; O-Slurry Out; S-Screen; R-Rotating agitator; A-Glass beads, sand or shot).

Perhaps the easiest of these processes to carry out is the dissolution of a fairly large size, smooth-faced solid, such as salt. The initial incorporation of each crystal into the liquid involves the complete replacement of the air-solid surface with a liquid-solid surface. This may be considered to be a three-stage process of adhesion, immersion and spreading Fig. 18.12. Immersion is complete when all the air has been displaced and the surface of the crystal has been completely wetted by the liquid. This process is aided by a low surface tension and low contact angle between the liquid and solid.

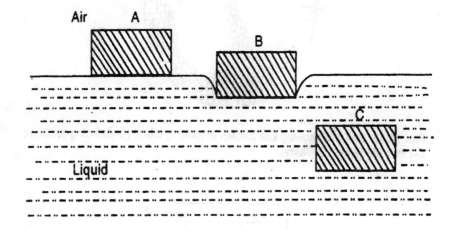

Fig. 18.12 Immersion of a solid in a liquid.
(A) Adhesion (B) Immersion (C) Spreading).

Not all powders used in cosmetics, however, have such favourable size and surface characteristics. The majority are of extremely small particle size and, as has already been noted, highly agglomerated. Each agglomerate will have a complex structure with an uneven surface and will be perforated by cavities of irregular shape. The complete wetting of such structures, involving the penetration of liquid into all the crevices and cavities together with the expulsion of air, is very much more difficult. It should be noted, for example, that penetration into cavities requires a low contact angle but a high surface tension – in conflict with conditions for easy wetting.

Powders that are small enough in particle size to form agglomerates are by far the most commonly used in cosmetics processing. In the dry state they entrap an enormous quantity of air (a bag of cosmetic-grade titanium dioxide, for example, contains only 25 per cent of powder together with 75 per cent of air). The majority of this air must be expelled if a smooth uniform mixture is to be obtained.

Immersion is only the first stage in the production of cosmetic quality dispersions. Even if the agglomerates were evenly distributed, the larger of them would give rise to 'grittiness'. Further, for pigments maximum colour can only be developed when these agglomerates are broken up and the maximum possible surface area of pigment is exposed. Disagglomeration is therefore the next step in the production process.

In cosmetic processes, the disagglomeration of solid particles in liquid media can be brought about by a variety of machines. In lipstick processing, for example, pigments are 'ground into' castor oil by preparing a coarse mixture which is then passed over a triple roll mill, or further ground in a colloid mill, ball mill or sand mill. These machines are used specifically because they will deal effectively with media of lipstick-paste viscosity.

For less viscous media (for example, the dispersion of pigments into the aqueous phase of an emulsion), a high shear device of the rotor-stator type is frequently used. In this case, processing time can be shortened by ensuring that the whole contents of the vessel are brought into the catchment area of the shearing head by secondary stirring. As with all disagglomeration, shear stress is largely responsible for the partial disintegration of the agglomerate.

For soluble powders, the enormous increase in the solid-liquid interface brought about by immersion and disagglomeration will ensure that the actual process of dissolution can proceed at the maximum possible rate. For insoluble powders, however, there remains the problem of maintaining a good stable dispersion.

Disagglomeration is usually a reversible phenomenon and it can usually be assumed that the opposite process—'flocculation'—will be simultaneously taking place.

It was noted when considering powder-powder dispersion that stabilisation could be achieved by the introduction of particles of larger size to which the disintegrated agglomerates could adhere. In some cases this can be applied to solid-liquid systems — for example, by pre-extending pigments onto talc before adding them to a liquid foundation base — but in many instances all the solid particles are of too small a size for this to be done. Under these circumstances rules similar to those used in emulsion technology can be applied. Thus the rate of flocculation can be slowed by some or all of the following means. :

1. The use of surface-active agents (sometimes as polymer coating of the powdered solid) to inhibit flocculation by steric hindrance.

2. The manipulation of electrostatic charges on the surface of the powder particles.

3. The manipulation of the viscosity of the dispersion.

Surface-active agents have a part to play at two stages in the process of manufacturing a stable dispersion. It has already been seen that the lowering of the solid-liquid contact angle speeds up the wetting process. In practice, the best results are often achieved not with a surfactant, which measurably lowers the surface tension of the liquid, but with what is sometimes described as a 'surface activator' which reduces the interfacial tension between solid and liquid. These surface activators (which are also described as 'dispersants' or 'wetting agents') can, if correctly chosen, cause an immediate improvement in the quality of the dispersion which is made manifest by a sudden increase in the colour intensity.

Suspension of Solids in agitated Tanks

If a particulate solid is dispersed in a liquid in which it does not dissolve and the suspension so formed is allowed to stand undisturbed in a vessel, provided that the densities of the two components are dissimilar some degree of settlement or flotation will eventually take place. Where the particles are present in sufficiently low concentration to have a negligible effect on the viscosity of the suspension, re-suspension can be achieved by the establishment in the liquid of flow patterns of sufficient turbulence. The suspension of solids in agitated tanks is frequently encountered in cosmetics processing, as an aid to dissolution or as a means of obtaining a good dispersion of particles prior to a change of viscosity of the liquid medium by gelling or cooling.

Three conditions can be recognised during the production of a suspension, namely complete suspension, homogeneous suspension and the ;formation of bottom or corner fillets.

Complete Suspension

Complete suspension exists when all particles are in motion and no particle remains stationary on the bottom or surface for more than a short period. Under these conditions, the whole surface of the particles is presented to the fluid, thereby ensuring the maximum area for dissolution or chemical reaction.

Homogeneous Suspension

Homogeneous suspension exists when the particle concentration and (for a range of sizes) the size distribution are the same throughout the tank. The homogeneous suspension speed is always considerably higher than 'complete suspension speed' and more difficult to achieve and to measure. Nevertheless, homogeneous suspension is very desirable for certain types of cosmetics applications and particularly so for continuous processing. In practice, for such processes the requirement is only that the particle size distribution and concentration in the discharge and the vessel are the same.

Sometimes heavier particles are allowed to collect in corners or on the bottom of the vessel in relatively stagnant regions to form *fillets*. This may have the practical advantage of very large saving in power consumption compared with the energy that may be needed to achieve complete suspension (provided, of course, that this saving offsets the loss of active solids in the fillets).

In general, it may be said that propeller or $45°$ - angle turbines offer the best advantage for rapid suspension for low power consumption – particularly if draught tubes are introduced. If, on the other hand, radial flow agitators need to be used, these should be of relatively large length-to-diameter ratio, be placed close to the bottom of the tank and have turbine blades extending to the shaft to prevent problems with central stagnant regions.

LIQUID-LIQUID MIXING

As indicated by Table 18.1, it is convenient to consider separately the case in which the liquid components are all mutually soluble and the case in which some or all of them can coexist as separate phases (that is to say, they are sparingly or partly soluble in each other).

Miscible Liquids

The mixing of miscible liquids (Blending) represents perhaps the simplest mixing operation in cosmetics manufacture. Several examples have already been cited and no further elaboration is needed except to reiterate that it is important to choose the mixing apparatus best suited to the viscosities of various components in order to carry out the operation efficiently.

Immiscible Liquids

Practically the only representatives of this category of mixing operation are emulsions. All cosmetic emulsions consist of two major immiscible liquids, one dispersed as fine droplets in the other and separated by a layer of surface-active agent at each liquid-liquid boundary.

The emulsification Process

The two major phases (these will be referred to as 'oil' and 'water') together with the emulsifier are brought together under turbulent conditions. Depending on the prevailing conditions, one major phase is broken up into droplets (predominantly by the action of shear stress imparted by turbulent eddies) and distributed throughout the other major ('continuous') phase.

While the droplets remain larger than the eddies, they will continue to break up into ever smaller droplets. Eventually a point is reached in this process when the available power giving rise to the turbulence cannot provide the shear stress necessary to reduce the droplet size any further. All this stage there exists an emulsion containing droplets of a certain mean diameter but over a range d_{min} to d_{max}. Provided that it is correctly chosen, the emulsifier prevents the rapid coalescence of these droplets and a stable emulsion is formed.

Orientation of Phases

In any emulsion the orientation of the phase (that is, whether the oil or the water phases is continuous) is determined principally by the choice of emulsifier and the volume ratio of oil to water. Usually, however, there is a range of volume ratio over which either phase may be dispersed, depending upon the method of manufacture. If a quiescent mixture of two phases coexisting as two simple layers (one upon the other) is agitated, the phase into which the agitator is placed is most likely to form the continuous phase in the resulting emulsion. In other words, drops are drawn into the phase in which the impeller is placed. If initially only one phase is present in the mixing vessel containing the impeller, an added second phase will inevitably form the disperse or discontinuous phase. If, however, the continued addition of the second phase combined with the choice of emulsifier eventually leads to a volume ratio at which the system is more stable with the added phase being continuous, then the emulsion will spontaneously invert to achieve this end result. When inversion takes place, it is very often accompanied by a change in droplet size. Where this change is a decrease, then inversion leads to a more stable emulsion and gives rise to a valuable method of manufacture.

Addition of Surfactant

In a batch manufacturing process for emulsions, there are four possible methods of adding the emulsifier. The first of these involves dissolving (or dispersing) the emulsifying agent in water, to which the oil is added. An oil-in-water emulsion is initially produced but inversion to water-in-oil may take place if more oil is needed.

Alternatively, the emulsifier may be added to the oil phase; the mixture may then be added directly to water to form an oil-in-water emulsion or water may be added to the mixture to form a water-in-oil emulsion. Many emulsions, on the other hand, are stabilised by soaps which are formed at the interface between the two phases. In this case, the fatty acid end of the soap is dissolved in the oil and the alkaline component is dissolved in the water. The two phases can be brought together in any order.

Finally, a less used method is one in which water and oil are added alternately to the emulsifying agent. Usually, the improvement in product quality obtained by the use of this method does not warrant the complication it causes in the manufacturing procedure.

Batch Processing Equipment

It will be evident from the discussion so far that there are at least two important elements of emulsion processing, namely shear (for the emulsification and particle size reduction process) and flow (in order to bring the whole contents of the vessel through the region of the high shear). Flow is also important in the heating and cooling of the emulsion. Most emulsion processing vessels are equipped with a jacket through which steam or hot water can be circulated to heat the contents and cold water circulated to cool them. Evidently then, to be effective, the mixing circulated to cool them. Evidently then, to be effective, the mixing mechanism must be able to provide adequate flow and from the vessel walls.

For these reasons, most emulsion batch processing vessels contain a high shear turbine or rotor-stator device (typically bottom or side entry rather than top entry, to decrease the likelihood of air entrapment) and a high flow, low shear mixing device which may be driven by a separate motor. This high flow device is of variable design, the most popular being a gate stirrer in which the arms are inclined at about 45° to the horizontal so as to give an element of axial flow. In more complicated designs, a central shaft carries more blades which sweep the area between the first set, the sets of blades rotating in opposite directions. Whatever the design, the frame holding the outer blades normally carries spring-loaded plastic scraper blades to prevent the build-up of product on the inner vessel wall, which would interfere with efficient heat exchange across the surface (Fig. 18.13).

The main motor may be driven electricity or by air (up to about 100 psi or 9 bar). The advantages of air-driven motors are that they are infinitely variable in speed, torque-sensitive (and therefore less likely to become damaged when subjected to sudden loads), they do not constitute a hazard in the processing of low flash-point materials and generally they require less maintenance. Electric motors can be built to match some of these advantages (with slipping clutches and flameproofing), but only at considerable expense.

Equipment used in the Manufacture of Cosmetics

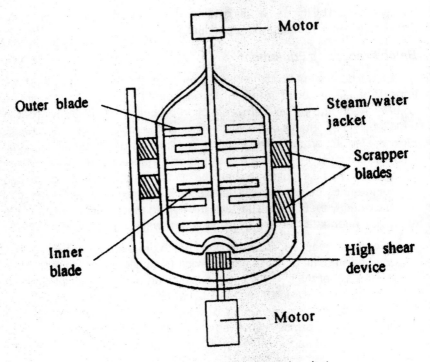

Fig. 18.13 Batch emulsion processing plant

This traditional gate-type impeller system suffers from the grave disadvantage of limited axial flow. This is not noticeable in smaller vessels (below 600 liters capacity) but becomes a major problem in large tanks. One approach to the problem is to provide top-to-bottom transfer for the contents by means of a pump and an external pipe. A more satisfactory arrangement for the manufacture of emulsions of medium and low viscosity is to replace the gate stirrer by one or more axial flow impellers mounted centrally on a single central shaft. Although it becomes more difficult to provide wall-scrapers, the excellent flow around the vessel walls makes scraping less necessary.

The problem of ensuring that all the product passes through the region of high shear has led to the idea of passing the batch through an external circuit containing an in-line homogeniser; this may be a rotor-stator device, colloid mill or valve homogeniser.

Continuous Processing

In view of the difficulties encountered in manufacturing large batches of emulsion, a logical extension of an external circuit with in-line homogeniser is a continuous processing plant. A simple form of such a plant is illustrated diagrammatically in Fig. 18.14. Such a plant is more correctly referred to as 'batch-continuous' since in essence a single batch is manufactured at a time. For long-run products, a truly continuous plant would be suitable, such as that illustrated in Fig. 18.15. In this case, the addition of second vessels A' and B' (which are exact duplicates of A and B respectively) together with the three-way valves V_1 and V_2 means that a second batch of each phase can be prepared while the first is being used. In this way, a continuous supply of each phase is assured by the turning of a valve. In reality, continuous plants tend to be slightly more complex than is illustrated in the diagrams with the inclusion of take-off points for sampling and other sophisticated features. Nevertheless, continuous manufacture is a very practical and, for some applications, extremely economical method of processing emulsions.

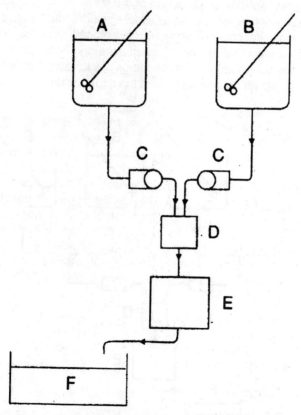

Fig. 18.14 Simple continuous-processing emulsion plant. (The two phases are prepared separately in tanks A and B, then pumped in correct proportions via metering pumps, C, into an in-line premixer, D (such as a static mixer), and then through a

Equipment used in the Manufacture of Cosmetics

homogeniser, E. Finally, the formed emulsion is pumped into F, which may be a storage tank or the hopper of a filling vessel. A heat exchanger can be incorporated between E and F for rapid cooling.)

Emulsion Temperature

The primary reason for raising the temperature of the phases during emulsion manufacture is to ensure that both are in the liquid state. In particular, the oil phase may contain fats and waxes that are solid at room temperature; there is very little point in raising the temperature of the oil phase much above that at which these liquefy. Excessive heating of the phases during manufacture prolongs the manufacturing time and wastes energy.

If the water phase is liquid at room temperature, it is customarily heated to approximately 5°C above the temperature chosen for the oil phase (so as not to cause the sudden solidification of the latter on blending). There is, however, an interesting alternative – namely, emulsification between hot oil phase and cold water phase. The plant for this procedure is illustrated in Fig. 18.16, which shows that mixing of the phases and homogenisation take place simultaneously. The obvious advantage of such a method is the saving of time and energy in not having to heat the aqueous phase.

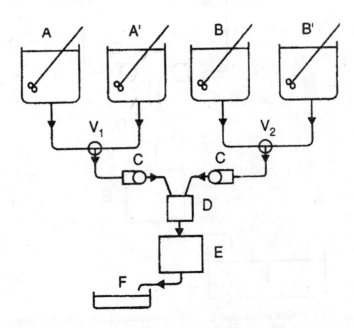

Fig. 18.15 Continuous-processing emulsion plant for long-run products.

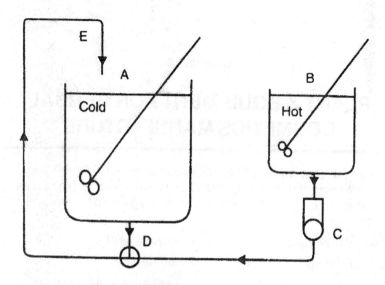

Fig. 18.16 Hot/Cold processing emulsion plant.

(The hot oil phase from tank A and the cold water phase from tank B are pumped into an in-line homogeniser at D and thence into the main tank B at E).

Storage of Cosmetic powders

Two factors have an important effect on stored cosmetic powders : moisture and pressure. It is not always appreciated that a small increase in relative humidity can give rise to sufficient moisture in the stored powder to change the main mechanism of particle-particle bonding, increasing the bond strength of agglomerates by a factor of 2 or more. Such an increase in cohesiveness can make the handling and flow problems already inherent in cosmetic powders perceptibly worse and can change the processing characteristics of (say) an eyeshadow to the point where all the pressing machine settings may have to be altered to compensate.

In the same way, powder bulk that has been stored in large vertical containers exhibits increasingly difficult flow characteristics as the container gradually empties. The lower layers, having been compressed by the weight of powder above them, become increasingly cohesive as the bottom is approached. For this reason it is far better to store powder in a large number of small well-sealed containers than in loosely covered large bins.

Chapter - 4

PLANT & EQUIPMENT FOR HERBAL COSMETICS MANUFACTURE

For the preparation of herbal cosmetics of different kinds, as detailed earlier, different processes or combination of processes are adopted. Some of the basic process and equipment required for it are as under :

S. No.	Processes	Equipment
1.	Heating	Immersion heater, jacketed & non jacketed kettles
2.	Grinding or size Reduction	Micropulverisers, Grinders
3.	Sieving & granding	Sifter
4.	Mixing (dry)	Paddle mixer, drum mixer
5.	Mixing (wet)	Universal mixer
6.	Homogenization	Homogenizer
7.	Emulsification	Emulsification equipment
8.	Straining/filtering/	strainer/filter
9.	Filling/sealing form	Automatic liquid filling Machines
	fill & seal machines for pouches	
10.	Labelling	Labelling Equipment

Plant & Equipment for Herbal Cosmetics Manufacture

These processes and equipment are described as under :

1. Heating Equipment

a. Immersion heaters

An accurately controlled, electric immersion heater is fast becoming recognized in the preparation of cosmetic products of different kinds as heating applications.

Each application usually presents a separate problem in the selection of the correct immersion heater. For most cosmetic mixtures containing oils, fats, and waxes, standard heaters with steel sheaths are satisfactory; for use in materials where steel would be corroded, heaters can be supplied with the enclosing sheath of a special corrosion resisting alloy such as stainless steel.

The required heater capacity will depend upon the amount and physical constant of the material being heated, the temperature to which the material is to be heated, and the time allowed for heating, as well as upon the size and construction of the container. As a rough approximation, 30 watts of heater capacity will raise the temperature of 1 lb of a substance. similar to wax, approximately 100° F. in a period of one hour.

b. Jacketed / non-jacketed kettles

In good cosmetic practice heat (gas burner or stove) is rarely applied directly to a container. The only time direct gas heat may be used is in dissolving substances in water or similar inert solvent.

Many small manufacturers do not use water baths claiming that heating is too slow and that scorching is averted by constant attention. True heating is somewhat slower in one respect but a more even heat over the sides of the kettle is obtained in this way. Also the savings and assurance resulting from slower heating on a water bath more than repay the effort expended.

Small batch heating may be accomplished by using inexpensive aluminium jacketed kettles of the double boiler type. The removable pan is easy to handle and is suitable for small scale production.

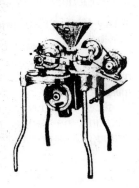

2. Grinders / Micro Pulverisers

The process of reducing a material to finer particles is called comminution or disintegration, sometimes loosely referred to as grinding. It is one of the most important chemical engineering process in industry. The fineness of finished product determines if the process shall be called grinding, pulverizing or micropulverizing.

Fine pigments as well as pigment mixtures are prepared by grinding. Commonest form of grinding is accomplished with a mortar and pestle.

Pulverizers and micropulverizers are being used more in the manufacture of face powder, eliminating a sifting operation.

Only a rough premixing is required, the material which passes through the machine is finely ground and quite uniformly mixed. If not sufficiently uniform, it may be passed through the machine again.

Grinding can also be accomplished by the use of ball or pebble mills specially in preparing uniform blends.

3. Sieving & Grading Equipment

Next to grinding operation is the sifting process the separation of large particles from small ones. Sifting is accomplihsed by means of suitable screens and the products to be sifted must be mixed to assure uniformity. The lighter particles pass through the screen first, the heavier particles last.

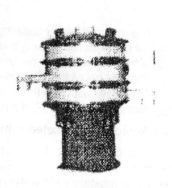

Face powder and certain make-up cosmetics are sifted atleast once before being packed. Cosmetics as a group require that a product pass through a 200 mesh sieve if they are to be considered satisfactory for consumer use. The term 200 mesh means that there are 200 holes per lineal inch. Simple sifting devices are like silk cloth of 120-160 mesh, conveniently held in position by two wooden rings, one of which fits over the other. Similarly a sieve of 25 cm diameter is suitable for small batches. With mesh sieves can also be used but as metal affects the colour of the product, silk sifter is more suitable.

4. Dry-Mixing Equipment

The dry powers commonly mixed are face powders horizontal, round bottom mixers are the most frequently used for mixing powdered ingredients in cosmetic practice. It has two twisted paddles for agitating the central mass effecting thorough mixing of the ingredients.

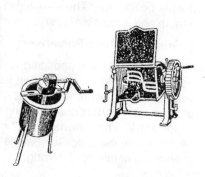

Plant & Equipment for Herbal Cosmetics Manufacture

5. Wet mixing Equipment

Mixing-Paste, Creams and Emulsions is readily accomplished with a push-pull type of portable agitators.

Simplicity of construction, ruggedness and adaptability of this kind of agitation makes it a common sight in cosmetic plants. It can be used successfully in making liquid emulsion, emulsified cold creams and other medium-heavy mixers.

Not as commonly seed as the "push-pull" or propeller type of mixing machine but very popular indeed is a blade type mixing machine. In these machines agitation and mixing are very thorough. The adaptability of the machinery will make it useful for any mixing operation.

6. Homogenizing Equipment

The principle upon which all homogenizers are based is the forcing of substance under pressure, through a minute opening regulated by a spring needle valve. The substance passes the needle valve into discharge chamber where the pressure is released. The material in effect "explodes," producing a very fine dispersion.

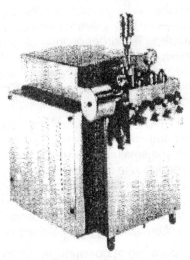

A complete unit of universal vacutherm mixer comprising of mixer kettle, mixing baffle, dosing funnel & valves, jacket heating vacuum condensor is used for efficient mixing of different ingredient in liquid state.

7. Emulsification Equipment

An emulsion consists of two immiscible liquids, one being dispersed in the other. These are known as the internal and external phases respectively. Cosmetic emulsions are generally creams.

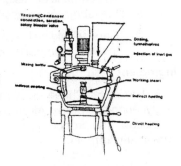

Most cosmetic emulsions are oil and water systems, of which there are two types. The type of emulsion obtained depends on the proportion of oil and water used. When the oil or fatty phase is dispersed in the aqueous or water phase, it is known as an oil in water (O/W) system. When the aqueous phase is dispersed in the oil phase it is referred to as a water in oil (W/O) system

The two types of emulsions may be distinguished by several means. An oil in water emulsion is less greasy than a water in oil emulsion because water is the external phase. An oil in water emulsion is dispersible in water. It is also more easily washed than a water in oil emulsion, which is not so readily water dispersible. Again because water is the external phase, an oil in water emulsion will conduct electricity, whereas a water in oil emulsion will not conduct electricity unless an electrolyte has been added.

An emulsion of oil in water should consist of oil dispersed in the water. If a very small amount of oil is added to water it is comparatively easy to reduce it to very small droplets. Once in this state the droplets do not readily coalesce. This is due to electrical charges which form on the surfaces of the droplets. If a larger quantity of oil is required, it is less easy to mix with the water, and once mixed there is a tendency for the phases to separate. To prevent this an emulsifying agent is used. The emulsifying agent stabilizes the emulsion by forming a thin film over the droplets and preventing them from coalescing.

Thus there are two main conditions which must be satisfied in the preparation of emulsions. The first is that the droplets of the internal phase must be small. This is ensured during the process of mixing, which should be designed to make the emulsion, homogenous throughout. Homoegenizing the emulsion can be done by shaking the phases in a bottle, by stirring them in a beaker or by using a mortar and pestle, depending usually on the nature of the oil phase. The second condition is that the droplets should have a thin film of emulsifying agent around them.

Preparation of cosmetic emulsions

1. All cosmetic emulsions should be prepared in glass containers. In the laboratory, glass beakers are the most suitable.
2. Care should be taken to follow the correct formula. The will ensure that the preparation is of the right consistency.

Ingredient

The Water Phase should contain all the water soluble materials such as glycering and borax. All preparations must contain a preservative and an antioxidant. The proportion of water in a stable emulsion should not fall below 50% in any formula.

Some oil phase ingredients :

1. Liquid paraffin : This is one of the major oils used either as an ingredient in cleansing creams, or as a diluent for other fatty materials.
2. Almond oil : This is the best oil for cosmetic emulsion.
3. Sesame oil : This can be substituted for olive oil.
4. Petroleum jelly : This is sometimes used as an oil-thickening agent and emollient.
5. Fatty acids - oleic acid : This is the chief oil phase ingredient in vanishing and shaving creams.
6. Esters : Isopropyl myristate, iropropyl palmitate, isopropyl stearate - these are in liquid form and promote skin penetration.
7. Spermaceti : This is an excellent emollient.
8. Carnauba wax : This is the thickening agent for the oil phase.
9. Beeswax : This acts as an emollient and emulsifier.

Perfumes and insoluble powders are not added until after the phases have been mixed.

The choice of an emulsifying agent : The first emulsifier to be used was soap, but nowadays oil soluble materials such as fatty alcohols (e.g. cetyl alcohol) and esters (e.g. glyceryl monostearate) are used. The choice of the emulsifying agent depends on two important factors :

1. The nature of the emulsion - that is, whether it is to be an oil in water or water in oil emulsion.
2. The computability of the emulsifying agent with the rest of the substances in the emulsion.

Most emulsifying agents produce oil in water systems. Some examples are wool fats, beeswax-borax mixture, wool alcohols and triethanolamine.

If a surfactant (i.e. a surface active agent) is used to make oily or waxy substances mix with water, the resulting emulsion may be either opaque or clear. Many detergents are classed as surfactant and are often used to stabilize oil and water emulsions. A detergent molecule has a long hydrocarbon part which is insoluble in water but soluble in oil (hydrophilic and lipophobic). The ionic end group is insoluble in oil but soluble in water(hydrophilic and lipophobic). If a small amount of detergent is added to water, a colloidal suspension is formed. The hydrocarbon ends of the detergent molecules cluster together and leave their ionic and groups in contact with the water. If oil is then introduced and the whole stirred together, the hydrocarbon parts of the detergent molecules enter the oil droplets, leaving the ionics end groups in the water. Thus round the oil droplets is formed a film which is partly in the water and partly in the oil.

Method of preparation

The phases. As most cosmetic emulsions are preapred from waxes and other substances that are numerally solid at room temperature, the two phases must first be heated separately. The waxes and oils should be heated to about $10^{\circ}C$ above the melting point of the highest melting wax, taking care not to overheat. This usually means heating the waxes to about $70^{\circ}C$ above that of the oil phase, to allow for cooling when the phases are mixed.

Mixing and cooling. Generally the water phase should be added to the oil phase. An exception to this is made in the case of high oil content (80-90%). There must be continuous stirring with a glass rod as there is a tendency for the phases to separate if stirring is stopped. The rate of cooling should be slow, to avoid coarsening of the emulsion. Stirring should continue unitil temperature reaches about $40^{\circ}C$. Perfumes should be added whilst stirring, when the emulsion is partially cool ($35^{\circ}C$). If there are may insoluble powders to be used in the preparation they should be heated to $75^{\circ}C$ and added soon after the phases have been mixed.

The finished preparation should be smooth and creamy. If this has not been achieved during the mixing process, it may be necessary to completely homogenize the emulsion at the this stage. This may be done by using an ordinary whisk or, if the emulsion is semi-solid, by using a mortar and pestle. Homogenization helps to prepare a most stable emulsion by breaking up the drops of oil into smaller droplets.

O/W emulsions. In preparing these emulsions it is best to make a preliminary mixture containing a portion of the water and emulsifier with an equal amount of oil. This should be stirred with a glass rod and homogenized slowly while the remaining oil is added. When the remaining water is added slowly to the oil phase, a very heavy W/O emulsion is formed. This will thin out suddenly to the O/W type of emulsion. When this happens the water can then be added more rapidly.

Control of the thickness of emulsions

Liquid emulsions tend to thicken. They then no longer pour. This increase in viscosity may be due to one or more of the following :

1. Too high a concentration of waxes in the oil phase
2. Too much emulsifying agent.
3. Too much homogenizing

To lower the viscosity of the emulsion any of the following methods

Plant & Equipment for Herbal Cosmetics Manufacture

may be used :

1. Increase the proportion of the external phase.
2. Decrease the proportion of the internal phase.
3. Use a lower melting point ingredient in the internal phase.
4. Add a water soluble emulsifier.

To raise the viscosity use one of the following methods :

1. Increase the proportion of the internal phase.
2. Add thickeners such as emulsifiers or gums.
3. Include a higher melting point ingredient in the internal phase.

Cause of failure of emulsion preparations

1. Insufficient emulsifying agent. this is rarely the cause of trouble as the tendency is to add too much emulsifier.
2. Decomposition of the emulsifying agent. This could be due to chemical reaction or the activities of micro-organisms. The emulsifying agent may be destroyed by chemical reaction with one of the ingredients.
3. Temperature changes. An increase in temperature can cause the two phases to separate, if the emulsifier is susceptible to temperature variations. Freezing can also destroy an emulsion by the formation of ice crystals on the surface.
4. Presence of electrolytes. Occasionally, small quantities of electrolytes (e.g. calcium salts) are added to emulsions containing triethanolamine soaps. This cause the phases to separate.
5. The concentration of the phases. The concentration of the phases should be in the region of 60% water and 40% oil. A higher phase volume ratio than 60:40, i.e. too much water, tends to cause separation of the phases.
6. Rancidity of the oil. Some animal and vegetable oils may become rancid on prolonged storage and cause the phases to separate. Rancidity may be prevented by the addition of an antioxidant.

Emulsification process for preparation of herbal creams.

Creams are an emulsion of oil and a water soluble liquid, allowing the final product to be readily absorbed by the skin. The easiest way to make a herbal cream is to buy an emulsifying cream from the drugstore, and heat the desired herb plant material in it.

1. To being, melt approximately 2 tablespoons of emulsifying cream in a bowl placed over a pot of boiling water.

2. Add one large tablespoon of dried herbs to the mixture, and stir slowly until the cream takes on the color of the herbs.
3. Remove from heat, strain, and squeeze the remaining liquid from the clamp.
4. Let cream cool in a glass bowl, and spoon into small, dark bottles.
5. Store jars in a cool, dark place for up to one year.

8. Straining, Filtering & Clarifying

In straining only the bigger undesirable particles are removed, as through the ordinary kitchen or tea strainer. In making mucilages, with quinee seed for example, the seeds must be strained off in due time. Mucilages of most gums are too thick to filter, but can be partially cleaned by straining. Further polishing requires centrifuging.

Filtration is "more perfect strainging." The more closely woven the strainer, the more nearly it approaches a filtering device.

For greater production filtering machines are now used. The material to be filtered is pumped through the discs by means of an attached pump. Such machines give good production for small as well as moderate scale manufacture.

9. Filling liquids

After manufacture, filling of the cosmetic into containers becomes an important problem, Liquids may be filled by gravity, siphon or vacuum. Small manufacturers perfer the gravity filler as it is most useful for all round liquid filling.

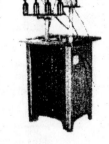

Gravity fillers are best for shampoo and foaming bath preparations because vacuum filling tends to produce foam in the bottle.

Siphon fillers are based on a wll known principle going back before the time of the ancient Egyptians.

Economical and simple fillers for limited production are used for "touching up" purposes. Hundreds of these little fillers are in use throughout the country in large and small manufacturing plants alike. These are available at a price within the reach of the smallest manufacture. It may also be used for filling creams in the liquid state.

Filling Pastes - Creams

Heavy creams, ointments or pastes present an entirely different problem in filling.

Ordinary pastes, such as tooth paste, can be filled with a hand operated machine. In the case of tubes, they can be folded over and crimped with inexpensive hand operated machinery.

10. Labelling Equipment

Attaching the labels is the next step in completing a package, most manufacturers prefer to buy labels printed on plain paper stock and apply glue at the time of labelling.

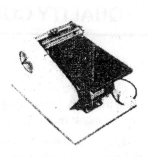

This requires a lot of labour or the purchase of gluing equipment. Simple machines are available for the purpose of applying a thin, even film of glue. The lable is then placed on the package and smoothed on by hand. Machines of this sort are very inexpensive. The speed of labelling is dependent on the operator.

OTHER USEFUL PUBLICATIONS

★ HANDBOOK OF SYNTHETIC & HERBAL COSMETICS
★ COSMETICS PROCESSES & FORMULATIONS HANDBOOK
★ HAND BOOK OF PERFUEMS WITH FORMULATIONS
★ ESSENTIAL OILS PROCESSES & FORMULATIONS HAND BOOK
★ HAND BOOK OF ESSENTIAL OILS MFG. & AROMATIC PLANTS
★ HANDBOOK OF PERFUMES & FLAVOURS
★ HAND BOOK OF HERBS, MEDICINAL & AROMATIC PLANTS CULTIVATION

AVAILABLE AT :

ENGINEERS INDIA RESEARCH INSTITUTE

Regd. Off. : 4449, Nai Sarak (S1), Main Road, Delhi-6 (India)
Ph. : 3918117, 3916431, 3960797, 3920361 Fax : 91-11-3916431
E-mail : eirisidi@bol.net.in Website : startindustry.com

Chapter - 5

QUALITY CONTROL OF COSMETICS

INTRODUCTION

Quality is the totality of features and characteristics of a product or service that bear on its ability to satisfy a given need ! Thus, quality is seen not as a single factor, but as a concept made up of several criteria.

Quality is the sum of all factors which contribute directly or indirectly to the safety, effectiveness and acceptability of the product !

Quality means conformance to requirements. Quality department personnel cannot be concerned with the various mystical aspects of quality – beauty, elegance, value for money, or even fitness for purpose (unless this means conformance to a defined purpose). The emphsis on conformance throws the responsibility on the marketing and technical departments to define the requirement and the product, such that a product specification is produced. This specification should define the environmental and reliability characteristics that the product must have, the workmanship standards that are applicable, and so on. The quality department are responssible for checking conformance to this specification.

The traditional view of quality requires modification, and that a new philosophy of quality is needed. The terms quality and productivity are not only to be related to the production of goods but also to process. For this reason, these concepts of quality must encompass every level of a business organisation – from administration, sales, to financing and marketing. The new concept of quality "built in" instead of 'tested for' emphasises prevention in all phases of the production cycle and beyond that in every work process within a business, rather than verification or post-improvement procedures. In this chapter, we discuss this new conception of quality.

The Analytical Laborator – Its Significance for Raw Materials/Active Ingrdientws and the Finished Preparation

All the raw materials and ingreients needed for cosmetic preparations are tested for usability in an analytical laboratory. The finished cosmetic preparations are also tested here.

The prerequisites for optimal chemical control (optimal is used here to signify the lowest expenditure that provides the highest degree of protection) are the msot modern technical aids, such as IR, Uv, AAS spectrometers as well as gas chromatography and personal computers. Qualified and experienced technical personnel are also indispensable.

The Microbiological Laboratory – Assurance of Purity and Hygiene

It is the task of microbiological laboratory to control mould or bacteria in cosmetic preparations. During production of a cosmetic preparation it must already be known which micro-organisms the preparation is exposed to; the germs discovered must be analysed and tested to ensure that a precisely fixed germ count is not exceeded.

Sterile working conditions are not required for cosmetic preparations, buy hygiene regulations must be observed during the production process. The Good Manufacturing Practice (GMP) and Good Laboratory Practice (GLP) guidelines are generally regarded as the applicable regulations. Cleaning and disinfecting are just as essential as the provision of hygiene education to personnel. Only informed employees can gurantee that all regulations are adhered to. Disinfecting machines and machine components is normally cost and time-intensive. The "clean in place" system is an example of innovative attempts in this area, which no business can ignore.

"Clean in place" refers to washing, cleaning and disinfecting machines by an installed system of pipes, without having to take apart machine components or pumps.

Raw Material Inspection

The inspection of cosmetic ingredients is based on specifications. It takes into consideration the specific requirements of the company as well as legal guidelines. Each detail of the specification must be coordinated with the producer of the raw materials. An inspection certificate which is given to the user with each delivery makes it easier for laboratory administrators to decide which properties of the specification need to be sujected to chemical analysis. It is not necessary to analyse every property of each delivery. The decision regarding how often to test is dependent upon the frequency of delivery, coordination of all specification properties between supplier and buyer, the inspection certificate accompanying each deliery, the histroy of the raw material in question, the degree of trust between buyer, supplier, and the complete documentàtion of all data. A sensory test of smell, colour and/or appearance, together with an IR spectrum is often sufficient to identify a delivery accurately. The decision as to whether a full analysis of all specific values needs to be carried out on every third, fourth or fifth delivery is made by the laboratory administration. It is also absolutely

Quality Control of Cosmetics

necessary to store allanalytical data in a personal computer. An evaluation of the raw material or supplier can be made at any time with the help of this data.

Inspection of the Finished Product

Specific manufacturing instructions are essential for the production of the finished preparation. Instructions regarding temperature, mixing speed, instruments or the order in which ingredients are incorporated make it easier to keep to the specification. here too an in-process control which registers the actual values (temperature, mixing speed, etc.), in relation to the specified values should be adopted.

A particular risk can be bound up with the weighing of the individual raw materials. However great the inspection expenditures are (for example, the additional presence of a psecialist from the analytical laboratory while weighing in active ingredients), mistakes by personnel cannot be excluded. For example, too much of an active ingredient (such as a preservative) could cause fatal effects. For this reason active ingredients are often inspected again by the analytical laboratory as to their proportion in the final preparation. This doubled or tripled safe guarding is cost-intensive and hence not justifiable according to modern conceptions of quality. In the search for preventative test characteristics, the use of computerised weighing controls has therefore become prominent. A preparation manufactured under these conditons will generally meet the prescribed standards.

Inspection of Containers and Packaging Materials

It would not be possible to inspect each of bottles delivered for packaging purposes. Yet it must be guaranteed that they are all in flawless condition. Breakage and structural faults which would lead to leakage or glass splinters must be totally excluded. it is impossible to compromise on this issue. the problem can be resolved with the help of statistics. Probability statements regarding the specific quality of a delivery can be made through the use of spot tests and fault evaluation methods that practically eliminate error. The results of tests on a small representative sample of a total delivery are used to decide whether an entire delivery of an item should be acepted or rejected. In terms of cost-benefit analysis, this is the only practicable system for inspecting large lot quantities, from the view point of both buyers and manufacturers of packaging materials.

Skip Lot Inspection

The cosmetics industry also makes use of packaging materials which are relatively simple to produce. They have therefore retained consistently good quality over the years, but each delivery must nevertheles be thoroughly inspected. If the history of the packaging component has remained unchanged, it is sufficient to tinspect every third, fourth, or fifth delivery (hence the term skip lot). Precise knowledge of the packaging components and the supplier are however essential prerequisites for using this method of inspection. For deliveries which are not inspected, an identity check (appearance, potential transport damage, code number and so on) will sufice.

Source Inspection

Packaging materials that are produced in large quantities and ordered in partial lots also do not require comprehensive inspection of each delivery. This is especially important when using the just-in-time inventroy method, where small quantities of the material are ordered with greater frequency. Source inspection requires that the total amount be statistically checked once by the producer. An identity check is then sufficient for all deliveries of partial lots. In this case too, cooperation beteween supplier and buyer is necessary, especially regarding the lot size per order.

Vendor Certification

There are suppliers whose preparations have proved themselves over the years to be of exceptional quality. Packaging components supplied by them do not need to be routinely checked with every deliver, since the risk remains small. A control can be made via skip lot or source inspection methods at any time.

Computer-Assisted Delivery Testing

An exact record and evaluation of all available data is an essential prerequisite of the above mentioned tests employed in less frequent quality inspection methods. A computerised system of measurement at the packaging delivery point makes this possible. Such a system is organised so that it contains all the basic data regarding a supplier and a component, and the data from every further test procedure, regardless of whether it is a skip lot or routine test method, is fed into its memory. The results of attributive tests (of appearace, colour and so on), are entered manually. The analysis of a number of these tests shows immediately whether there is a tendency towards deviation from the norm, or whether the values remain constant within the specifiction. The computer is "queried" every time goods arrive. It provides the decision on whether to test that particular delivery. This system has proved its reliability in practice and can therefore be recommended for use in every business.

In-Process Control

Prevention is the only possible means of recognising and correcting errors, and cutting costs. In-process controls are preventative technical-operational procedures which monitor the work process by means of measurement devices intergrated into that process. An example of this is the computerised weighing control of ingredients. In this system, the quantity of an ingredient which is given in the formulation instructions is stored in memory and automatically compared with the actual amount weighed. Each deviation is communicated immediately by a signal or a print-out. The sum of the individual weitht readings must correspond exactly to the quantity of the formulation. Projections of the actual amount of a basic ingredient used in relation to the target amount with reference to the amount in stock provides additional security.

Integrated Inspection Processes in the Manufacture of the Finished Product

Different companies offer memory-programmed management and ispection systems. Their purpose is to automate a mixing process with computer assistance according to predetermined specifications. This optimises effective time management of a facility and consistent reproducibility of the finsihed preparation, as well as the storage of formulation data. Control systems continually monitor temperature, mixing speed and process duration.

These systmes also help in prevention, or advance inspection (in-process control procedures). The check weigher belongs to this group of systems, for example. This is a weighing system which is intergrated into the production line and automatically checks the weight of each individual preparation. A computer evaluates the measurement results. In production facilities which cannot implement check weigher, weight inspection takes place during the production process by means of spot checks (computer assisted inspection of fill quantities). The evalutaion and projection of individual results at a central point provides certainty that the proper fill quantities are always contained. Torque measurement, an ongoing check for container leakage, and inspection of the finished product with automatic removal of faulty items - those with missing labels or lot codes, empty containers, containers without lids, or insufficiently filled containers - are also possible in this way.

Finished Goods Control

The systematic prevention of error encompasses errors related to machines on the one hand and to human error on the other. In production of the finished product, this is especiall important because it is the last opportunity to spot and rectify errors before the product is released. Specifications features for the packaged preparation are prescribed by the Cosmetics Decree, the Finished Package Decree, and the Guidelines for

Aerosols, as well as by the specifications. The "in-process controls" are employed as a rule in this inspections. The manufacturer msut estblish the extent of inspection activities in such a way that every preparation which reaches the consumer fully meets all legal requirements.

Good Laboratory Practice (GLP) and Good Manufacturing Practice (GMP)

Good Laboratory Practce (GLP) and Good Manufacturing Practice (GMP) are used widely for the production of cosmetic preparations.GLP offers guidelines for laboratory investigations of chemical substances in terms of their characteristics and/or safety. The guidelines cover the direction of laboratory tests, the responsibilities of the laboratory administration, and quality assurance .Similarly, GMP provides fundamental advice concerning hygienic production practices in the cosmetics industry, including recommendations concerning raw materials and packaging materials, disinfection, microbiological quality control, personnel and preservation.

Environmental Protection

In accordance with regulations regarding waste products, tariffs are levied on companies in proportion to the burden they place on the waste disposal system.

The determination of disposable substances and of the chemical oxygen demand (COD) should be part of the routine of a laboratory concerned with environmental protection. Expenditure on such controls is justifiable and inspection can be restricted to 2 or 3 times per year once values have been standardised. The biological oxygen demand (BOD) must as a rule be determined by an independent body. The quality of the air should also be known, at least for the prodution facility. With the help of this kind of data, a company can have an influence on air and waste water quality and thus keep these costs under control.

Quality promotion

Improvement of quality is an attitude which every level of a company needs to adopt, because the goal of improvement demands that every work procedure, every service and product meets the norms of quality every time. The process of improving quality and productivity is an ongoing process which has in view nothing less than the approach and the engagement of all co-workers. This approach requires a philosophy of quality whose goal is to encourage employees in the direction of improving quality within the framework of the company's strategy.

The following plan is based on bringing the classic works proposal system together with an innovative quality team.

Works Proposal System

The works proposal system, which is usually regulated by agreements between managment and the works committee, is an instrument of the employees for voluntarily improving current conditions.

A transitional stage from the works proposal system to quality team is offered by the group proposal. The regulation stipulates that "suggestions for improvement may be prepared and submitted by individual workers (individaul proposals), or by a group of workers (group proposals)." Employees are thus motivated to develop new ideas and initiatives that lie outside of their immediate assignment areas.

It may seem strange to intergrate the classic works proposal system into the general category of "quality assurance." However, a modern conception of quality must concern itself with systems of improvement that ultimately secure success through implementation of quality standards.

Chapter - 6

DETAILS OF PLANT, MACHINERY & EQUIPMENTS.

MIXER:

With all contact parts made our of mixing S.S-304 quality with two mechanical seal ends to prevent outside lubricants from entering into mixing chamber. The paddles on the shaft are so arranged as to give thorough and uniform mixing. The unit is supplied with dust proof stainless steel cover, tilting and safety device to prevent any accident. Complete with motor, gear box and starter etc.

MULTIMILL

The Multimill is useful for various purposes like granulation, shredding, pulverizating etc. The unit consists of vertically mounted 3 HP motor which drives the shaft through bearing housing. The motor has Nos. swinging type type knife blades and 2 Nos. scrapper blades. All contact parts are made out of S.S. complete with motor, DOL starter with reversible switch and one No. stainless steel sieve.

HERBS GRINDER

The unit is suitable to reduce the size of the herbs as per your requirement. All contact parts of body made of stainless steel. The S.S. body is fitted with 1 HP single phase motor D.P. switch for ON/OFF, with provision for affixing mesh of different sizes as per the nature of the material to be grinded, supplied with different sizes perforated sieves.

HOT AIR OVEN/TRAY DRYER

Complete in all respect with electrically heated drying chamber, suitable for drying granules, with double wall body, housing heavy fibre glass wool insulation, with special U type heaters, air circulation fan, thermostat, panel box etc. Machine duly painted and finished inside with heat resistant aluminium paint complete body made out of m.s. sheet of 16 swg thickness. The unit is with aluminium trays of 18 swg sheet material.

PORTABLE MECHANICAL SHIFTER

Machine complete in all respects, will all contact part of SS-304, suitable for bolting of free-flowing powders and granules, with flanged type motor, flywheel mechanism giving gyratory vibrations, with one S.S.-304 screen/sieve of given mesh, discharge chute, screen loading channel and hoisting clamps etc. fitted with heavy duty castors, machine duty castors, machine duly painted and finished etc.

OSCILLATING GRANULATOR

Machine complete in all respects, with all contact parts of SS-304, horizontal type, suitable type, suitable for wet and dry granulation process, complete with suitable electric motor, reduction gear box, quick opening and locking arrangement for changing the sieves, machine duly painted and finished.

SEMI AUTOMATIC-2-TRACK STRIP PACKING MACHINE

Complete with one set of change parts, feeding Fibre Disc, Chute Rollers, complete with batch printing attachment, with 0.5 HP Electronic motor stainless contact part etc.

AUTOMATIC 4 TRACK STRIP PACKING MACHINE

Complete with vibrator, S.S. feeding disc, Set of Rollers, chute, cutter etc. with batch printing attachment complete with 0.5 HP Motor, starter etc.

PACKING CONVEYOR BELT

Compete in all respects, designed for packaging /transportation operations of the inspected strips, cartons packs, etc. with 9-inch width superior quality, P.V.C. coated belt at the center having 12-inch width sunmica top working table on both sides of the conveyor belt, with HP/3 phase electric Motor reduction gear DOL starter and roller, with MS pipe legs, height adjustable between 30" to 36" standard 10-ft. length machine.

DOUBLE CONE BLENDER

Double cone blenders are useful for mixing dry powders or granules and are especially useful for small portion of One Product Mix with larger Portion of other. The blender is made of stainless steel and is mounted on mild steel stand. Unit is driven by a motor, through a gearbox with sliding angular blades for efficient mixing complete in all respects.

FOIL SEALER/TAGGER SEALING MACHINE

The machine is complete in all respect, all covered with stainless steel, with thermostatically controlled heaters of 1 KW enclosed in a heating plate. The heater works on single phase. The machine can seal lid size of various plastic PET & PVC container of dia-1 inch to 5 inch.

BATCH PRINTING MACHINE (MOTORISED)

This is small printing unit and is most suitable for over printing labels, cartons, etc. for printing details like mfg. Date batch no. Expiry date, retail price etc. The unit is supplied with composing block, set of words, ink, roller, L.N. Key etc. and Motor of 1/4 HP.

PULVERIZER S.S.

The unit is to reduce the size of the herbs, medicines powder etc. All contact parts of made of stainless steel 304 quality. The S.S. body is fitted with 2 HP/3 phase motor, the size of main body is 6" dia.

The unit is provided with provision for affixing mesh of different size as per requirement and nature of material to be pulverized.

PULVERIZER M.S

With contact parts of milk steel.

-capacity 50 Kg/hr./3HP/3 phase Motor

-capacity 75 Kg/hr./3 phase Motor

LABEL GUMMING MACHINE MOTORISED

Fitted with Crompton motors, Base Plate of stainless steel with Gum pot fitted on wooden mica Board, Cord and Plug, Roller size 6" with 3 brass label lifter.

DEHUMIDIFIER

The unit is a versatile, wherever excess humidity must be removed from the air. One ton hermetically sealed compressor of **'Kirloskar'** mini starter etc. suitable etc. suitable for approx. 2000 cu. ft. area with 3/4 occupants. The unit is fully mobile indegendently without attendant.

PLATE FORM BALANCE

This is a versatile and general weighing machine. It is strictly manufactured according to weights and measures, specifications and rules.

Capacity Steel yard graduation Plate form size

200 Kg. 10 Kg x 100 gms. 370 mm x 550 mm

300 Kg. 10 kg x 100 gms. 500 mm x 625 mm

S.S.SIEVE

Fitted in S.S. frame size 22" x 18" complete with one sieve fitted with out bolt system.

S.S.SIEVES: MOUNTED IN NON FRIABLE WOODEN FRAME

Stainless steel sieve of different meshes size 24" x 18" all mounted in teak wood friable wooden frame.

STAINLESS STEEL SCOOPS S.S 304 QUALITY

With handles highly polished

-Small sizes 300 gm.

-Medium size 700 gm.

-Bigger size 1200 gm.

-Extra bigger size 2 kg.

BOTTLE WASHING MACHINE

Complete in all respects with ss-304 brushing heads, 1/2 HP electric Motor, with suitable covering, duly painted & finished etc.

BOTTLE DRYING OVEN

Complete in all respects with 8 M.S. crates to hold 240 bottles/lb., size/per loading with 1 HP/3 phase electric Motor, uniform heat distribution fan, starter, indicators, thermostat, 6kw special tubular heaters, complete body made out of m.s. sheet of 16 swg thick and its double wall housing heavy fibre best quality glass wool insulation, machine duly painted and finished with inner chamber given heat. resistant aluminium paint.

AUTOMATIC VOLUMETRIC LIQUID FILLING MACHINE

Complete in all respect with all contact parts and suitable covering of ss-304, double head filling system with filling capacity of 15-125 ml on one side and 90-260 ml on the other side, with adjustable nozzle 1 HP/3 phase electric Motor, starter, suitable reduction gear box, quantly adjustment device, and no-bottle-no fill device, etc. with attached ss-belt chain conveyor of 7-ft. length. The conveyor belt is driven by a separate 1 HP/3 phase electric Motor coupld to a sturdy reduction box and starter, etc. Output 26-30 bottles per minute.

SEMI AUTOMATIC VOLUMETRIC LIQUID FILLING MACHINE

Complete in all respects with two filling heads and all contact parts of ss-304, with filling capacity of 15-125 ml on one side and 90-260 ml on the other side, with adjustable nozzle, 1 HP/3 phase electric Motor, starter, suitable reduction geat box and quantity adjustment device etc. with filling speed 26-30 bottles per minute/single stroke. Standard Table Model machine.

SEMI AUTOMATIC ALL-PURPOSE FILLING MACHINE (SINGLE HEAD)

For filling liquids, semisolids etc. in filling range of 15 ml/gm to 125 ml/gm, with ss-304 hopper of 22 kg kg/Lt. capacity and all contact part of ss-304, 1/2 Hp standard electric Motor suitable reduction gear box, one filling nozzle etc. machine all covered with ss-top and heavy duty castors, etc. with filling speed of 16 to 20 counts per minute/single stroke.

FOOT/HAND OPERATED ALL PURPOSE FILLING MACHINE

With all contact parts and 15 Lt/Kg capacity hopper of ss-304, liquid valve, m.s. angle frame stand, ss-304 filling nozzle & culinder, etc. suitable for filling 5 ml/gm to 50 ml/gm range in all types of liquid/semi-solids, creams pasts, inks in tubes, jars cans and bottles etc.

BOTTLE INSPECTION TABLE (SIZE 18"X36")

With flourescent tube and shaded background, provision for attachment of conveyor at any later stage

HIGH SPEED DISSOLVER & STIRRER MACHINE

Self balancing type with 3 variable speed complete in all respects with all contact parts of ss-304 mechanical height adjustment system, suitable electric Motor, heavy m.s. base & pipe stand complete with motor starter etc.

STAINLESS STEEL MIXING/STORAGE TANKS

These vessels are fabricated out of imported stainless steel sheet of 304 quality with M.S. frame legs mounted on wheels. Wheels provided are special type, with two ball bearing for effciently working especially rounded from circumference for easy rotation. Vessels are with removable type lid at the top having hinge lever arrangement, so that during mixing. The unit is also provided 'Internal Marking' in liters at various levels, complete with ball valve for solution removal. The vessels are given mirror finished polish.

PRIMARY SYRUP VESSELS

Stainless steel primary syrup vessels with 16 SWG 304 quality body-14 SWG base with handle bars on both sides, complete with removable type lid.

- Capacity : 50 ltrs.
- Capacity : 100 ltrs.
- Capacity : 200 ltrs.

P.P.CAP SEALING MACHINE (FLOOR MODEL)

For pilfer proof capping, capacity to seal 900 to 1200 cap/hr. depending upon the efficiency of the operator, complete with bottle resting tray and dies of 22,25 & 28mm, easy & adjustable, according to requirement

STAINLESS STEEL CHAIN CONVEYER MACHINE (10 FT. LENGTH)

Complete in all respects, with 1HP/3 Phase electric Motor, suitable reduction gear box, starter and height adjustable between 28" to 34" from the floor level, with suitable s.s.covering etc.

PACKING CONVEYER BELT MACHINE

Complete in all respects, designed for packaging/transportation the inspected bottles, carton packs, etc, with 9-inch width superior quality pvc coated belt at the centre having 12-inch width Sunmica top working table on both sides of the conveyer belt, with 1HP/3 Phase electric Motor, to a sturdy reduction gear box, DOL starter, tension idler and roller, with coupled m.s.pipe legs, height adjustable with between 28" to 34" from the floor level with the help of guided screws, machine duly painted and finished (standard 10-ft length).

EMUILSIFIER/HOMOGENISER WITH LIFTING SYSTEM

Complete in all respect with all contact parts of s.s-304, mounted on heavy m.s. angle Frame hanger, arrangement for height adjustment, with impeller of specially design to suit the HP of the drive, motor protected with four studs, rotor encaged with four studs, rotor encaged with four bars, complete with motor, starter and one classifying screen of any desired mesh.

-100 lt. Mixing capacity, with 1 HP/3 Phase motor

-200 lt. Mixing capacity, with 2 HP/3 Phase motor

-300 lt. Mixing capacity, with 3 HP/3 Phase motor

-500 lt. Mixing capacity, with 5 HP/3 Phase motor

HORIZONTAL PLATE FILTER PRESS MACHINE

Complete in all respects with all contact parts of s.s-304, with 8" dia, transfer gear pump of s.s-304, 1HP/3 Phase electrict. motor, 6-Plate (7-Filter pad) model machine, with s.s.-filter holder, Plates assembled in a cartridge with interlocking kin cups, mounted on m.s. pipe trolley with s.s-top portable unit.

WATER DEIONISER PLANT

To produce Deionised water output depends on the PPM of the total hardness of in-feed Raw Water. The unit is complete with Anion & Cation column, conductivity meter, cell, etc.

Details of Plant, Machinery & Equipments

H.D. PURIFIED WATER STORAGE TANK

Vertical high density polyethylene, made, purified water storage tank, wide mouth complete with removable type lid.

DOUBLE CONE BLENDER

Double cone blenders are useful for mixing dry powders or granules and are especially useful for small portion of One Product Mix with Portion of other. The blender is made of stainless steel and is mounted on mild steel stand. Unit is driven by a motor, through a gearbox with sliding angular blades for efficient mixing complete in all respects.

PORTABLE MECHANICAL SHIFTER

Machine complete in all respects, with allcontact parts of S.S-304, suitable for bolting and sifting of h free-flowing powders and granules, with flanged type motor, flywheel mechanism giving gyratory vibrations, with one S.S-304 screen/sieve of given mesh, discharge chute, screen loading channel and hoisting clamps etc. fitted with heavy duty costors, machine duly painted and finished etc.

DEHUMIDIFIER

The unit is a versatile wherever excess humidity must be removed from the air. One ton hermatically sealed compressor of 'Kirloskar' refrigeration type to operate on 230 volts, single phase, complete with trolley, water collecting tank, mini starter etc. suitable for approx. 2000 cu. ft area with 3/4 occupants. The unit is fully mobile works independently without attendent.

THREE SPEED PLANETARY MIXER

Complete in all respects with all contact parts of ss-304 suitable for mixing, kneading and emulsifying creams, ointments, pastes, powders, wet mass, chavanaprash, gums and duplicating inks, etc. with ss-bowl, suitable locking plug for fixing the bowl to the machine, with specially designed slow speed beater rotating planetarly ensuring effecient and uniform mixing, with specially designed slow speed beater rotating planetarly ensuring efficient and uniform mixing, driven by an electric motor coupled to a 3-speed gear box with belt and pulley arrangement, hand operated mechanical up & down lifting device etc. Planetary movement speed-18,27 & 36 r.p.m. Beater movement speed 54,8 and 108 r.p.m. approx.

DOUBLE SPEED PLANETARY MIXER (SPECIAL TYPE) MACHINE

Complete in all respects with all contact parts of ss-304, with double speed (960/1440 rpm) TEFC motor for most efficient working, with suitable reduction gear box, panel box and DOL changing switch and starter, etc. with a fully jacketed bowl of ss-304 housing, thermostatically controlled suitable capacity heaters for cooling/heating of material, with hand operated mechanical up and down lifting devices.

DOUBLE SPEED PLANETARY MIXER (SPECIAL TYPE/HEAVY DUTY) MACHINE WITH MOTORISED LIFTING.

Complete in all respects, with all contact parts of ss-304, fully jacketed bowl of ss-304 with thermostatically controlled suitable capacity heaters for cooling/heating of materials, with two electric Motor, one dual speed (960/1440 rpm) TEFC motor with suitable reduction gear box coupled through belt and pulley arrangement for driving the agitation assembly and the other single speed (1440 rpm) motor with suitable reduction gear box, belt and pulley arrangement, for lifting the drive assembly for up and down, height adjustment of the drive assembly.

VACUUM PLANETARY MIXER MACHINE

Complete in all respect with all contact parts of ss-304, with a fully jacketed bowl of ss-304 housing thermostatically controlled suitable capacity heaters for cooling/heating of materials, suitable for products where air entrapment is problem, machine complete with dual speed (960/1440 rpm) TEFC motor, suitable reduction gear box belt and pulley arrangement for driving the main agitation assembly, flexible pipe for vacuum application through suitable vacuum pump and provided with a light & light & sight glass, etc. with hand operated mechanical up and down lifting device.

SEMI AUTOMATIC ALL-PURPOSE FILLING MACHINE (SINGLE HEAD)

For filling liquids, semisolids etc. in the filling range of 15 ml/gm to 125 ml/gm, with ss-304 hopper of 22 kg kg/Lt. capacity and all contact parts of ss-304, 1/2 Hp standard electric Motor suitable reduction gear box, one filling nozzle etc. machine all covered with ss-top and heavy duty castors, etc. with filling speed of 16 to 20 counts per minute/single stroke.

FOOT/HAND OPERATED ALL PURPOSE FILLING MACHINE

With all contact parts and 15 Lt./Kg capacity hopper of ss-304, liquid valve, m.s. angle frame stand, ss-304 filling nozzle & cylinder, etc. suitable for filling 5 ml/gm to 50 ml/gm range in all types of liquids/semi-solids, creams pasts, inks in tubes, jars can and bottles etc.

HOMOGENIZER

Complete in all respects, specially designed to grid the mixture of ointment, pastes, suspensions, ink, etc. up to the required fitness through regulation of emulsion head, hardened rotor etc. with 1 HP/3 phase electric Motor, starter and suitable reduction gear box, suitable for 15-25 kg/hr. capacity output.

LABORATORY EQUIPMENTS

HOT AIR OVEN:

Outer body is made of M.S. finished in hammerton spray stoving white enamel paint, with superior quality glass wool insulation in a gap of 65 mm, between the two walls. Heating elements are placed in ribs at the bottom and sides, adjustable air ventilator at top, built in horizontal L shaped thermometer 0 to 250 C, supplied complete with two pilot lamps, thermostate, perforated shelves adjusted at any level to work on 220/230 volts. A.C.main.

VACUUM OVEN

Double walled vacuum chamber made of Al/stainless steel, top lid of thick aluminium sheet with glass window and rubber gasket, vacuum gauge nozzles for suction release valves. Thermometer pocket at top, tempr. from C to 150 C accuracy + 2 C for 220 volts 50 cycles A.C. main. Outer body mild steel with stoving enamel paints wool insulation, complete with perforated aluminum/stainless steel, but without VACUUM PUMP.

STAINLESS STEEL WATER DISTILLATION APPARATUS

Wall type electrically operated on 220/230 volts, AC main complete.

AUTOCLAVE VERTICAL

Inner chamber made of SS outer of M.S. top lid of GUN METAL fitted with pressure gauge safety valve, steam release cock, pressure adjustable upto 35 lb sq. inch, complete with Al/stainless steel basket for sterilizing culture media, glass ware, utensils, instruments etc. In steam under pressure. Also with plug and cable to work on 220 volts AC main. Single rod-locking device with cladding.

FRIABILITY TEST APPARATUS

Used to determine the durability of tablets from the production to the time of use. Acrylic plastic drum has plastic handles, which carries the tablet along with it up to a predetermined height. The rotation period is determined by a timer to work on 230/220 volts, complete with wire & plug.

HERBS GRINDER

The unit is suitable to reduce the size of the herbs as per your requirement. All contact parts of the body made of stainless steel. The S.S. body is fitted with 1 HP single phase motor D.P. switch for ON/OFF, with provision for affixing mesh of different sizes as per the nature of the material to be grinded, supplied with different sizes perforated sieves.

HOT AIR OVEN/TRAY DRYER

Complete in all respect with electrically heated drying chamber, suitable for drying granules, with double wall body, housing heavy fibre glass wool insulation, with special U type heaters, air circulation fan, thermostat, panel box etc. Machine duly painted and finished inside with heat resistant aluminium paint complete body made out of m.s. sheet of 16 swg thickness. The unit is with aluminium trays of 18 swg sheet material.

PORTABLE MECHANICAL SHIFTER

Machine complete in all respects, with all contact parts of SS-304, suitable for bolting and sifting of free-flowing powders and granules, with flanged type motor, flywheel mechanism giving gyratory vibrations, with one S.S-304 screen/sieve of given mesh, discharge chute, screen loading channel and hoisting clamps etc. fitted duty castors, machine duly painted and finished etc.

DOUBLE CONE BLENDER

Double cone blenders are useful for mixing dry powders or granules and are especially useful for small portion of One Product Mix and larger Portion of other. The blender is made of stainless steel and is mounted on mild steel stand. Unit is driven by a motor, through a gearbox with sliding angular blades for efficient mixing complete in all respects.

PULVERIZER S.S.

With all contact parts of stainless steel.

The unit is to reduce the size of the herbs, medicines powder etc. All contact parts of the made of stainless steel 304 quality. The S.S. body is fitted with 2 HP/3 phase motor, the size of main body is 6" dia.

The unit is provided with provision for affixing mesh of different size as per requirement and nature of material to be pulverized.

PULVERIZER M.S.

With contact parts of mild steel.

The unit is for size reduction of herbs, medicinal powders etc. with all parts made of mild steel (M.S) all mounted on M.S. stand with extra heavy duty cyclone type.

Details of Plant, Machinery & Equipments　　　　　　　　　　**103**

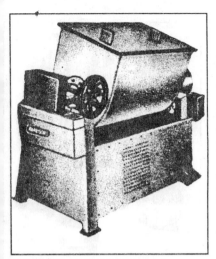

POWDER & MASS MIXER :
All contact parts of stainless steel. Capacity : 25 Kg to 200 Kg. with motor, gear box, starter etc.

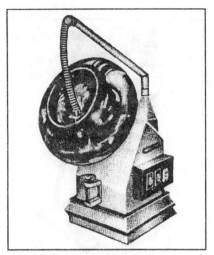

COATING PAN MACHINE :
Pan Dia 12", 36" & 42" with motor, hot Air Blower etc.

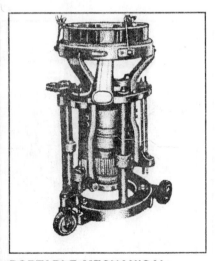

PORTABLE MECHANICAL SHIFTER
All contact part of S.S. with motor of 1.5 H.P. Size of sieve 22" dia. Unit is with one sieve

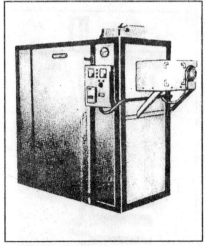

POWDER DRYER :
Model for 12, 24, 48 trays. size of tray 16" x 32" x 1¼"

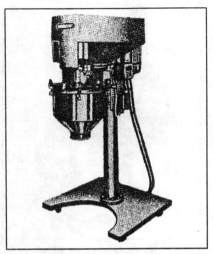

MULTIMILL :
For granulation and pulverization of dry & wet material.
All contact parts of S.S. with motor of 3 H.P./3 Phase.

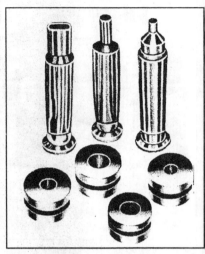

DIE PUNCH :
For all sizes and shapes for type of tablet compression machine

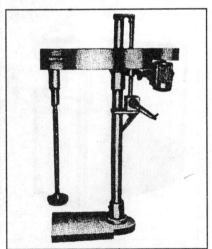

HIGH SPEED DISSOLVER :
With three variable speed and mechanical arrangement for increase and decrease in height.

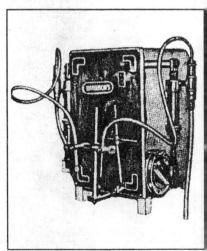

VOLUMETRIC LIQUID FILLING MACHINE :
All contact parts of stainless steel. Filling Range 2 CC to 540CC filling accuracy ± 1%
Capacity 1200 bottle/hr

Details of Plant, Machinery & Equipments

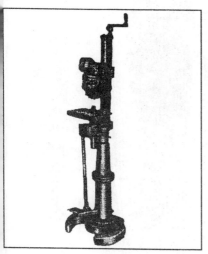

P.P. CAP SEALING MACHINE :
With bottle resting tray and dies of 22, 25 & 28 mm. size.

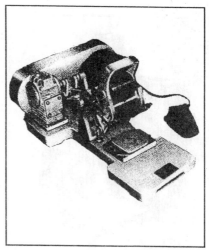

BATCH PRINTING MACHINE :
(Hand operated & motorised)
for over printing mfg. date batch No, etc. with composing block, set of words, Ink, Roller complete.

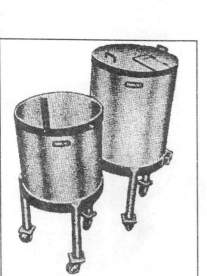

STAINLESS STEEL MIXING/ STORAGE TANK :
Fabricated out of S.S. sheet, with hinge lever lid, INTERNAL MARKING, ball valve capacity 50 ltr. to 2000 ltr

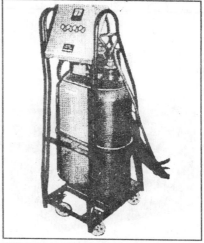

WATER DEMINERALISER :
To remove minerals from the raw water available in various capacity.

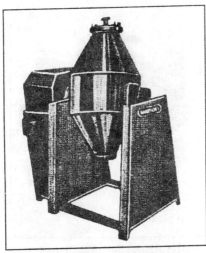

DOUBLE CONE BLENDER :

Contact parts of stainless steel. Capacity : 25 Kg. to 200 Kg./batch size

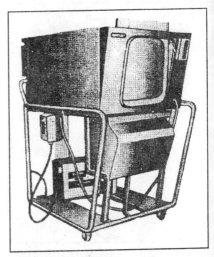

DEHUMIDIFIER :

Refrigeration type with Hermatically sealed compressor, motor fan, Voltage stabilizer, trolley through humidistate etc.

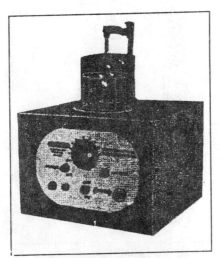

DISINTEGRATION TEST APPARATUS :

As per I.P/B.P/U.S.P. specification Frequency 30/32 cycles/min. with six glass tubes, disc beaker etc.

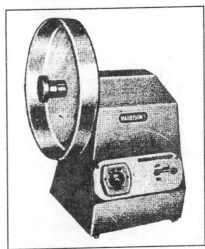

FRIABILITY TEST APPARATUS :

With transparent plastic drum, timer, wire & plug.

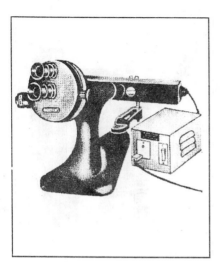

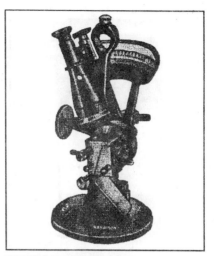

POLARIMETER :
Complete with sodium lamp assembly
Both angular & sugar scale.
Range: On ISS scale from -30° to +130°

REFRACTROMETER ABBE TYPE :
Accuracy 0.001 by direct reading and 0.0001 by estimation.
With refractive and sugar index.

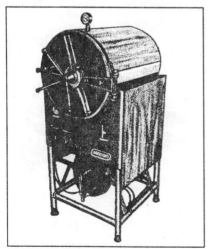

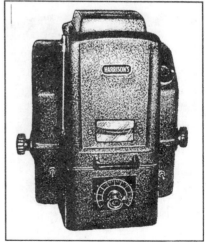

AUTOCLAVE :
(Horizontal/Vertical)
Suitable for rapid sterilization of culture media, utensils, glass ware etc.
Avaliable in various sizes.

INFRARED MOISTURE BALANCE :
Capacity from 5 gms. to 25 gms.
Accuracy 0.2% by direct reading & 0.1% by estimation.

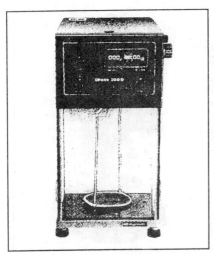

SINGLE PAN BALANCE :
Weighing range 100 gm, 160 gm and 200 gm. electrical operated

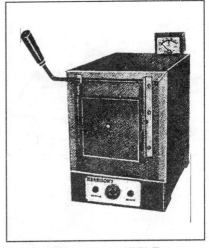

RECTANGULAR MUFFLE FURANCE :
Max. Tempr. 1000°C working tempr. 900°C Available in various sizes.

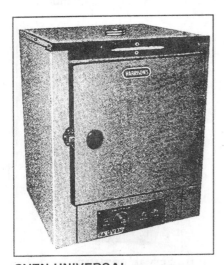

OVEN UNIVERSAL : (Mammert Type)
outer body of M.S. and inner chamber of Al/S.S.
Available in various sizes

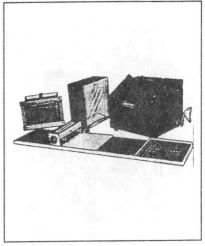

THIN LAYER CHROMATOGRAPHY KIT :
With applicator spreading board, rack, Micropipette & ultra violet lamp assembly.

Chapter - 7

SKIN CREAMS & LOTIONS

Skin creams & lotions described here cover following :-

   (i)   Cleansing creams

   (ii) Cold creams

   (iii) Vanishing creams

   (iv) Skin tonics & moisturizers

   (v) Face lotions

These skin creams and lotions are described in details with formulations and producers for manufacture.

(i) Cleansing Creams

The purpose of a cleasing cream is the removal of facial makeup, surface grime and oil from the face and throat. A properly formulated cleansing cream or lotion will quickly and efficiently remove such applied cosmetics as face powder, rouge, foundation bases, cake makeup and lipstick.

Although the use of soap with adequate washing will perform the same function with soft water, a cleansing cream has certain inherent advantages. The chemical nature of facial makeup is such as to allow more ready removal by a cleansing cream. The latter is specifically formualted to dissolve or lift away the greasy binding materials holding pigments or grime on the skin. A cleansing cream is conveniently applied and used. A positive consideration of importance is the low irritation factor in the use of a cleansing cream. A well balanced modern cleansing cream upon use will leave an emollient residual film on the skin which is proteective in a dry skin condition. The property would suggest the avoidance of such a cleansing creams for oily skins. However it is a common practice with many women to use a cleansing cream first for makeup removal and then to complete the cleansing process by using soap.

In addition to the primary function of cleaning a multipurpose character can be given to a cleansing cream by appropriate formulation. By the addition

Skin Cream & Lotions

of modifying ingredients such properties as softening, lubricating and protective are obtained and claimed for some modern cleansing creams.

Cleansing creams are used not only to lift the dust, but also remove stale makeup. Make-up has a waxy base which cannot be properly penetrated and cleansed simply by using soap and water. A cleansing cream is essential for this. Cleanser should be applied with an upward movement and kept on the skin for about half a minute, so that it could dissolve the make-up. Then remove with a tissue or damp cotton wool. State make-up and days's dirt and grime not only clog the pores of skin causing blackheads, but also eventually coarsen the skin. Here are a few cleansing creams. formulations and manufacturing procedure :-

Formulation for cleansing cream

Ingredients	Quantity
Bees wax	3,25 litres
Emulsifying wax	15.00 litres
Baby oil	60.00 litres
Water	30 litres
Preservative	—

Formulation for Cucumber Cleansing Cream

Ingredients	Quantity
Bess wax	15 litres
Coconut Oil	20 litres
Mineral oil	25 litres
Cucumber Juice	60 litres
Glycerine	5 litres
Borax & Preservative	

Manufacturing Procedure :

Melt the oils and wax in double boiler. Simultaneously, cucumber juice, glycerine, colouring and borax is separately heated. Both the contents are mixed and water is added slowly, alongwith the preservatives.

Formulation for rosewater Cleansing Cream

Ingredients	Quantity
Bees wax or white paraffin wax	22.5 litres
Emulsifying wax	15 litres

Mineral oil	60 litres
Rose extract	9 litres
Borax	90 litres
Rose oil	1 kg

Manufacturing Procedure :

The typical steps involved in cleansing cream manufacture are : (a) Preparation of oil phase; (b) Preparation of water phase; (c) Addition of water phase to oil phase; (d) Milling of cream if necessary; (e) Filling and packaging.

The equipment for the manufacture of cleansing creams and lotions is not very complicated but proper layout and good engineering and necessary to achieve a low processing cost and the best quality of product. The equipment normally used consists of mixing kettles, strainers, pumps, colloid mills or homogenizers and filling and packing machinery.

The equipment may employ tin-coated copper, mantel metal, glass lining or stainless steel. Production requirement and properties of the product control the type and size of equipment to be used. For smaller operation, a mixing kettle of the Hobert type is suitable. For larger operations stock kettles are requires, agitation being a most important factor. Stock kettles can be obtained with up to 500 gallon capacity. Larger kettles are made to specifications.

The mixing kettles should be equipped with jackets to allow heating with steam and subsequent cooling with water. The most suitable agitator is usually a heavy duty anchor type, well baffles with cross arms and driven at moderate speed. Spraprers on the sides of the agitator are effective in promoting good heat transfer in both the heating and cooling stages. Generally the action desired is a "smoothing" rather than a "milling action."

Where hardroom is available in simple and effective layout calls for the placing of the two feeding kettles above the batch mixing kettle. In one kettle waxes are melted. Cutting the waxes into smaller blocks saves both steam and time. Raw materials such as lanolin and petroleum can be melted by storage in a "hot room" or by use of heating coils in the drums to aloow easier transfer to the melting kettle by pumping. The melted oil phase is strained by gritty through unbleached muslin or an edge filter into the mixing kettle. The borax water solution is prepared in other tank, brought to the proper temperature and strained by gravity into the oil phase in the batch mixing kettle. This arrangement of kettles allows the best control of the entire process.

Where headroom is not available the two phases can be pumped into the batch mixing kettle.

After the addition of perfume and cooling of the batch to the filling temperature (approximately 42°C) the cream can be fed to filling equipment by a logged pipe. This applies to formulations which do not require milling or homogenizing.

The use of a colloid mill or homogenier improves the appearance and stability of some creams particularly those of the water-in-oil type.

Temperature at filling is an important factor from the standpoint of appearance and quality of the product. The optimum temperature for filling or puring is approximately 42°C for most formulations of cleansing creams. Creams filled or poured at higher temperatures may have less surface gloss; they may set to a more rigid consistency or have a tendency to shrink in the center when cool. Sometimes moisture will condense on the under side of the jar cap or liner.

In some cases a long travel on the conveyor belt prior to capping is given to the filled jar. The practice of "topping' is often used. Approximately three quarters of the cream is filled into the jar and gently swirled to leave a continuous film up to the rim. The remainder of contents is then filled into the jar and the jars are set aside to cool before being capped. This practice allows the cream to set with a smooth and even top.

The actual finishing method used depends upon the formula and upon available equipment.

(ii) Cold Creams

Cold cream is an emulsion in which the fat predominates, but the cooling effect produced when it is applied to the skin is due to the slow evaporation of the water contained. The base in general use in white beewax, and traces of borax are occasionally added to aid emulsification. The perfume generally used is rose-either as aqua rose or by the addition of otto. The method of manufacture is simple when borax is used, and consists of melting the wax on a water bath, adding the oil, and warming the whole to about 80° C. The equeous portion containing the borax is heated to this temperature and stirred in slowly. The perfume is added when cool, and the cream is potted liquid if a brilliant white surface is desired.

Formulation for Cold Creams

I

Ingredients	quantity
Almond oil	550
white wax	145
Borax	10

Water	290
Rose otto	5

II

Ingredients	Quantity
Peack Kernel oil	600
Spermaceti	20
White wax	150
Borax	5
Triple rose water	215
Phenylethyl alcohol	5
Geranium oil-French	5

III

Ingredients	Quantity
Almond oil	560
White wax	180
Lanolin, anhydrous	20
Borax	10
Zinc oxide-finely sifted	20
Water	200
Rose rogue	5
Rose-geranium oil	5

IV

Mineral Cold Creams may be prepared with petroleum oil of 860 sp. gravity as follows.

Ingredients	Quantity
Paraffin liquid	570
White wax	160
Lanolin	50
Borax	8
Water	200
Geraniol	8
Phenylethyl alcohol	4

Skin Creams & Lotions

V

Procedure : Melt 60 parts of white wax and 100 parts of spermaceti over a water bath, then add 1,000 parts of almond oil leaving the whole on the water bath. Next add 10 parts of castor oil, then 300 parts of rose water, stirring continuously. Finally incorporate 2 parts of oil of rose, 2 parts of oil of geranium and 10 parts of oil of bergamot and place in jars. A trace of methyl violet may be added to ensure that the preparation retains its whiteness.

VI

Procedure : Melt 1 oz. of white wax and 1 oz. of spermaceti; add 8 fl. oz. oil of sweet almonds in which 1 oz. of camphor has been dissolved with very gentle heat; then gradually add 5 fl. oz. of rose water in which 4 dr. of powdered borax has previously been dissolved, beating constantly with a wooden spatula until cold. Finally add 10 drops of oil of rose. This will yield comphorated cold cream.

VII

Procedure : Take petroleum oil 600 gr., white wax 60 gr., paraffin 140 dr., Eau de Cologne 30 gr., water 200 gr., rose water 200 gr., tincture of benzoin 10 gr., oil of ose geranium 10 drops. Mix the solid matter in the warm oils and pour into the mixture little by little, stirring at the same time Eau de Cologne and the perfumes. Stir well to get perfectly white.

VIII

Procedure : Mix together oil of almonds 425 parts, lanolin 185 parts, white wax 62 parts, spermaceti 62 parts. Make a solution of 4.5 parts of borax in 300 parts of rose water. Incorporate the solution to the solid ingredients.

IX

Procedure : Take spermaceti 4 1/2 iz, white wax 3 oz; fresh oil of almonds, 18 oz; melt over water bath and pour in a slightly warmed marble mortar and stir briskly to prevent granulation. When the mixture becomes of the consistency of butter, triturate until it has a white, cream appearance; add little by little, under constant stirring, a mixture of double water or rose, 1 1/2 oz; odourless glycerine, 1 1/2 oz; mix for 20 minutes, then add 15 drops of essence of rose and beat for about half an hour, when it will be ready for use.

X

Procedure : Melt 6 oz. of spermaceti and 4 oz. of white wax on a water bath. Add fresh oil of almonds 24 oz. and pour the whole into a slightly warmed mortar under constant and lively stirring to prevent granulation until the mass has a white, creamy appearance and is about the consistence of butter of ordinary temperature. Add little by little, under constant stirring, 2 oz. of rose water and 2 oz. of pure glycerine, mixed together, and fianally add oil of bergamot 24 drops, rose oil 6 drops, oil of bitter almonds 8 drops and tincture of ambergr is 5 drops. Continue the stirring for 15 to 20 minutes; then immediately pur into containers.

(iii) Vanishing Creams

Vanishing cream is so called becuase it disappears when rubbed into the skin. It consists of stearic acid partially saponified with alkali, the bulk of the fatty acid being emulsified by the soap thus formed. The main constituents is, of course, water and mucilage of tragacanth or agar-agar to prevent the collapsing of the cream and the whole is preserved with a trace of an aldehyde.

Some of the Formulations and Procedures are detailed as under :-

I

Procedure : Melt 60 grams of stearic acid in a tared vessel of about 2 litres capacity, over a waterbath, and add 9 grams of sodium carbonate, dissolved in the minimum amount of hot water; to this add 7 grams of glycerine. Keep the mixture on the waterbath for one hour, stirring constantly, but not vigorously; add sufficient water to bring the preparation to 300 grams; then add 300 grams of the Hamamelis water. Return the mixture until perfectly smooth. Pour into a warm mortar and beat to a foam. Let it stand for 12 hours, stir with a spatula and packs.

II

Precedure : Mix agar-agar 180 gr., distilled water 8 ft. oz., distilled solution of Hamamelis B.P. 12 ft. oz. and allow to stand for few days with occasional stirring until softened. Strain through muslin. Now heat together stearic acid 360 gr., oil of the obroma 360 gr., sodium carbonate 240 gr., distilled water 12 ft. oz., on a water-bath stirring constantly until combination is completed; transfer to a large jar and whip in the first solution with an egg whisk until a white foamy product results. Perfume to taste. Allow to stand for 14 days so that air bubbles may escape, mix gently and bottle. Large quantities may be made in an emulsifying machine. The preparation will not show any grit and will keep long.

III

Procedure : Bring 1 lb. of glycerine and 1½ pint of water to a boil and add ½ oz. of carbonate of potash. Strain through a piece of cloth and heat the whole mass again. In the meanwhile have ¼ lb. of stearine melted over a water bath and our this slowly over the first liquor. Continure heating till the mass is completely saponified. then remove it and add 15 drops of oil of bitter almonds and 20 drops of oil of lavender. beat the whole until cool and pack.

IV

Ingredients	Quantities
Glycerine	8.25 lbs.
Stearic acid (pure)	4.75 lbs.
Distilled water	224 fl. oz.
Spirit	16 fl. oz.
Liquid ammonia (Sp. Gr. O. 888	4.75 oz.
Terpineol	2 oz.
Synthetic Jasmine otto	0.5 oz.
Synthetic Musk Crystals	10 gr.
Phenyl acetaldehyde	6 minims.

Procedure : Melt the stearic acid on a water bath at 75.8°C. Heat 2 lbs. of the glycerine with 192 oz. of the water to the same temperature, add ammonia, and pour into the melted stearic acid slowly, with constant stirring. Mix the rest of the glycerine and water and heat to 80°C, pour this into the first mixture with constant stirring, and continue the heat stirring for about 15 minutes. Remove from the fire and heat till cold. Mix perfumes with the spirit, and add slowly, with constant stirring to the cream.

Owing to the air and water present, these creams sometimes dry up. To avoid this add glycerine, grease, agar-agar and tragacanth.

V

Ingredient	quantities
Stearic acid, triple pressed	200
Potassium hydroxide-sticks	14
Water	800
Carbitol	40
Perfume	10

Procedure : Dissolve the perfume in the carbitol and beat it into the cream at 20° Centigrade. To obtain a softer cream decrease the fatty acid and increase the potash.

VI

Ingredients	Quantities
Stearic acid	180

Ingredient	Quantity
Potassium carbonate crystals	12
Glycerine	50
Water	750
Bergamot oil	2
Lavender oil	1
Ylang-ylang oil	1
Vetivert oil	1
Geranium oil	3

Procedure : Maintain the temperature at least 20 minutes, with vigorous stirring from the commencement of saponification. This will allow the greater part of the carbon dioxide to escape.

VII

Ingredients	Quantities
Stearic acid	180
Caustic soda-stick	9
Glycerine	50
Water	750
Coumarin	2
Sadalwood oil	2
Vetivert oil	1
Methyl ionone	6

Procedure : dissolve the cuastic soda in 30 parts of the hot water and add to the fatty acid. Mix the glycerine with the remainder of the water at the same temperature and stir in.

VIII

Ingredients	Quantities
Stearic acid	200
Fresh lard	20
Strong solution of ammonia 880	10
distilled water	750
Linalol	5
Terpineol	8

Skin Creams & Lotions

Ingredients	Quantities
Ylang-ylang oil	2
Coumarin	4
Oakmoss resin	1

Procedure : Add the ammonia to the hot water, stir, and pour the solution rapidly into the melted fats, triturating briskly all the time.

IX

Ingredients	Quantities
Stearic acid	130
Borax crystals	58
Sodium carbonate crystals	12
Water	740
Glycerine	50
rose-geranium oil	9
Patchouli oil	1

Procedure : Pour the melted stearic acid into the boiling solution of glycerine, water, borax, and soda. Contnue to boil until the mixture gelatinises. Cool and add the perfumes.

X

Ingredients	Quantities
Stearic acid	180
Spermaceti	20
Triethanolamine	20
Carbitol	70
Perfume compound	10
Distilled water	700

Procedure : Melt the fats and heat the liquid to the same temperature. Mix and stir until cool-add the perfume.

Witch-hazel Foams are made on the same lines as vanishing creams, excepting that a proportion of the water is replaced by distilled extract of witch-hazel, which is added to the already saponifed fatty acid:

Ingredients	Quantities
Stearic Acid	180

Potassium hyroxide	12
Water	260
Distilled solution of witch-hazel	500
Glycerine	50

Perfume with rose otto if desired.

XII

Peroxide Creams contain hydrogen peroxide at the time of manufacture, but it seems doubtful if this exists as such when they are used. The only means of securing the presence of available oxygen is by stabilising the peroxide with methyl parahydroxy benzoate.

Ingredients	Quantities
Stearic acid	120
Lanolin, anhydrous	20
Borax	30
Glycerine	100
Water	670
Hydrogen peroxide-20 volumes	50
Jasmine	6
Bois de rose oil	3
Styrax R.	1

Add the hydrogen peroxide while the cream is cooling.

(iv) Skin Tonics & Moisturizers

Basically skin tonics freshen the skin. Skin tonics are generally composed of infusions of hersbs, flowers, vinegar, rosewater and witch-hazel. Stronger skin tonics or astringents dry and skin removing all traces of oil on the skin. they are suitable for greasy skins.

The herbs that are particularly good as skin tonics are :

yarrow	:	for greasy skin
Camomile	:	helps eliminate wrinkles
Rosemary	:	for healing and firming
Parsely	:	contains Vitamin C and is very useful for spotty and pathy skins

Skin Creams & Lotions

Tansy	:	Lotion helps get rid of freckles
Mint	:	for stimulating
Comfrey	:	especially good for clearing up spotty skins
Fennel	:	makes a mild tonic.

Formulations for Skin Tonic

I

Ingredients	Quantities
Elderflower water	15 litres
Cucumber Juice	7.5 litre
Eau-del-colonge	6 litres
Tincture of benzoin & preservative	1.5 litres

II

Ingredients	Quantities
Elder flower water	5 litres
Rose water	5 litres
Witch hazel	5 litres
Boric acid & preservative	900 gms

Marigold, hollyhock, honey, vinegar, orange, lemon, apple tree bark, Rose etc. can be used in tonics.

Moisturizers & Nouishing Creams

When the body supplies of harmones and other vital elements slows down. Creams and lotions containing hormones and other special extracts and serums, rich creams containing vitamins and concentrated oils, help to give the skin a more youthful appearance. here are a few easy to make simple misturizers & nourishing creams :

Moisturizers

I. Herb Cream

Ingredients	Quantities
Lanolin	1.5 litres
White Emulsifying wax	30 litre

Besswax	9.0 litres
Almond oil, herb lotion or in fusion	9.0 litres

II. Sunflower Cream

Ingredients	Quantities
Lanolin	2 litre
Emulsifying	1 litres
Beeswax	10 litres
Sunflower oil	9 litre
Glycerine	1 litre
Borax	250 gms

III. Avocado and Almond Cream

Ingredients	Quantities
Beeswax	1.5 litre
Emulsifying wax	1.5 litre
Almond oil	12 litre
Avocado Oil	6 litre
Rose Water	4.5 litre

IV. Jasmine mositure cream

Ingredients	Quantities
Emulsifying wax	3 litre
Almond oil	3 litre
Lanolin	500 gms
Borax	250 gms
Witch Hazel	500 gms
Glycerine	750 ml
Water	12 litre
Jasmine Oil	As required

Skin Creams & Lotions

Nourishing Creams

Nourshing preparations include all the skin foods whether they are oil based or of the moisturizing type, whether they are light and immediately absorbed or heavy and sticky needing to the massaged into skin. Harmone creams and lotions, vitamin products, serum ampoules, anti wrinkle creams and lotions, biologically active preparations all come into the nourishing group. Some of the easy to make nourishing recipes are give below.

I. Cocoa Butter Cream :

Ingredients	Quantities
Cocoa Butter	3 litre
Emulsifying Wax	3 litre
Beeswax	1.5 litre
Sesame Oil	6 litre
Almond Oil	1.5 litre

II. Elder Flower Cream:

Ingredients	Quantities
Almond Oil	4.5 litre
Eldeflower Blossom	6 litre
Lanolin Warm Water	1.5 litre

III. Wheat Germ Cream :

Ingredients	Quantities
Beeswax	500 gms
Emulsifying Wax	500 gms
Lanolin	7.5 litres
Sesame Oil	4.5 litres
Wheat Germ Oil	3 litres
Water	7.5 litres
Witch hazel	1.5 litres
Borax Perfume	250 ml

IV. Vitamin Cream :

Ingredients	Quantities
Beeswax	1.5 litre
Emulsifying Wax	1.5 litre
Lanolin	1.5 litre
Wheat Germ Oil	4.5 litre
Carrot Oil	4.5 litre
Distilled Water	9 litre
Borax, tincture of benzoin & Orange flower oil	250 ml.

V. Mixed Vegetable Cream:

Ingredients	Quantities
Beeswax	3 litres
Emulsifying Wax	6 litre
Lanolin	1.5 litre
Almond Oil	6 litre
Sesame Oil	6 litre
Adocado Oil	3 litre
Safflower Oil	3 litre
Sunflower Oil	3 litre
Water	7.5 litres
Borax & Amber Oil	250 ml

VI. Oily Nourishing Cream :

Ingredients	Quantities
Coconut Oil	4.5 litre
Olice Oil	3.00 litre
Almond Oil	1.5 litre
Beeswax	7.5 litres

Skin Creams & Lotions

Borax & treated water — as per requirement

VII. Orange Flower Skin Food

Ingredients	Quantities
Beeswax	1.00 litres
Emulsifying wax	1.00 litres
Almond Oil	4.00 litres
Lanolin	2.00 litres
Coconut Oil	2.00 litres
Organge Flower water	3.00 litres
Tincture of benzoin & orange Oil	200 ml

Besides above, few other nourishing and special creams such as Lime Juice Cream, Lime Juice Glycerine and Wrinkle Removing Creams are described below :-

Lime Juice Cream

I. Procedure : dissolve by gentle heat white wax 1/2 oz; oil of sweet almonds, 8 oz. Gradually; add glycerine, 1 oz; lime water (aqua calcis B.P.), 32 gr. with 1 oz. water; also add rectified spirit, 1.5 oz; essence of lemon, 2 dr.; essential oil of almonds, 5 minims.

II. Procedure : Take white wax 1 part, oil of sweet almonds 20 parts, lime water 22 parts, glycerine 2 parts, oil of lemon part. The advantage of this preparation is that it does not become rancid; on the other hand, it exerts a stimulating effect on the roots of the hair.

Lime Juice Glycerine

I

Ingredients	Quantities
Almond Oil	25 oz.
Glycerine	1.5 oz.
Lemon Oil	1.25 oz.
Lime Water to make	80 fl. oz.

Procedure ; Mix well by shaking.

II

Ingredients	Quantities
Almond Oil	2 oz.
Glycerine	4 dr.
Tincture of Senegal	1 dr.
Lime Water	2 oz.
Rose Water	4 oz.
Oil of Bergamot	10 drops
Oil of Lemon	20 drops

Procedure : Shake well the oil of almond and tincture of senegal and then add the glycerine, lime water and rose water. Lastly perfume with essential oils. If the cream becomes rancid, add 4 grains of salicylic acid to each pint of the cream.

Wrinkle Removing Cream

Procedure : Take white petrolatum, 7 av. oz.; paraffin wax, 1/2 av. oz.; lanolin, 2 av. oz,; water 3 fl. oz.; oil of rose, 3 drops; vanillin, 2 gr.; alcohol, 1 fl. dr. Melt the paraffin, add the lanolin and petrolatum, and when these have melted pour the mixture into a warm mortar, and with constant stirring incorporate the water. When nearly cold add the oil and vanillin, dissolved in the alcohol. Preparations of this kind should be rubbed into the skin vigorously, as friction assists the absorbed fat in developing the muscles, and also imparts softness and fullness to the skin.

Anti-Acne herbal Preparation
herbal Extracts Composition

1. Extract of Arjun Bark (8:1)   -17.50 %

2. Extract of Randia dumeterium Fruits (5:1) - 20.75 %

3. Extract of Ferula galabanifula (2:1)   -09.75%

4. Extract of orange peel (4:1)   -42.00%

Suggested Formulation

Extracts of four herbs mentioned above	-30.00 gms.
Honey-I.P. Grade	-30.00 gsm.
Acetic Acid (Glacial) I.P. Grade	-2.00 gms.
Water - sufficient to soften	

The above formulated product is used for external applications only.

Skin Creams & Lotions

the spot of skin is cleaned with soap, preferably at bed time and the product is applied.

(V) Face Lotions

I. Procedure : Dissolve 10 gr. of alum and 1 gr. of zinc sulphate in a little water; mix 1 fl. dr. of glycerine with the bulk of water and pour in 1 fl. dr. of tincture of benzoin and 30 drops of essence of EAu de Cologne. Finally add distilled water to make 1 pint and mix well. The result should be a non-separable milky lotion.

II. Procedure : Mix 40 oz. of lactic acid and 80 oz. of pure glycerine in 5 gallons of distilled water. now add 3 oz. of tincture of benzoin. Then colour with 40 grains of carmine and pour gradually a mixture of 1 oz. of commercial glycerine, 1/2 oz of ammonia solution in 3 oz. of distilled water. Heat the whole to drive off ammonia and mix intimately. Shake well and set aside for a day, filter and add 1 drachm of solution of ionone and a small quantity of kaolin. Finally filter until clear.

III

Ingredients	Quantities
Lactic acid, syrupy	5 c.c.
Glycerine	100 c.c.
Tincture Benzoin	10 c.c.
Tincture of Styrax	10 c.c.
Patchouli R.	1 c.c.
Rose Synthetic	4 c.c.
Rose water to produce	1000 c.c.

Procedure : Dissolve the perfumes in the tinctures and add to the glycerine. Shake with 800 c.c. of water and then add the aicd. Make up to volume with more rose water.

IV

Ingredients	Quantities
Hydrogen Peroxide 10 Vols.	100 c.c.
Tincture Benzoin	10 c.c.
Muguet Synthetic	5 c.c.
Rose Water to produce	1000 c.c.

IV

Ingredients	Quantitites
Hydrogen Peroxide 10 Vols.	100 c.c.
Tincture Benzoin	10 c.c.
Muguet Synthetic	5 c.c.
Rose Water to produce	1000 c.c.

Sun Burn Lotion

Ingredients	Quantities
Zinc Hydroxide (25 p.c.)	100 grams
Zinc Carbonate	70 grams
Corn Starch	30 grams
Glycerine	50 c.c.
Tincture of Benzoin	50 c.c.
Benzyl Cinnamate	2 grams
Heliotropin	5 grams
Tuberose Absolute	1 gram
Water to produce	1000 c.c.

Procedure : Dissolve the perfumes in the tincture of benzon. tint the powders with Armenian bole if desired be called a baby shampoo.

Shampoos for all hair types :

Lime Shampoo :

Ingredients	Quantity
Amla	1kg
Shikakai	2 kg
Char	1 kg
Charilla	1 kg
Khus	1 kg
Reetha	2 kg

Chapter - 8

POMADES & BEAUTY MASKS

The pomades are much in favour as toilet articles. The chief ingredient in all pomades is a soft white basis of white wax, spermaceti, lard, suet, vaseline, etc. when lard, suet, vaseline, etc. are used they should be previously refined and made free of all impurities and obnoxious matters. Other fats such as olive oil, almond oil, etc. may also be employed in conjunction with the above to serve as the basis.

The Mode of Preparation

To prepare the pomade the first step is to melt the pomade stock on a water bath and then add the olive and almond oil.

Now the pan is removed from fire and when it begins to thicken stir in various scents in proportions at discretion.

In preparing pomades the manufacturers may note that an addition of soap improves pomades. before perfuming add about 250 parts of soap dissolved in hot water and about 1.75 parts of borax to 12,500 parts of pomade stock. This renders the pomade as white as snow and very emollient, which is very difficult to attain by an addition of stearine. This pomade will bear an admixture of one third water.

In colouring pomades use in generally made of alkanet root, annatoo, gamboge root, chlorophyll, etc. It is usual to tie up the drug in a piece of coarse cloth and dip in a part of the pomade stock, Gentle heat may be applied and the whole squeezed from time to time. The strongly coloured stock may be diluted with ordinary stock to bring it to the desired shade.

Formulation I

Procedure : Prepared suet, olive oil, each 8 ounces, lard 4 ounces. Melt on a water bath, then remove the vessel, and, when it begins to thicken, stir in the following scents, in quantity at discretion: Oil of cloves, sixty drops; oil of neroli, twenty drops; oil lavender, sixty drops; oil of bergamot, ninety drops; essence musk, fifty drops; mix. A slight colour may be given to it, according to the fancy of the manufacturers with alkanet root or gamboge root.

Formulation II

Procedure : Melt 250 parts of freshly rendered lard and 25 parts of white wax at moderate heat and mix well with 200 parts of vaseline. Add 15 parts of bergamot oil, 3 parts of lavender oil, 2 parts of geranium oil and 2 part of lemon oil, mixing well.

Formulation III

Procedure : Strained suet, ten pounds white wax three quarters of a pound. Melt, their stir wiell in bergamot oil, and ounce; lemon oil, half an ounce; oil of rosemary, quarter of an ounce; oil of lavender, quarter of an ounce; rose water, one pint.

Formulation IV

Procedure : Clarified lard, twelve pounds; clarified suet, two pounds; essence of bergamot, one ounce; essence of lemon, half an ounce; oil of lavender, quarter of an ounce; rose water, eight ounces. Melt the first two, then take the pan from the fire and stir in the essences.

Formulation V

Procedure : Digest 20 parts of coconut oil and 1 part of benzoin, in coarse powder, in a waterbath for 2 hours. Now have 1 part of carnauba wax, 1 part of ceresine and 5 parts of liquid paraffin melted over a waterbath. Strain the benzoated oil into the molten mass of paraffin. The product may be perfumed as desired with essential oils.

Formulation VI

Procedure : Melt 2.50 oz. of refined wax over a slow fire and then add 8 oz. of coconut oil On cooling add 15 drops of oil of bergamot and 9 drops of oil of henna and stir well.

Formulation VII

Procedure : Take refined coconut oil 8 oz., white wax 2.05 oz., oil of bergamot 15 minims, oil of heena 5 minims and proceed as above. Add alkanet root to colour.

Formulation VIII

Procedure : Take white wax 2 oz., refined coconut oil 12 oz., rose geranium oil 5 minims and proceed as above. Add tincture carmine to colour

Formulation IX

Procedure : Take pure castor oil 8 oz., white wax 3 oz., otto of rose 5 minims, and proceed as above. Add tincture grass to colour.

Pomade A La Rose

Procedure : Lard, four pounds; suet, I pound; alkanet root q.s. Macerate with heat to give a faint colour, then allow it to cool and before it sets, stir in five ounces of rose water and add otto of rose to perfume.

Pomade A La Jasmine

Procedure : lard, suet, each one pound; oil of almonds, four ounces. Mix, then add spirit of jasmine, one ounce and a half.

Beauty Masks

There are numerous classification systems employed in discussion of beauty masks, perhaps the least combersome of which is based on viscosity. Mask preparations can be divided roughly into two groups--those with sufficiently high viscosities as to be considered nonmobile or pastes and those with low viscosities and which flow or are capable of being poured from their containers. This second class of prepartion has become more popular in recent times, probably due both to the greater availability of suitable raw materials and to the desire of the marketing personnel to provide products which can be used quickly and easily. Both classes of masks can be modified by the inclusion of "special purpose" components to gain certain unusual or specific features. All well-formulated products should, however have some characteristics in common, which may be summarized as follows.

1. They shoul produce a noticeable tightening effect on the skin after application.
2. They should possess sufficient absorbent power to achieve a cleansing effect.
3. They should allow ease of application and removal.
4. They should achieve their results without undue time requried for drying or hardening.
5. They should be non irritating to normal skin.

High-Viscosity or Paste Masks

High-viscosity or paste masks are exemplified by the "clay facial packs" and the fashionable "mud packs". In general they contain a rather high percentage of colloidal clay, Kaolin or other suitable solid dispersed in a liquid vehicle. the concentration of solids varies with both the type of solid used and the composition of the liquid vehicle. The plasticity desired in the finished product will also determine this concentration of solids.

Low viscosity of liquid masks

Liquid beauty masks are currently accounting for a significantly increased share of the dollar sales volume in these preparations. this probably can be attributed to their greater ease of application and in general their more rapid drying time. The advertising value of these products is apparently almost limitless, and the fact has aided in the attainment of their present position in the market.

Liquid masks are usually formulated around the film-forming characteristics of one or more of the hydrophilic colloids. The colloids like the clay-type components in the paste preparations, dimnish in size upon the loss of significant quantitties of solvent or diluent; their modus operandi then is based upon the same mechanical astringency as is manifested by the dispersed solids in the high viscosity products. Most liquid preparations as compared with the pastes, suffer one major shortcoming namely a pronounced dimiution of cleanising properties. As pointed out, the cleansing effect of the paste mask is due primarily to the adsorption efficiency of the dispersed solids employed.

Manufacturing Procedure

Because these paste mask preparations constitute heavy, compact masses upon the completion of processing. It is necessary that the mixing equipment chose have sufficient power to provide thorough blending. In general, planetary action dough mixers are suitable since they have ample power and their wide bowl tops allow easy loading of the bulky dry materials. In additions most equipment of this type has detachable mixing bowls which can be wheeled to the tilting device for removing the finished product.

The accurate weighed dry materials are suitably pre-blended, a process which can be accomplished by the use of ribbon-powder mixed or directly in the planetary action mixer itself. If a pigment is used to achieve the desired colour in the finished product his pigment must be well dispersed in a portion of the dry materials. This is best done by incorporating the pigment in the desired amount of dry solid and then passing this mixture through a hammer mill. If the liquid phase contains a humectant or other water-miscible components they may be mixed together with the water prior to addition to liquid phase to the solids. Samll additions of liquid are made to the dry solids, with mixing continued between additions. This intermittent addition of liquid produces initially a very viscous paste which ensures the thorough wetting of the dry components. As the liquid phase is added, the viscosity of the paste decreases and the liquid additions can be made with shorter time intervals separating them since the mass absorbs these subsequent additions more easily than it did the initial ones. If the formulations contains solid esters of waxes these must of course, be added while molten, and this necessitates heating of the aqueous solids dispersions as well. In general, under theses circumstances the manufacturing procedure employed should closely parallel that used in the production of any emulsion containing dispersed solids.

Efficay of masks :

Despite their transient action, masks are frequently used. Sometimes the face is surprisingly rejuvenated by the treatment, and then it is hoped the excellent effect will remain.

It is manufacturer's object to prepare an unctuous or greasy mass which cannot only be easily applied in successive layers, but can also be easily removed or cleaned off.

A gelatine mask is the most efficient. When it is applied warm by means of a brush, it will readily set on cooling and it can then be lifted like a rubber membrane. The behaviour of the mask does not only depend upon the nature of the added materials. It also depends on pH of the gelatine; the iso-electric point of gelatine is lower than that of the skin keratin.

Formulation for Gelatine Mask

Ingredients	Weight in Grammes
Powdered or granulated gelatine	40
Hot water (for dissolving)	900
Glycerine (for addition)	30
Titanium or zinc oxide	30

A pink or flesh-tinted lake can be used to colour the preparations. It should only be perfumed with aromatic distilled waters, according to their purpose, detailed below :

1. Rose water as astringent.

2. Orange flower water as hypnotic and sedative

3. Lavender water as soothing agent

4. Hyssop water as anti-herpes agent's. Garden sage as perspirant

5. Cypress and hammamelidis waters as vasomotors.

6. Camphor or rosemary water as sedative

Aromatic masks :

Aromatic masks are prepared by adding 400 grammes of the aromatic water to the gelatine dissolved in 500 grammes distilled water. The flower water is added just before the mask is used.

A gum e.g. gum tragacanth, or agar-agar can be used in place of 1 part of the gelatine. The first two suggested alternatives are acid, the third is neutral. Alkaline alginates should not be avoided. Glycerinated starch is not excluded. Tapioca or arrow root can be used instead of starch. Glyverine gives it the hydration which is useful in the treatment of dry skins.

The formulations are as under :

Ist Formulation

Ingredients	Quantities
Powdered gelatine	25
Hot water	500
Gum Tragacanth	20
Glycerinated Starch	100
Titanium oxide	15
Distilled floral water	340

The titanium oxide leaves a pearl like shine on the skin and forms a porcelin like foundation for further make-up. The gelatine is sometimes replaced by casein, which is also acid. One hundred and fifty grammes casein is required per 1 litre of water. A mixed formula gives good results.

2nd Formulation

Ingredients	Quantity
Powdered gelatine	15
Casein	100
Glycerine	25
Zinc Oxide	840

The absorbent effect of masks is very important. They tend to dry normal skins and still more dry skins (fat-free). This disadvantage can be almost countered by the action of the monoesters of glycerine or glycol emulsified into the gelatinous or clay containing masses. Moreover, these esters give a stainy effect on the skin and also provide deeply penetrating fatty nourishment.

3rd Formulation - Fatty Masks

Ingredients	Quantity
White gelatine	35
Dissolved in hot water add	900
Self-emulsifying glycol monoester	50
Titanium oxide	15

This can be added to the masks indicated above whether they contain case in or clays.

4th Formulation-Fatty Mask (Almond)

Ingredients	Quantity
Osmo-Kaolin	200
Glycol monomyristate T.G.	50
Hydrophilic almond oil	20
Distilled hot water	400

After emulsification and immediately before use, 280 grammes of Laurel or almond water is added.

The old preparation based on balanced almonds can be replaced by this mask. For acid masks, containing egg, fruit juices, a pure monoester emulsified with a small quantity of sulphonated fatty alcohol is used.

5th Formulation - Acid, Cleaning Mask

Ingredients	Quantities
Osmo-Kaolin	175
Pure glyceryl monostearate	20
Sulphonated fatty alcohol	5
Water	525
Fruit Juice	270

The fruit juice can be expressed from the fruit just before it is used or it can be prepared from a concentrate. It will of course, be diluted according to its acidity.

6th Formulation - Neutral fatty Mask

Ingredients	Quantities
Kaolin	120
Oleocetyl alcohol	20
Zinc Oxide	40
Lavender Water	400
Orange flower water	420

Lecithin can be added to all the formulation in the above the lecithin is taken up in the fatty material and added to other ingredients immediately before use.

Chapter - 9
FACE POWDERS & TALCUM POWDERS

In manufacturing face powders the materials should be ground to a very fine state of sub-division and then passed through sieve of at least 100 mesh. For perfect results 120 mesh sieve is recommended.

After grinding and sifting, the ingredients are taken in specified proportion and a small quantity of such a mixture is put in a mortar and rubbed with suitable colour and then mixed with the whole lot and sifted twice to make sure that sub-division of the basic pigments has been accomplished.

Perfumes are next added by spraying the liquid perfumes on to the powder as it falls thorough the silk sifter. The amount of perfume used should be reduced to a minimum.

Formulation I

Procedure : Mix zinc white 5 parts; English precipitated calcium carbonate, 30 parts; best white steatite, 5 pars; wheat or rice starch, 10 parts; triple extract of white rose, 3 parts; triple extract of jasmine, 3 parts; triple extract of orange flower, 3 parts; triple extract of cassia 3 parts; tincture of musk, 8 parts. The whole is to be mixed thoroughly be repeated siftings. Orris root in powder may be substituted for the perfumes.

Formulation II

Procedure : Take pearl or bismuth white and Frech chalk, equal parts. Reduce them to fine powder and sift through cloth. Lastly add some artificial perfumes, as desired.

Formulation III

Procedure : A face powder of rosy hue may be prepared as follows: Starch 1,000 grams, carmine 20 grams, otto of rose 15 grams, otto of hus khus 15 grams, sandal oil 15 grams.

Formulation IV

Procedure : Take oxide of zinc 1 oz,; starch 8¼ oz.; essence of rose 5 to 10 drops; and carmine, as much as required for producing the desired tint.

Formulation V

Procedure : Mix 32 parts of bergamot ol, 10 parts of lemon oil and 6 parts of musk infusion with 500 parts of magnesium carbonate. Then triturate 5000 parts of rice starch, 3500 parts of calcium sulphate, 1000 parts of talc and 200 parts of powdered orris. Finally pass through a fine sieve.

Formulation VI

Ingredients	Quantity
Rice Starch	600 grams
Maize Starch	200 grams
Talcum	100 grams
Zinc Stearate	50 grmas
Zinc Oxie	50 grams

Formulation VII

Ingredients	Quantity
Rice Starch	500 grams
Zinc Oxide	400 grams
French Chalk	100 grams
Magnesium Stearate	100 grams

Talcum Toilet Powder

Procedure : Talc, to be used as a toilet powder, should be in a state of very fine division. Antiseptics are sometimes added in small doses. As a perfume, rose oil may be employed, but, on account of its cost, rose geranium oil is probably more frequently used. A satisfactory proporation is 1/2 dr. of the oil to 1 lb. of the powder. In order that the perfume may be thoroughly disseminated throughout the powder, the oil should be triturated first with a small portion of it; this should then be further triturated with a larger portion, and if the quantity operated on be large, the final mixing may be effected by sifting. Many odours besides that of rose would, of course, be suitable for a toilet powder. Ylang-ylangwould doubtless prove very attractive, but its use is rather restricted on account of its high price.

Chapter - 10
HAIR WASHES & SHAMPOOS

Function of A Shampoo & hair Wash

A shampoo can be defined as " a preparation of a surfactant (i.e. surface-active material) in suitable form-liquid, solid or powder-which when used under the conditions specified will remove surface grease, dirt and skin debris from the hair shaft and scalp without affecting adversely the hair, scalp of health of the user". A good shampoo should " Cleanse hair and scalp thoroughly without staining or irritation and should not remove too much of the natural oil from the scalp."The success of shampoos in replacing a cake of soap, lies in the fact that the shampoo is not only a detergent but a cosmetic as well, and that it must impart luster, beauty and manageability. A success ful shampoo may be defined as a product having some cleansing and foaming action which leaves the hair soft, lustrous and manageable.

Shampoo Types and Forms

Shampoos are available in may types and forms which lend themselves in classification according to their physical appearance or insome instances according to their special ingredients or properties. These forms are liquid clear shampoos, liquid cream or cream lotion shampoos, cream paste shampoos, egg shampoos, herbal shampoos, dry shampoos, lizuid dry shampoos, colour shampoos and aerosol shampoos. In addition one of several of these types amy be based on special raw materials or have special additives, that would make a given product an antiseptic or antidandruff shampoo, or would render it particularly suitable for use infants and young children, and hence permit it to be called a baby shampoo.

Shampoos for All hair Types :

Lime Shampoo :

Ingredients	Quantity
Amla	1 kg
Shikakai	2 kg
Char	1 kg
Charilla	1 kg

Hair Washes & Shampoos

Khus	1 kg
Reetha	2 kg
Water	25 litres
Glycerine	4.00 gms
Lime Juice	200 kg
Sodium Benzoate	75 gms

Lavender Shampoor

Ingredients	Quantity
Amla	1 Kg
Shikakai	2 kg
Henna	1 kg
Khus	1 kg
Char	1 kg
Charilla	1 kg
Reetha	2 kg
Sodium Benzolate	75 Gms
Lavender Oil	400 ml
Water	25 litres

Procedure of making : Soak Amla, Shikakai, henna, Khus, Charilla & Reetha for one night for 12 hours. Boil till the mixture remains half. Strain and add lavender oil & sodium benzoate.

Methi Shikakai Shampoo

Ingrdients	Quantity
Methi	2.5 kgs
Shikakai	10 kgs
Orange peel	1 kg

Crush all the ingredients into powdery form to make dry shampoo.

Coconut Oil Shampoo

This is made by saponifying odourless oil with potash. Sometimes other fixed oil are added and these include palm, peanut, etc., but they have a tendency to decrease the foaming properties of the product and are only used in cheaper grade articles. Usually 1,000 parts of coconut oil require for complete saponification about 300 parts of potassium hydroxide. This is dissolved in 1 litre of water at about 75° C and added to the oil at the same temperature in a steam pan. Saponification can be tested by using phenolphthalein as indicator. If the liquid remains white, further additions of alkali are necessary whereas when it turns red more oil should be added. The heat is continued until saponification has taken place and the product is neutral. It is then dluted to 5 litres with ditilled water in which some carbonate of potash has been dissolved.

Formulation

Ingredients	Quantity
Coconut Oil	1000 parts
Potassium hydroxide	300 parts
Distilled Water	1000 parts
Potassium Carbonate	30 parts
Distilled Water	2970 parts

It is now perfumed with any of the stable synthetics, such as linalol, terpineol, methyl acetophenone, etc., or such oil as lavender and rosemary.

Hair rinses, hair wash & hair setting preparations

hair Rinses :

1. Chamomole hair rinse	Proportion
a) Chamomile flower powder	50%
b) Kaolin Powder	50%
2. Rosemary Chamomile hair rinse	
a) Rosemary Tops (powder)	50%
b) Chamomile flower (powder)	50%

Cantharides Hair Wash

Acetum Cantharides	15 parts
Alcohol	150 parts
Rosemary Oil	15 parts
Bergamot Oil	10 parts
Lavender Oil	5 parts
Rose Oil	5 parts

Glycerine   50 parts
Water   700 parts

Procedure : Dissolve the oils in the spirit and the rest in water. Mix the two solutions and volume with water. Filter bright, using talc or Kieselguhr.

Hair Setting preparations.

Ingredients	Quanity
Clove hair setting	Proportion
Almond oil	1 kg
Palm oil	100 ml
Benzoated lard	5 kg
Lemon Extract	100 ml
Oil of cloves	50 ml

Chapter - 11
HAIR OILS & HAIR LOTIONS

Hair oils are combination of oils and suitable perfumes. The base oils like Castor oil, coconut oil and seasamum oil are mostly used vegetable based oils. besides vegetable based oils another class of base oils which are used in Hair Oils are florol oils such as bela oil, chameli oil, Henna oil etc. which posses most delicate fragrances. Vegetable oils are refined before using it in the Hiar Oil formulations. the antural scents added to hair oil such as balsom peru, cantharidin and fly cantharides help to invigorate the growth of hairs and prevent baldness.

Herbal Hair Oil

Some of the important herbal hiar oils are based upon following :

1. Amla
2. Brahmi
3. Bhringraj
4. Bhangra
5. Kaddu Seeds
6. Soya Lecithin
7. Henna

Herbal Hair Oil Extract

Herbal well known for use in Hair oils are processed into thick pulp which is soluble in both vegetable and mineral oils. These are :

Common Name	Sanskrit Name	Botanical Name	Part used
Amla	Amarphalam	Emblica officienalis	Dried Fruit
Amalakam		Phyllanthus emblica	
Brahmi	Mandukaparni	Centella asiatica	herb

(Cont'd)

Hair Oils & Hair Lotions

Bhringraj	Bringraja	Ecliptica alba/eracta	Herb
Bhangra	Kesaraja	Wadellie calandulacea	Herb
Kaddu seeds	Alabu	Legenarie sinceraria	seeds

Efficacy of Herbal Hair Oils

Hair oil containing any one or combination of herbs mentioned above have been used in India since time immemorial and are highly spoken of in folklore and books on indigenous drugs.

Amla - Fruits are rich in tannins; Fixed oil in berries strengthen and promotes growth of hair.

Brahmi - Local stimulant useful for skin erruption, Eczema. The extract is a remedy in ulcers, eczema and Psoriasis.

Bhringraj - Antispetic; excellent for head; renders hair black and promotes luxurious growth; paste of herb in oil is useful for skin diseases, itch, headache and also for dying hair black.

Bhangra - Contains oil soluble dye use fule in alopecia and skin diseases.

Kaddu seeds - Have Fatty oil which is applied in headache, oil of seed is cooling and emolient.

Henna leaves - Have colouring matter, for external application in headache; astringent; detergent and deodorant, applied to hair to promote growth.

Typical Formulation & Procedures for Hair Oil

A few typical recipes for making scented hair oils follow :

Formulation I

Ingredients	Quantity
Refined Cocoanut of Sesamum Oil	5 seers
Balsam Peru	2.50 oz.
Fly Cantharides	5 dr.
Sandal Oil	15 dr.
Alkanet Root	15 dr.
Otto of Henna	5 dr.
Oil Rosemary	10 dr.

Procedure : Firts of all the oil is treated with alkanet root and allowed to remain undisturbed for 2 days for colouring. Then strain the oil through cloth. The fly cantharides are next fried in about one chhatak of fresh coconut or sesamum oil and when these are well fried and discoloured, these are allowed to cool. Afterwards add the previously coloured oil, and the Balsam Peru (after melting it over a slow fire) Finally add the other ingredients one by one with constant shaking.

Formulation II

Ingredients	Quantity
Refined Seasamum Oil	24 oz.
Alkanet Root	2 dr.
Oil Bergamot	6 dr.
Oil Lemon	3 dr.
Oil Rosemary	2 dr.
Oil Neroli	1 dr.
Oil Lavender (English)	2 dr.
Oil Orange	1 dr.
Oil Rose Geranium	2 dr.
Cantharidin	3 grains
Balsam Peru	2 dr.

Procedure : The best quality of refined sesamum oil is taken and into it is added 2 dr. of alkanet root previously cut into small pieces. The whole is then allowed to stand undisturbed for 2 days and then filtered through a piece of fine cloth. Next add the other ingredients one after another in the order they appear in the recipe and shake the whole for 15 minutes after each such addition. Balsam Peru, the last ingredient, is to be melted over a slow fire before incorporation. When the ingredients are all incorporated, the whole is kept aside air-tight in a vessel for a fortnight and then packed.

Formulation III

Ingredients	Quantity
Chameli Oil	2 litre
Almond Oil	1 litre
Alkanet Root	1 oz.
Cantharidin	12 grains
balsam Peru	5 oz.

Hair Oils & Hair Lotions

Sandal Oil	3 oz.
Flora Jasmine	12 dr.
English Lavender	2 oz.

Procedure : Mix the Chameli and almond oil together and drop into this the alkanet root in small pieces and let the oil remain undisturbed for 2 days. Then strain through a piece of cloth and add the ingredients one after another with constant shaking. While adding the balsam peru take care that it is melted over a slow fire before addition. When all the ingredients are well incorporated, pack in a vessel with the mouth well-covered and put in the strong sunlight for 20 days together. Finally strain and pack into phials.

Formulation IV

Ingredients	Quantity
Sesamum Oil	6 litre
Alkanet Root	2 oz.
Otto Keora	1 oz.
Oil Lavender	2 oz.
Oil Rosemary	1 oz.

Procedure : The sesamum oil is first of all treated with animal charcoal and put in the sun for a fortnight. This is then filtered through a filter paper or through flannel. To the oil thus refined add the alkanet root in small bits and strain after two days. Then incorporate the other ingredients one after another with constant stirring and let the wholestand for 7 days in a vessel tightly corked. Finally strain again and pack into phials.

This oil keeps the brain cool and stimulates the growth of hair.

Formulation V

Ingredients	Quantity
Coconut Oil	12 ch.
White Oil	4 ch.
Oil Lavender	3 dr.
Oil Sandal	3 dr.
Oil Bergamot	3 dr.
Alkanet Root	1.5 dr.

Procedure : First refine the coconut oil and add the alkanet roots. The whole is left for colouring for 2 days. Now filter and add the essential oils one by one and shake well before the addition of the next one. The whole is left well corked for 7 days for ripending, then phial.

Formulation VI

Ingredients	Quantity
Til, Coconut or Castor oil	500 parts
Balsam Peru	15 parts
Oil of Jasmine	60 parts
Oil of Roses	30 parts
Oil of Bitter Almonds	30 parts
Oil of Vanilla	60 parts
Oil of Ambergris	30 parts
Oil of Musk	30 parts

Procedure : The balsam Peru is first of all digested for 14 days in the oil, shaking the vessel frequently. When the mixture is clear, add the essential oils one by one. The oil keeps for a long time and resembles verymuch the heliotrope oil in odour.

Formulation VII

Ingredients	Quantity
Benzoated Oil	20 oz.
Otto of Rose	25 minims
Heliotropin	20 dr.

Procedure : the benzoated oil is made by digesting an ounce of bruised benzoin, prefereably of Siam, in a pint of almond or olive oil for three hours, and filtering through filter paper. Finally add the scent, shake and phial. The oil does not become rancid.

In the prepartion of these scented hair oils, precautions are to be taken that procedures are to be followed strictly so that desired quality is achieved. The addition of scents and colouring of hair oil are two important steps.

Addition of scents

The addition of the perfumes also must be methodical. They should be added one after another in the order they are put in the recipes. The order should not be changed by any means. Moreover a few minutes time should be allowed to the fixation of one scent before the next one is incorporated and if possible the whole mass should be agitated carefully so that the scent may be intimately incorporated, absorbed by the oil itself and sweetly tempered. After the whole preparation is finished, the mass is recommended to be set aside for a certain period of time before final bottling. This is a most

Hair Oils & Hair Lotions

important matter that should not be overlooked by the manufacturers. It is found that on keeping the preparation substantially improves in quality, and hence whenever excellent quality is desired to be attained, the preparation should be allowed to stand for a number of days before final packing.

Colouring Hair Oils

The coloration of the hair oils is not a difficult affair. For red, the alkanet root is mostly in vogue. This is cheap and being of vegetable origin is perfectly non-neurosis. For yellow shade saffron may be added but this is rarely done as this is rather costly. Now-a-days all tints in hair oils except red are produced by the incorporation of aniline dyes. But from hygienic point of view these are not non-injurious to health and their use should be as much restricted as permissible.

Packaging

Finally for poackaging the hari oil, decent phials should be used. These should be nicely corked and capsuled and balelled and put in decent paper cartons.

Herbal Hair Dyes

Hena dyes give dark hair a reddish colour. But the exact colour result is very difficult to predict so a test dye is very essential. Henna dye can be made following the undermentioned method.

Henna powder	2 cups
Hot water	2 cup
vinegar	1 tsp

Stir them all to a thick paste and let this stand for 1 hour. Pourt it into a bowl and put this bowl in a saucepan filled with water. Keep the paste stirring till the water in the bottom of the saucepan bubbles freely. Let the mixture stand for another hour, then apply the mixture into each strand of the hair by parting hair with a comb. Start applying henna from one side of the head and working to the other end. Leave the henna on your head for 3-6 hours.

Some of the formulations for Heena and other herbal hair dyes are described as under :-

Henna Hair Dye

Henna	200 gm
Coffee powder	1 tsp
Egg yolk	1 egg
Rum/Brandy	1 tbsp

Procedure : Mix coffee powder in the water and make a paste of henna with this water. Beat the egg yok and mix this into henna. Also add brandy to it. Apply the paste and leave it on for 3-4 hours before washing it with lukewarm water.

Saffron Hair Dye

Saffron	1 pinch
Boiling water	500 ml

Soak saffron in water for 10 minutes. Strain and use it on the hair. Grey hair will acquire a rich golden tint.

Walnut Hair Dye

Walnut husk	500 gm
Water	500 ml

Boil husk in the water for 15 minutes. Then strain and use this liquid to dye your hair. It will colour brown hair to a darker shade.

Chapter - 12

AROMATIC & TOILET WATERS WITH COSMETICS FOR MAKEUP

Natural aromatic & toilet waters are based upon Rose, Keora, Lavender, Sandal, Bergamot etc. Rose water or Keora Water is prepared by butting cleaned flower petals in an earthen pot and pouring boiling water on the petals, closing the vessel and straining after one hour.

The formulation and procedure for making commerce rose water is as under :-

Commercial Rose Water

Ingredients	Quality
Rose Oil	2.5 grams
Clove Oil	0.25 gram
Alcohol to make	100 c.c.
Distilled Water	10,000 c.c.

Procedure : Mix the first two ingredients and add alcohol to make 100 c.c. Now mix the spirituous liquid with 10,000 c.c. of boiling distilled water and allow to stand unitl it has undergone the viscous fermentation and blend producing a stuff superior to most of the commercial rose water.

The above recipe obviates the necessity of distilling rose petals and yields rose water of satisfactory quality on simply mixing the ingredients mentioned in the receipe.

Toilet Water

Some of the formulations and procedures for making toilet waters are as under:-

Lavender Water

Ingredients	Quantity
Oil Lavender (Burgoyne)	3 dr.
Oil Bergamot	3 dr.

Otto de Rose	5 minims.
Oil cloves	6 minims.
Musk	2 gr.
Oil of Rosemary (true)	1 dr.
Honey	1 oz.
Benzoic Acid	2 scruples
Rectified Spirit	1 pint.
Distilled Water	3 oz.

Procedure : mix together and allow to mature for 6 months.

Violet Water

Ingredients	Quantity
Oil of Sandal	4 dr.
Oil of Bergamot	4 dr.
Oil of Rose Geranium	1 dr.
Oil of Neroli	1 dr.
Oil of Bitter Almonds	15 drops
Musk	1 gr.
Tincture of Benzoin	4 dr.
Powdered Orris Root	2 dr.
Water	60 oz.
Alcohol	100 oz.

Procedure : Macerate 30 days and filter. The product is coloured with just a trace of green dye.

Eau De Cologne

Ingredients	Quantity
Oil Bergamot	1 oz.
Oil Lemon	0.5 oz.
Oil Rosemary	2 dr.
Oil Neroli	30 minims.
Oil Lavender	4 dr.
Oil Orange	2 dr.
Rectified Spirit	2 lbs.

Aromatic Toilet Waters with Cosmetics for Makeup

Procedure : The ingredients are mixed with brisk shaking one by one. Set the whole aside in a stoppered vessel for a fortnigh and during that period shake the vessel thrice daily at a time. Fianally filter and pack.

Cosmetics for Make-up

Some of the cosmetics for make-up which can be made using herbal ingredient are as under :-

Finger-tip colouring

Alkanet	0.5 oz.
Rectified Spirit	12 oz.
Rose Water	4 oz.

Procedure : macerate for a week, add 10 drops of otto of rose, shake and filter.

Bindi Stick

Wax	1.1125 dr.
Almond oil	3 dr.
Carmine	6 gr.
Otto of rose	6 drops

Procedure : melt the wax over a water bath, then incorporate the almond oil. Now dissolve the carmine in just enough solution of ammonia, put in a warm mortar, and add the bases. next remove from the water bath and add the otto. Lastly pour the mass in tin moulds.

Taral Alta

Taral Alta is the Bengali name for a kind of fluid rouge, like lip-salve, for imparting a rosy hue to the skin. It is a universal custom in bengal and elsewhere amongst Hindu women to paint their feet, palms of hands, finger tips, etc., periodically with indigenous lac dye. This decoration adds to the grace of feminine beauty. And for this purpose the service of the female barber has got to be requisitioned. But with the help of ready-made Taral Alta a lady can paint herself by simply applying the liquid dye with a swab.

Taral Alta is, therefore, now in great vogue. It commands a wide sale specially during marriage season and in times of festivities. Its manufacture will, therfore, be found remunerative.

Method of preparation comprises of soaking freshly blown scented flowers in distilled water in a covered vessel for 24 hours by which time it will absorb their fragrance. The perfumed water is strained through a flannel sheet, and a solution of scarlet dye in this water yields Taral Alta as before.

the fragrances of Rose, Lily, henna, Khus, violet, Bela, jasmine, Champaka or Bakul can be used, a typical formulation using Rose otto is as under :-

Formulation for rose based alta

Rose Otto	30 Minims.
Magnesium Carbonate	1 oz.
Distilled Water	12 quarts
Perfumed Water	1 quart
Scarlet Dye	2 oz.

Procedure : Macerate the essential oil with magnesium carbonate in a stone mortar with a stone pestle. Stir in the distilled water and filter. To the perfumed water thus prepared add the scarlet dye when good scented Alta will be obtained.

Packaging of Taral Alta

The final products should be bottled in decent phials and corked and capsuled. A sponge swab with a wire holder should be inserted in every packet. The label should be printed in attractive design. Instructions should be given first to wash the skin and then to apply uniformly with the swab and finally to allow to dry up.

Chapter - 13

HERBAL COSMETICS

HEALING WITH HERBS

Beauty and health are, two sides of the same coin. If nature has the qualities of a cosmetologist, its therapeutic treasure is equally vast and abundant. Unfortunately, till recently, ayurveda was never considered a mainstream method of healing. The reason, of course, is that the emphasis has been more on symptomatic healing than curing the disease from its roots.

A time when herbal cosmetics are taking over the cosmetic market, it seems that herbal medicines still have to make a noticeable impact. And that can happen only if you are prepared to see the same doctor again when he prescribes Dashmolarishta intead of Vitamin C for you.

HERBAL OR PLANT MATERIALS

Some of the herbal ingredients which are being commonly used in cosmetics are given below.

Almond

Fixed oil obtained form almonds is emollient in nature. It has extensive applications in cosmetics. A white milk used in cleansers and astringents is obtained by soaking ground almonds in milk or water and then by milling. Ground almonds are used in facial and body scrubs.

Apricot

Apricots contain highly nourishing oil and rich in vitamin A. It is believed to improve condition and elasticity of skin. The pulp of both fresh and dry fruit is used in face masks. Finely ground shell and kernel of the stone is used in facial and body scrubs.

Avocado

Oil of Avocado is rich in vitamin A. Its uses are similar to apricot oil.

Azadirachta (Neem)

Neem leaves are antiseptic. Neem fruits yield an oil called neem oil. Nimbidin is the chief bitter principle of Neem oil. Neem oil is used in soaps. Extract of leaves can be used in toothpastes and skin care products.

Cabbage

Cabbage is chiefly valuable for its high mineral and vitamin contents. It has wonderful cleansing and reducing properties. Its juice can used in skin care products.

Camomile

Camomile flower contains a dye hence used with henna in herbal hair dye. Infusion of flowers can also be used for astringency in cleansers, conditioners and hair rinses.

Carrots

Carrots are rich source of vitamin A. These are good for irritated or sunburnt skin. The raw grated vegetables and juice make excellent cleanser. Carrot juice can be used in masks and tonics.

Comfrey

Decoction of root and infusion of comfrey leaves have antiseptic and healing properties. These can be used in creams and lotions.

Common Basil (Tulsi)

Flowers and leaves of tulsi yield an essential oil which is considered antiseptic. Juice of its leaves can be used in skin creams and lotions.

Cornflower

Infusion of flowers can be used in skin tonics and freshners.

Cucumber

Cucumber juice is used in cosmetics. Cucumber juice is soothing healing and slightly astringent. It can be used in masks, cleansers and toners.

Dandelion

Infusion of dandelion flowers can be used in masks, cleansers. Sap from the stem can be used in bleaching creams.

E. Alba (Bhringaraja)

It is a source of black stain and is used in hair preparations.

Elderflower

Infusion of flowers are mildly bleaching and therefore can be used in skin cleansers, conditioners and creams. Decoction of leaves of elderflower is healing and can be used for sun-burnt or wind-burnt skin.

Eucalyptus

Decoction of leaves of eucalyptus is antiseptic and invigorating. Decoction can be used in skin care products.

Fennel

Infusion of chopped leaves is soothing and stimulating. Infusion can be used in masks, cleansers and toners.

Funegreek

Funegreek (Methi) is a traditional, component of hair care products. It is used for its Cleansing and softening activity. It promoters scape health. It can be used in hair care, skin care products.

Garlic

Garlic juice is considered antiseptic. Its juice can be used in antiseptic and smoothing creams.

Geranium

Geranium yields an essential oil which is used in perfumery. Geranium leaves and flowers can be used for healing or rejuvenating. Alternatively, geranium oil can be added in healing and cleansing creams.

Henna

Henna leaves contain a dye. Henna leaves are used in herbal hair dyes. Henna can be used with camomile flowers for dyeing the hair. Leaves and flowers yield an essential oil.

Indian Gooseberry (Amla)

Fruits, bark and leaves of India Gooseberry are rich in tannins. Fruits are used in herbal hair dyes, particularly with henna. Dried fruits are also used for washing the hair.

Indian Nard (Jatamansi)

Indian nard yields an oil, called spikenard oil. Oil is considered to improve hair growth and is also believed to darken hair. Spikenard oil can be used in hair preparations.

Jasmine

Flowers of jasmine yield an essential oil, called jasmine oil. Jasmine oil is used in traditional hair oils.

Lady's Mantle

Juice of leaves of lady's mantle has healing and mild bleaching properties. Its juice can be added to tonics for oily skin or to the creams for dry skin.

Lavender

Flowers and leaves of lavender yield an essential oil called lavender oil. Infusion of leaves and flower is considered antiseptic. Infusion can be used in skin creams and toners.

Lemon

Peel of lemon yields an essential oil which is used in perfumery and soaps. Infusion of leaves of lemon has soothing and mild astringent properties which can be used in skin tonics and cleansers.

Lime

Infusion of flowers and young leaves can be used in healing and moisturising creams and lotions.

Marigold

sInfusion and decoction of flowers and leaves can be used in skin creams and lotions. These can also be used for hair lightening rinses.

Marsh Mallow

Infusion of flower of marsh mallow and decoction of its roots have antiseptic properties. These can be used in skin creams and cleansers.

Nutmeg

Nutmeg butter or fat obtained from nutmegs is used as external stimulant in hair lotions. Nutmeg oil is also used in spicy perfumes in soaps.

Orange Blossom

Its essential oil is soothing and can be used in creams to soothe dry skin.

Parsley

Crushed leaves or juice of parsley can be used in poultices. Juice or infusion of leaves can be used in skin creams, lotions or cleansers. Also has antidandruff and deodorising properties. It can therefore be used in hair preparations also.

Peach

The pulp of fresh peach is used in face masks, cleansers and moisturisers. Peach nut oil is fragrant and rich and is used in nourishing cream.

Rose

Rose petals yield an essential oil, called rose oil. Infusion of petals can be used in skin toners, cleansers moisturisers and colognes.

Rosemary

Flowers and leaves of rosemary have antiseptic and anti-dandruff properties. Infusions of flowers and leaves can be used in skin cream and lotions. Herbal oil made from leaves can be used for the hair.

Safflower

Flower heads are a source of red and yellow dye called safflower. This dye is used in rouges.

Sage

Infusion of flowers and leaves of sage is healing and mild stringent. The intrusion can be used in skin tonics and cleansers.

Sandal

Sandalwood oil is extracted from heart-wood of sandal tree. Sandalwood oil is used in perfumes.

S. Racemosa (Lodhra)

Decoction of lodhra is used to prevent bleeding of gums.

Thyme

Leaves of thyme make astringent infusion. Leaves also make strongly perfumed herbal hair oil. Thyme also has deodorising anti-dandruff properties.

Turmeric

Turmeric has been long used in poultices and scrubs in India. Its water extract has antiseptic properties. It can be used in skin creams.

Wheatgerm

It is rich in vitamins and minerals. It is extremely beneficial in face masks and body scrubs. Wheatgerm oil is rich in vitamin E which is considered good for skin.

Witch Hazel

Steam distillate of bark is astringent and antiseptic and can be used in skin creams, lotions and toners.

HOW TO USE HERBS

In earlier times, herbs were used for both medicinal purposes as well as for beautification. They have been used in fresh form and dried form. These can be used by mashing and directly applying to the body with or without using other ingredients. In fact, in earlier times these were used this way. But now-a-days, their extracts, decoctions, infusions, tinctures, steam distillates etc., are used rather than herbs themselves. Whenever these are prepared, preservatives should be added to them as these are perishable.

Infusions

Infusions are basically strong teas of herb(s) and can be prepared either in china clay pots or stainless steel vessels. Aluminium vessels should not be used as these can taint the infusions. The process of preparation is as follows :

Pour freshly boiled water in the vessel containing herb (coarse powder). Cover and leave for at least three hours. Strain and filter. The quantity of herb and solvent (water) may vary depending on whether herb is fresh or dried. Usually, for 100 gm of fresh herb or 50 gm of dried herb 575 ml of water can be used.

Decoctions

Decoctions are prepared by boiling the herb with water. The following is the process :

Place the herb (coarse powder) in stainless steel or enamel pan, add sufficient water and cover the pan. Gently boil and continue boiling on gentle heat till the water is reduced to one quarter. This may require boiling for about 2-3 hours. Strain and filter. The same proportions of herb and water can be used as recommended in case of infusions.

Extracts and Tinctures

Extracts are generally prepared with hydro-alcoholic solvents and tinctures are prepared with either alcohol or hydro-alcoholic solvent with high percentage of alcohol. The following method can be used for preparing extracts and tinctures :

Herbal Cosmetics

Place in a macerator crushed herbs or flowers. Add alcohol or alcohol-water mixture to cover the herb. Close the macerator tightly with lid and leave overnight. Add more solvent and further macerate for 2-3 days. Sometimes maceration may be as long as a week. Strain the mixture firmly with a strainer and filter the extract/tincture. Depending upon the constituents this extract/tincture could be used or it could be used as solvent for maceration of fresh herb. The recommended proportions are 100 gm of fresh herb or flowers and 575 ml. Extracts/tinctures should be stored in tightly closed containers.

Flower Waters

Flower waters are made in the same way as infusions. The same proportions of herbs and water can be used. However, the difference in infusion and flower waters is that solvent is allowed to remain in contact with flowers overnight in case of flower waters. Flower waters can also be prepared by using flower essence (essential oil) and purified water.

Oil Soluble Extracts

Oil soluble extracts are prepared by extracting herbs with petroleum ether. The herb (coarse powder) is left in contact with water overnight. More water is added next day. This herb-water mixture is placed with oil in a vessel and the vessel is heated till all the water has been removed. The oil is allowed to cool and is then filtered. In this way oil soluble principle of herb go into oil.

Some herbal extracts are available commercially. Balsara Herbal Products (Pvt.) Ltd. are making herbal extracts under the trade name Folicon. Some of the extracts are oil extracts and some are aqueous-glycol extracts. A list of these extract and the products in which these can be used is given below in table 41.1.

Table 41.1.

Folicon Herbal Extracts (Cosmetic grade)

Application	Type	Code	
AMLA	Aqueoust extract	C 3101	Hair Care
AMLA	Oil extract	C 3101	Hair Care
ALOE	Aqueoust extract	C 3102	Skin & Hair Care
BHRINGRAJ/MAKA	Aqueoust extract	C 3103	Hair Care
BHRINGRAJ/MAKA	Oil Extract	C 3103	Hair Care
BRAHMI	Aqueoust extract	C 3104	Hair Care

(Cont'd)

BRAHMI	Oil extract	C 3104	Hair Care
HENNA/MEHENDI	Aqueoust extract	C 3105	Hair Care
HALDI/TURMERIC	Aqueoust extract	C 3106	Hair Care
HIBISCUS	Aqueoust extract	C 3107	Skin & Hair Care
KHUS	Aqueoust extract	C 3108	Skin & Hair Care
LEMON PEEL	Aqueoust extract	C 3109	Skin & Hair Care
METHI/FENUGREEK	Aqueoust extract	C 3110	Skin & Hair Care
NEEM	Aqueoust extract	C 3111	Skin & Hair Care
ROSE PETAL	Aqueoust extract	C 3112	Skin & Hair Care
SHIKAKAI	Aqueoust extract	C 3113	Hair Care
SANDALWOOD	Aqueoust extract	C 3114	Hair Care
TULSI	Aqueoust extract	C 3115	Hair Care

Recommended concentration in different preparations are shown in table 41.2

Table 41.2.
Folicon herbalextracts cosmetic products guidelines (use levels).

FOLICON Hair oil Herbal Extracts	Anti Perspi--rants	Cleansers, Freshners, and masks		Lotions, Creams	Hair Conditioners	Medicated sun-cream	shampoo Creams
%	%	%	%	%	%	%	%
Amla	-	5-10	5-10	5-10	-	1.5	-
5-10							
Aloe	5-10	5-10	5-10	5-10	10-15	1-5	-
Bhringraj/Maka	-	-	-	-	-	-	-
5-10							
Brahmi 5-10	-	-	-	-	10-15	1-5	-
Henna/Mehendi	-	-	-	5-10	-	1-5	-
Haldi/Turmeric	-	5-10	-	-	5-10	-	-
Hibiscus	-	-	-	-	-	1-5	-
Khus	5-10	1-5	-	-	-	-	1-5
Lemon peel	1-5	-	1-5	-	1-5	-	-
Methi/Fenugreek	-	-	-	1-5	-	1-5	-
Neem	5-10	-	-	-	5-10	-	-
Rose petal	-	1-5	-	-	-	-	-

(Cont'd)

Shikakai	-	-	-	5-10	-	-	-
Sandalwood	5	-	1-5	-	-	-	10
Tulsi	1-5	-	-	-	5-10	-	5

HERBAL COSMETICS FOR THE SKIN

Creams and emulsions are all basically mixtures of water, oils, waxes and fragrances perfumery products in varying proportions. A slight change in the quantities in the preparations changes the character of the preparation and one should be careful when measuring the ingredients. When measuring the following rough equivalents should be kept in mind while formulating the product.

- 1 Teaspoon + 60 drops = 5 ml.
- 3 Teaspoon = 1 Tablespoon = 15 ml.
- 2 Tablespoons = 1/8 cup = 10 ml.
- 4 Tablespoons = 1/4 cup = 20 ml.
- 8 Tablespoons = 1/2 cup = 40 ml.
- 16 Tablespoons = 1 cup = 80 ml.
- 15 4 grains = gm.
- 28 3 gms = 1 oz.
- 16 oz = 1 lb. = 454 gms.
- 1 kg. = 2.202 lbs.

Equipment Used for Herbal Preparations

(i) Enamel or pyrex bowls; (ii) One large frying pan; (iii) Measuring spoons; (iv) Measuring cups; (v) Electric heater or manual heater; (vi) A good strong sieve; (vii) A pipette or eye dropper; (viii) A wool of tissue paper for wiping jars, spoons, hands etc; (ix) Jars and Bottles and (x) Printed/plain labels.

Cleansing Creams

Cleansing creams are used to lift the dust. Also to remove stale make up. Soap can not remove waxy base of make-up thus, cleansing cream is used. The cleanser is generally applied with an upward movement and kept on the skin for about half a minute os as to dissolve the make up. Then it is removed with a tissue or damp cotton wool. The dirt and grime not only dogs the pores of the skin causing block heads but also coarsens the skin. A few formulations of cleansing creams are given below :

Formulation

Beeswax	1/2 Tablespoon
Emulsifying Wax (Petroleum)	1 Tablespoon
Baby oil	4 Tablespoons
Coconut oil	2 Tablespoons
Water	2 Tablespoons
Borax	1/4 Teaspoon
Witch Hazel	1 Tablespoon
Perfume	3-5 drops

Note : Witch hazel is made from twigs of hamamelis or alderbush.

Process of Manufacture

Melt the mixture of waxes and oil by transfering from enamel bowl to pan of boiling water. Prepare solution of borax in water in another bowl, add witch-hazel and heat it to dissolve. Mix solutions of both bowl in water with stirring cool to form, add perfume. It begins to thicken as it cools and beatens.

Rose Water Cleansing Cream

Formulation

Beeswax or white Paraffin Wax	1 1/2 Tablespoons
Emulsifying Wax (Petrolatum)	1 Tablespoon
Mineral oil	4 Tablespoons
Rose water	6 Tablespoons
Borax	1/2 Teaspoon
Perfume	3-5 drops

Cucumber Cleansing Cream

Formulation

Beeswax	3 Teaspoon
Coconut Oil	4 Teaspoons
Mineral oil or Olive oil	4 Teaspoons
Cucumber Juice	4 Tablespoons
Glycerine	1 Teaspoon
Borax	1 Pinch
Green Colouring	1 Drop

Violet Cleansing Cream

Formulation

Lanolin	1/2 Tablespoon
Petroleum Jelly	1 Tablespoon
Mineral oil	4 Tablespoons
Water	10 Tablespoons
Violet extract	5 drops

Masks

Masks have been used for beauty treatment of the face. They are applied and kept on the face, left on the same for ten to twenty minutes and then washed off. They have nourishing, healing, cleansing and an astringent effect. These masks whip up the circulation and temporarily iron out wrinkles. They freshen the skin and leave it glowing. A few formulations of simple home made face masks are given as under :

Milk Mask

This is one of the cheapest and simplest masks. Cotton wool is soaked in milk and rubbed on the face and left to dry for 10-15 minutes and then the face is washed.

Cleansing Mask

Formulation

Powdered Brewers yeast	1 Table spoon
Yogurt	1/2 Table spoon
Lemon Juice	1 Tea spoon
Orange Juice	1 Tea spoon
Carrot Juice	1 Tea spoon
Olive Oil	1 Tea spoon

Procedure

Make a paste by mixing above ingredients, then apply and keep on face for 15 mins. If the skin is very dry more oil is added and discarded if the skin is oily. The brewer's yeast stimulates the flow of blood to the skin and gives the complexion a healthy glow. The yogurt cleanses the skin and the fruit juices provide vitamins and minerals.

Butter Milk Mask

A cup of butter milk is heated and three tablespoons of elderflower blossoms are put into it. The mixture is simmered on a very low heat for about 30 mins. And then allowed to cool. It helps in bleaching and cleansing large pores.

Meal Mask

A paste of barley meal, pea flower and rose water is applied and left on the skin for several hours to make the skin soft and supple. One tablespoon each of finely ground oatmeal and milk along with a few drops of almond oil are allowed to form paste. The paste is applied and left on the skin for 15 mins. And then rinsed off.

Carrot and Turnip Mask

A paste is prepared by boiling carrot and turnip. It is applied for 10-15 minutes and then rinsed off with milk. This make leaves the skin feeling fresh and clean.

Oatmeal Mask

Formulation of Oatmeal mask is given below :

Dried orange peel	2 Tablespoons
Oatmeal	2 Teaspoons
Cold cream	2 Tablespoons

The above ingredients are mixed into a paste and then applied generously all over the face and neck. After 10 to 15 minutes when it is dry the same is rubbed off using an upward circular motion. This leaves the skin smooth and shining.

Potato Mask

Formulation of potato mask is given below :

| Potato juice | 1 Tablespoon |
| Fuller's earth | 1 Tablespoon |

The above ingredients are mixed to form a paste and applied on the face. Potatoes contain Vit-C and clear the skin of blemishes. Fuller's earth absorbs all the dirt and grease from the skin.

Paw Paw Mask

This is also known as Papaya Mask. Two tablespoons of ripe papaya flesh can be used as mask. Face is washed with water after applying mask.

Luxurious Cleansing Mask

Three strawberries are mashed into a paste and applied as a mask and then left on for 10 minutes and then washed off with rose water. Strawberries have slightly acidic properties and contain vitamin C, which cleanses the skin leaving it sparkingly clean. Another luxurious formulation consists of mashing and sieving the flesh of half a peach and then mixing it with a tablespoon of brandy.

Bath Salts

Two cups of ordinary washing soda are taken and two tablespoons of potassium carbonate is added to the same. A drop of an aromatic essential oil such as lavender or pine are added to the mixture and the mixture homogenised.

Bath Oils

Bath oil can be prepared by adding any vegetable oil such as almond, olive or sunflower to the bath water. Baby oil or mineral oil is not suitable as it cannot be absorbed by the skin and only remains on the skin surface. These basic oils can also be mixed with some of the herb oils or aromatic oil.

Bath Oil

Formulation

Eggs	2 Nos.
Almond Oil	1/4 Cup
Sunflower oil or Corn oil	1/4 Cup
Safflower oil or Olive oil	1/2 Cup
Honey	1 Teaspoon
Washing Detergent	2 Teaspoons
Vodka	1/4 Cup
Milk	1/4 Cups
Perfume	3-5 drops.

Procedure

The thick emulsified mixture is prepared by adding eggs, honey, oil and detergent. Continue beating with addition of Vodka slowly, also add milk and perfume.

Massage Preparations

This is a special recipe for brides to be used daily at the time of bath for ten days before marriage. The following ingredients are mixed to a paste and rubbed vigorously. They cleanse and stimulate the skin leaving it soft, supple and shiny.

Formulation

Dried, ground and sieved orange peel	1 Tablespoon
Dried, ground and sieved lemon peel	1 Tablespoon
Ground Almond	2 Tablespoons
Salt	1 pinch
Ground Thyme	1 Tablespoon
Ground all spice	1 pinch
Almond Oil	Sufficient to make a paste
Jasmine Oil (Perfume)	3-5 drops

Massage Paste

This consists of wheat flour or oatmeal mixed into a paste with double cream. The paste has a deep cleansing effect on the skin and removes dead cells and dirt.

Massage Oil

The oils are heated and then the heated water is slowly added along with a tablespoon of winter green or camphor oil to make a really invigorating massage cream.

Formulations

Almond Oil	1/2 Cup
Castor Oil	1/2 Cup
Camphor Oil	1 Teaspoon

Body Lotions

Mix three tablespoons of rose water, one tablespoon of glycerine and two tablespoons lime juice. This mixture is used after the bath if you suffer from dry skin. The proportion of this lotions is to suit this type of skin. The lotion no longer feels sticky and mixed into the skin easily. It has to be stored in a refrigerator.

Blue Ratin Body Lotion

Formulation

Soap flakes	3 Tablespoons
Glycerine	1 Teaspoon
Witch Hazel	1 Teaspoon
Olive Oil	4 Teaspoons
Water	5 Teaspoons
Blue Colouring	3-5 drops
Perfume	3-5 drops

Procedure

First soap flakes are dissolved in water with heating in a saucepan. Add glycerine, olive oil and witch hazel. Continue stirring until it cools, add blue colour and perfume. A lovely thin creamy blue mixture thus made is an ideal non-greasy, after-bath lotion which leaves the skin glowing like satin.

Lavender Body Lotion

Dissolve 1 teaspoon of borax in 1 cup of rose water and then add 2 tablespoons warmed olive oil with continuous beating. When all the oil has been added to the water and an emulsion has been formed the lavender water is added. The lavender water is made by infusing a handful of lavender flowers in 2 cups of boiling water. The above mixture is allowed to stand for an hour and then strained for use.

Almond body Lotion

The formulation of almond body lotion is given below :

Formulation

Lanolin	3 Teaspoons
Almond Oil	1 Teaspoon
Petroleum Jelly	1 Teaspoon
Vegetable Lard	1 Teaspoon
Glycerine	2 Teaspoons
Water	10 Tablespoons
Soap Flakes	1 Teaspoon
Cornflower	1 Teaspoon
Perfume or Almond Essence	q.s.

Moisturising Creams

Almond Oil Moisturising Cream

Melt two and one teaspoon of beeswax and emulsifying wax heating with water in a bowl and add five teaspoon almond oil. Now add hot water in melted mixture with stirring. Stop heating after sometime, cool and add lavender oil.

Herb Cream (Comfrey Cream)

A lanolin, white emulsifying wax and beeswax (1, 2 and 6 tablespoon) is melted. Add herb lotion or almond oil or infusion (6 tablespoon). This mixture is comfrey cream. Comfrey is a healing herb which is ideal for the sensitive skin or for skin having irritations or spots. A handful of comfrey is taken, liquidised and then strained. The comfrey residue need not be thrown away. A teaspoon honey may be added to tablespoon of this residue to form a paste and this can be used as a face mask.

Avocado Almond Cream

The formulation of avocado almond cream is given below :

Beeswax	3 Teaspoons
Emulsifying Wax (Petroleum Wax)	3 Teaspoons
Almond Oil	1/2 Cup
Avocado Oil	1/4 Cup
Rose Water	3 Tablespoons

Sun flower Cream

The process to prepare sunflower cream is as follows. The waxes, oil and lanolin are heated over a water bath till they melt. The water, glycerine and borax are heated separately till the borax gets completely dissolved. While the melted oils and waxes are still on the heat, the water is added drop-by-drop with continuous beating with a wooden spoon till a whitish thick and creamy textured rich cream is formed. This is a good moisturising cream leaving the skin looking soft and moist.

Jasmine Moisturising Cream

The composition of jasmine moisturising cream is given below :

Emulsifying Wax (Petroleum)	2 Tablespoons
Almond or Sunflower Oil	2 Tablespoons
Lanolin	1 Teaspoon

(Cont'd)

Borax	1/2 Teaspoon
Witch Hazel	1 Teaspoon
Glycerine	1 1/2 Teaspoons
Water	8 Tablespoons
Jasmine Oil	3-5 drops

Nourishing Creams

Preparations of this type include all skin nutrients whether they are oil based or of the moisturising type. They may be light and immediately absorbed or heavy and sticky requiring to be managed into the skin. The nourishing creams comprise of Hormone creams and lotions, vitamin products, screen ampoules, antiwrinkle creams and lotions, and biologically active preparations. A few formulations of nourishing creams are given as under :

Cocoa Butter	2 Table spoons
Emulsifying Wax (Petroleum Wax)	2 Table spoons
Beeswax	1 Table spoons
Sesame Oil	4 Table spoons
Almond Oil	1 Table spoons

Elderflower Cream

The process to prepare elderflower cream include mixing of almond oil, elder flower blossoms and lanoline (3, 4 and 1 tablespoon) in a bowl over a water bath and allowed to simmer together for an hour. It is then strained and then warm water is added slowly with constant stirring.

Wheat Germ Cream

The composition of wheat germ cream is given below :

Beeswax	1 Teaspoon
Emulsifying Wax (Petrolatum)	1 Teaspoon
Lanolin	5 Table spoons
Sesame Oil	3 Table spoons
Wheat Germ Oil	2 Tablespoons
Water	5 Table spoons
Witch Hazel	1 Tablespoon
Borax	½ Teaspoon
Perfume	3-5 drops

Honey Cream

Honey is a very useful ingredient creams used for dry, coarse and sensitive skin. For a nourishing cream for sallow skin melt lanolin, honey, lectithin (3, 0.5, 1, tablespoon) in a bowl with heating. Add slowly warm water (4 tablespoons) with beating and cool it.

Vitamin Cream

The composition of vitamin cream is given below:

Beeswax	1 Tablespoon
Emulsifying Wax	1 Tablespoon
Lanolin	1 Tablespoon
Wheat Germ Oil (or vitamin - E Capsules 2 No)	3 Tablespoons
Carrot Oil (or Vit-A Capsules -2 Nos)	3 Tablespoons
Borax	½ Teaspoons
Distilled Water	6 Tablespoons
Tincture of Benzoin	2 drops
Orange Flower Oil	3-5 drops

Mixed Vegetable Cream

Beeswax	2 Tablespoons
Emulsifying Wax (Petrolatum)	4 Tablespoons
Lanolin	3 Teaspoons
Almond Oil	4 Tablespoons
Sesame Oil	4 Tablespoons
Avocado Oil	2 Tablespoons
Safflower Oil	2 Tablespoons
Sun flower Oil	2 Tablespoons
Water	5 Tablespoons
Borax	½ Teaspoon
Amber Oil	3-5 drops

Water-in-Oil Emulsions

These are grooming preparations hence more popular. The emulsifiers like polyvalent soaps, bees wax and borax haven been used. The other emulsifiers for the water-in-oil emulsions which are used are calcium oleate, calcium stearate, zinc stearate, aluminium stearate. The composition of hair grooming preparation is given below, 1 to 5.

No. 1	per cent
Mineral oil	65.55
Beeswax white	2.5
Water	34.8
Borax	0.15
Perfume	q.s.

Formulations (Emulsified Hair Grooming Preparation)

Ingredients	per cent			
	2	3	4	5
Oleic acid	12	20	1.0	-
Beeswax	2	1	1.5	2.5
Mineral Oil	45	-	41.7	48
Lanolin	2	0.5	-	-
Lime Water	19	33.5	53.8	-
Saccharated lime water	20	5	-	-
Olive Oil	-	40	-	-
Magnesium sulphate(25%)	-	-	2.0	-
Stearic acid	-	-	-	1.5
Absorption base	-	-	-	5.0
Petrolatum	-	-	-	12.5
Magnesium oleate	-	-	-	2.5
Water	-	-	-	28
Perfume and Preservative	q.s.	q.s.	q.s.	q.s.

HERBAL COSMETICS FOR THE HAIR

The cosmetics having ayurvedic base with some medicinal compound yielding desired properties are implied as herbal cosmetics. The preparations like herbal hair oil, herbal shampoos are best examples. Hair Care products and cures comprising of herbal Hair Rinses, Hair tonics, Shampoos, Henna powders, are designed to restore beauty and health to the hair. They contain extracts known for their qualities of stimulating hair growth, improving hair texture and colour. The range of Market Products are :

Herbal Hair Conditioners

This is a powerful combination of invaluable herbal ingredients like Amla, sandalwood, Brahmi, Lichens and other precious herbs. It makes the hair strong, healthy and lustrous. Prevents hair loss and acts as a scalp deep cleanser while maintaining the natural moisture balance. It provides body to dull lifeless hair.

Herbal Hair Oil

This is an effective combination of Arnica, Henna, Shikakai and other herbal extracts, especially created to prevent hair loss and promote luxurious hair growth.

Herbal Henna

The preparation of herbal henna include combination of pure henna leaves and various herbal ingredients. They make the hair lustrous, manageable and silky. It also works as a powerful treatment for scalp disorders and gives a mild natural colour and sheen to the hair.

Herbal Hair Tonic

This preparation is for controlling hair loss/dandruff/greying hair. It stimulates hair growth and thickness. It is a specialised tonic treatment for revitalising the hair and generating a natural lustroics glow. It serves well for texturising rough brittle hair and split ends.

Herbal Henna Shampoo (for normal to oily hair)

This preparation is to cleanse the scalp and controls excessive secretion of scalp oils and imparts sheen to dull hair making it tangle free.

Herbal Amla Shampoo (for normal to dry hair)

This preparation is made from extracts of Amla, Dater and Arnica and Other rare herbs. This shampoo makes the hair lustrous, healthier and manageable and cleanses the scalp while retaining and stimulating its natural oil.

Hair Treatment Cream

This preparation is an effective, medicated antiseptic ointment for the treatment of dandruff scalp disorders, seborrhoea and sealy skin conditions and is used for the treatment of dandruff and falling hair.

Herbal Mint/Hair Gloss conditioner

It is used as a hair sheen and can be used just before shampoo for providing texture and conditioning to the hair.

Herbal Cosmetics

Herbal Hair Rinse

This is a combination of mint, brahmi and other herbal extracts and is an effective control for dandruff and scalp disorders and promoters hair growth.

Herbal Hair Oils (Medicated)

Medicated herbal oils are also used as scenting material for the hair. The base oil may be a mineral oil such as coconut oil, groundnut oil, castor oil, neem oil etc. To make an oil ayurvedic or a herbal product certain essential oils are added which provide certain specific characteristics of the individual used in the formulation

Base Formulation For Herbal hair Oil

Ingredient	Quantity
Til Oil	91 ml
Mollha Kankola	0.3 ml
whees Charrila	0.3 ml
Sailag Nagar	0.03 ml
Chander	0.04 ml
Long Dalchini	0.03 ml
Ratanjot	0.02 ml
Kapur Kachuri	0.05 ml
Satabar	0.02 ml
Tejpal	0.03 gms
Howber	0.03 gms
Balhere	0.06 gms
Amla	0.06 gms
Harral	0.03 gms
Chanpa	0.03 gms
Keora (keya)	0.06 gms
Gulabphul	0.03 gms
Alaichi (Big)	0.02 gms
Pudhina	0.4 gms
Perfume	0.3-15 gms
Quatah water	1.5 kg
Menthol	0.2

There is no unique formulations for herbal hair oil. The formulations of the manufacturers are trade secrets. However, the above formulation can be taken as a standard base and it can be changed according to requirements.

Herbal Shampoos

These products are more suitable in hard-water areas. *Quillaja saponania* is one of a whole class of Saponias widely distributed in nature. Commercially saponin is extracted with water and alcohol from the *Quillaja* bark or from the soap root. Preparations of saponin are generally intended to cleanse the scalp and to reduce scaliness. These are generally compounded with rosemary or celandine and in addition to its use in shampoos saponin has found some use in bubble baths. Some formulations for Herbal Shampoos are given as under :

	Ingredients	per cent
(i)	Quilaja bark, powdered	5.0
	Ammonium carbonate	1.0
	Borax	1.0
	Bay leaf oil	0.1
	Water	92.9
(ii)	Sodium carbonate anhydrous	19.4
	Powdered soap	79.0
	Saponin	1.6
	Perfume	q.s.
(iii)	Borax	20.0
	Sodium, sesquicarbonate	40.0
	Powdered soap	35.0
	Saponin	5.0
	Perfume	q.s.

Hair Dye

Henna is the only important vegetable dye. The presence of 2- hydroxy-1, 4-naphthaquinone gives henna a dyeing properties. It consists of the dried powdered leaves of Lawsonia alba, Lawsonia spinosa and Lawsonia inemis, which are removed from the plants prior to flowering. It is soluble in hot water and is, in acid solution, a substantive dye for Keratine. The powdered henna is mixed with hot water. Citric or adipic or other suitable acid is added to adjust pH 5-8. Then hair is dyed using this paste and kept for five to sixty minutes, then shampooed, rinsed and dried. The "Henna Pack" is kept in place by means of a towel and is allowed to remain on the head for the required time varying from five to sixty minutes after which the hair is thoroughly shampooed, rinsed and dried

Henna

The henna plant is shrub, *Lawsonia alba lans* of bears small, fragrant, greenish-white flowers, but as the only plant utilised for dye are the leaves and stems, the plants are frequently at back. For infusions, used as raises the leaves are usually left whole, but is the more common commercial form of henna, the leaves and stems are ground to a powder, about the colour of dark unstand and with characteristic earthy odour.

The principal advantage offered by henna as a modern hair dye is that it is harmless to the system and causes no irritations on the skin. A few applications impart a slight amount of colour to the entire hair shift and depending on the original colour of the hair, a whole range of reddish pure vegetable shades - tomato, beet, egg plant - can be produced. If it is plied often enough, therefore, hair of any and all original shades can be brought to the same characteristics orangered.

Applications of Henna

Despite the intense dark red shade of solutions of henna, the active dyeing principle, is only about 1% of it. This dye is used mostly in beauty shops, as a rinse or as a pack.

Henna Rinse

For slight change of colour, bring out highlights on dark hair, henna levels are steeped in boiling water until all the dye is extracted. This solution is then poured several times over freshly shampooed hair. Commercial preparations of a henna rinse should be acidified with 1 to 2% of some mild organic acid viz adipic acid, citric acid, tartaric.

Henna Pack

For a more decided, or more lasting, change in shade, powdered henna leaves are made into a paste with boiling water. This is applied to all the hair, which is allowed to remain covered and undisturbed until test on a single strand shows that the desired shade has been attained. The subsequnet treatment, the colour can be kept uniform by applying the paste to only the new growth of hair.

To prepare henna powder, the fresh leaves are ground extremely fine. Fresh powder is dark brownish-green, as it ages bearing yellowish red. It is usually packed in waxed paper in cans or boxes that can be tightly sealed.

Henna Mixtures

To modify the often unpleasing reddish shades that are the only ones possible with henna alone, this plant was long ago mixed with indigo. The dried and powdered leaves of indigo origin are either mixed with ground henna or applied alternatively with henna, to produce a good black. Shades from light brings to black can be produced by varying the proportions of henna and indigo.

Camomile

Camomile is another plants used for colouring the hair. Sveral varieties of related plants are found in U.K., Western Europe, and the U.S.A., of which only two - camomile and German or Hungarian camomile - are used to any extent. The essential oil distilled from camomile flowers in pale blue, due to the presence of some hydrocarbon azulien. Like henna, camomile can be used as rinse, a pack, or a shampoo.

Camomile Pack

Camomile pack is prepared by mixing 2 parts of its powder with Kaolin or 1 part of fullers. Boiler water is then added to make paste. The shade produced depends on the original shade of the hair and the time of contact, and the change in color lasts considerably longer than the glints produced by a rinse. As with the henna pack the paste must be kept hot during the entire application, and the operation should be completed as quickly as possible.

Camomile Shampoo

German camomile is usually prepared because it produces a slightly better colour and because it is considerably cheaper than Roman variety. Camomile shampoos are marketed as powders and as liquids. It constitutes : Camomile German Powdered (10%); Mild organic acid (5%); Sodium sulphate (85%); Oil of camomile (q.s. (for perfume).

A liquid shampoo is most effective when freshly prepared. Hence it may be made in concentrated form. It constitutes : Camomile infusion (10%); Sodium laurge sulphate (30-40%); Water (50-60%).

Camomile-Henna Mixtures

Pack of this type may be prepared to very good effect to produce a fair range of colours on hair of different basic shades as shown below.

Formulations for Camomile-Henna Mixture

Ingredients	1	2	3
Camomile	75	50	25
Henna	25	50	75
Orininal Colour	Shade Produced		
Blond	Golden-blond		
	Red - Gold		
	Gloden - Red		
Light brown	Light auburn		
	Auburn		
	Bright auburn		
	Chest Nut		
Dark Brown	Reddish - Brown		
	Dark auburn		

Henna Reng Dye

It is possible to produce other shades instead auburn. The blue black shade shade is obtained by the mixture of powered indigo and henna. It is known as henna renges.

Camomile Herbar Dye

Of the various species of camomile, only 'Anthemis nobilis' (Roma Camomile) and Matricaria camomile (German camomile) have been used in cosmetics and are useful in tinting the hair. The active ingredient of these flowers in 1, 3, 4-trihydronyflavore, known as apigenin. Either an aqueous extract or a paste of the ground flower heads are generally used. To lighten the hair a paste consisting of 2 parts camomile and 1-2 parts Kaolin mixed to a thin cream with hot water is applied to the head for a period varying from 15 minutes to 60 minutes depending upon the shade required. While making a formulation it is essential that at least 5% camomile or its equivalent in extract, must be present to produce any effect at all and the azulene also present in camomile contributes to the brightening effect.

Fresh Soap-Wort Shampoo

When water is added to soap-wort foam is produced due to saponina. All parts of the plant produce a gentle cleansing lather that does not sting the eyes or make the hair brittle. It can be combined with other herbs that suit particular types of hair and colour.

Formulation No. 1

Leafy Soapwort stems 6-8 long	10 Nos.
Water	500 ml.
Strong Herb or flower infusion	3 Tablespoon

For making an infusion use the following amounts. To each ½ litre of boiling bottled spring water add.

Dried Herbs :	14 gms for weak infusion
	28 gms for normal strength
	56 gms for strong infusion
Fresh Herbs :	1 1/2 handfuls for weak infusion
	3 handfuls for normal strength
	6 handfuls for strong infusion

Dried herbs of any of the flowers given below can be used.

– Camomile, Lime flower, yarrow.

– Rosemary, sage, comfrey, henna (powder).

– Marigold flowers.

– Lavender, peppermint, white, dead nettle.

– Marsh mallow, comfrey

– Southerriwood, stinging nettle.

– Elder flower, Uiyme, rosemary.

Procedure

The stems are cut into short lengths and put into an enamel saucepan. Then bruised lightly with a wooden spoon and water is added. The mixture is boiled and then covered and allowed to simmer for 15 minutes with continuous stirring, till cool Then the contents are strained and bottled for future use. A flower infusion is prepared and 3 tablespoon of strong herb or flower is added. The shampoo is covered and then allowed to cool and then strained. The whole of the above liquid is used for one hair wash.

Dried Soap-Wort

The process of preparation of dried soap wort root shampoo include soaking of dried soap-wort in a boiling water for 12 hours or overnight. Transfer it to enamel and, boil and simmered for 15 minutes. The dried herbs or flowers are then added, stirred, covered and left to cool. The mixture is then stirred into a fug and used for one hair wash.

Nettle Rinse and Conditioner

Nettle is an excellent hair conditioner. it is an acidic plant and promotes a healthy gloss. it is prepared by first cutting nettles, thenput it saucepan and add cold water and boil. Simmer for 15 minutes by covering it. Strain the mixture into a jug and allow it to cool.

Lotion for Unruly Hair

Formulation No. 2

– Herb or flower infusion of normal strength	– 8 Tablespoons
– Eau de cologne	– 1 Tablespoon
– Glycerien	– 1 Tablespoon

Horsetail Hair Rinse and Tonic

Herba hair tonics and conditioners help restore the scalps natural acidity and strengthen the circulation giving a healthy shine to the hair. Horsetail Contains saponins which create lather, flavour-glycosides which act on the scalps tiny blood vessels to stimulate the circulation and silica which provides body to the hair. The horsetail stems (long) are bruised with a spoon before adding the boiling water to make an infusion. They are then covered and left until lukewarm and then strained. After shampooing and rinsing, the infusion is poured on the hair and massaged on the scalp. Blot the mixture with towel and the hair is combed. Before dry hair cover the head with warm towel and wait for 10 mins.

Tonic Shampoo

Put 135 gms each of dried reetha, shikakai and amla into one litre water. Keep it for 24 hours. Boil and then allow to cool. Filter the mixture and use as a shampoo.

Herb Shampoo

Soak overnight in an iron pot 210 gms of dried olives and shikakai in cold water. Then boil for 10-15 minutes and strain liquidige the flesh that remains and use the paste to wash your hair. This shampoo leaves your hair soft and shining.

Chapter - 14

TESTING OF COSMETICS

INTRODUCTION

Cosmetic analysis is both specialised and diversified. The range of tests covered in this chapter reveals that it utilises the full gamut of modern analytical chemistry to identify and determine inorganic and organic components in extremely complex mixtures. However, as is often the case techniques developed by cosmetic chemists to solve their particular problems also have great utilitarian value in other areas of analytical chemistry.

A cosmetic is considered to be adulterated if it contains a poisonous or deleterious substance which may cause it to be injurious to users under customary conditions of use or if it is contaminated in a manner which may render it harmful to health. It is misbranded if its labeling is false or misleading, if it does not bear the required labeling information, or if it is not truthfully packaged.

The composition of cosmetic raw materials themselves requires increasing scrutiny by the analytical chemist for the support of safety testing programmes for ingredients and for the establishment of precise standards and specifications for such ingredients.

This chapter provides both specific procedures and general methods for approaching the analysis of cosmetics, toiletries, in a logical and systematic manner. The analyst must supplement this information with laboratory experience gained in the actual analysis of products. The chemist should have a good understanding of spectrophotometry and chromatography. It is hoped that the experienced cosmetic chemist will find this text a source of new ideas from which to increase the range and scope of his investigations.

SPECTROSCOPY IN COSMETIC ANALYSIS

Ultraviolet and visible, fluorometric, infra-red, mass, and nuclear magnetic resonance spectroscopy plays vital role in cosmetic analysis.

Ultraviolet and Visible Spectroscopy

Ultraviolet (uv) spectrophotometry plays an important role in cosmetic analysis for identifying and determining compounds which, through electronic transitions, absorb radiation in the region from 200 to 380 nm. Primarily this technique applies to aromatic compounds, although uv spectra are useful for characterising some aliphatic substances such as compounds with conjugated double bonds, ketones, and mercaptans.

Constituents that Absorb in the Ultra-Violet

The following partial listing of cosmetic raw materials which absorb in the ultra-violet :

Alkyl aryl polyether alcohols, Alkyl aryl sulphonates, Aminobenzoates, Aminophenols, Arylamines, Aryl sulphonamide-formaldehyde resin, Benzoyl peroxide. Camphor, Cinnamates, Coumarins, Dichlorophene, Furocoumarins, Hexachlorophene, p-Hydroxybenzoates, Nitroarylamines, Phenosulphonates, Phthalates, Quaternaries containing aryl groups, Salicylates, Silicons containing phenyl groups, Tricresyl phosphates.

For several cosmetic ingredients, e.g., sunscreens, preservatives, and arylamine oxidation hair dye intermediates, uv spectrophotometry is an invaluable analytical technique.

Visible spectrophotometry (colourimetry) is based on the same principles as uv spectrophotometry, except that the absorption range of interest extends from 380 to 800 nm. The substances to be determined appear coloured to the human eye. Many coloured inorganic and organic cosmetic materials have been investigated. For example, ethanol can be measured through its reaction with potassium dichromate; a coloured chromic complex is determined. The coloured Schiffs derivatives of citral and citronellal have been evaluated. Poloyvinyl pyrrolidone and its copolymers form a coloured complex with a red dye which enables their determination down to 0.1 ppm. As a final example, the amount of tartar emetic in certain toilet waters can be measured through its coloured iodonatimonous acid complex.

Infrared Spectroscopy

The infrared (IR) region of the spectrum most frequently studied by the analytical chemist lies between 4000 and 660 cm^{-1} (2.5 and 15 µm). Organic molecules selectively absorb energy at specific wavelengths within that region. A plot of the wavelengths where absorption occurs vs. their intensities provides an IR spectrum which can be useful for characterising or identifying a cosmetic ingredient.

Sample Preparation

Analysis of a cosmetic may be initiated by obtaining an IR spectrum of the non-volatile portion of the sample. Almost all preparations containing water (which absorbs IR radiation), such as creams, lotions, antiperspirants, depilatories, shampoos, and hair dyes, can be dehydrated by heating them on a steam bath or at 105°C in an oven. The IR spectrum of the liquid or solid residue may be obtained by placing the sample between salt plates either as a neat film or in mulls made with mineral and/or halocarbon oil. A neat film is deposited on a plate by evaporation of a volatile solvent, such as alcohol or acetone, containing the dispersed or soluble residue. Solids with low melting points may be placed on the plate, heated to the liquid state, and resolidified by cooling into thin glassy films. Alternatively, about 2 mg of a solid sample can be mixed with approximately 200 mg of KBr powder and pressed into a pellet in a die at 20,000–50,000 psi pressure.

IR spectra of solutions and gases are generated with the aid of sealed cells of various pathlengths. Spectra of volatile solvents in nail lacquers are obtained by dissolving a sample aliquot in carbon disulphide, a solvent which is transparent to most IR radiation, and adding the solution to a selected liquid cell. Gases, such as propellant mixtures in aerosol products, are allowed to flow into a previously evacuated gas cell. (If the concentration of gas in the cell is too great, it can conveniently be reduced by using a pipet to which a rubber bulb is attached to withdraw some of the gas.)

Characteristic Absorbances

A cosmetic sample IR spectrum should first be examined in the 2–9 μm region, where absorption peaks at specific wavelengths can be associated with given functional groups. Such a study can frequently provide a quick indication of the presence or absence of alcohols, amines, acids, esters, ethers, amides, soaps, nitriles, mercapto compounds, nitro compounds, alikyl sulphates, sulphonates, and sulphonamides. Frequently, closely related ingredients can be differentiated by comparison of the "fingerprint" region (9–15 μm) of the spectrum where secondary information may be provided. The relationship among the observed absorbances at the various wavelengths is studied for an estimation of the relative amount of each ingredient.

Structural Elucidation

Infrared spectrophotometry is a helpful too for structural elucidation of previously uncharacterised compounds which may be encoutered in many of the complex raw materials used in cosmetic formulation. When IR spectra of pure substances differ to only a minor degree, the substances are very similar chemically. On occasion, the absence of a key absorption peak can provide important in formation which may be used to reduce the number of suspected compounds.

Fluorometry

When selected excitation wavelengths of uv light impinge upon certain types of chemical substances, characteristic light emissions occur at longer ultravioler or visible wavelengths. Usually, an excitation wavelength which elicits a maximum emission response is chosen for a given compound in order to achieve the greatest sensitivity. The most appropriate emission wavelength is the one with the greatest intensity whose maximum is well removed from that of the excitation band. Fluorometric sensitivity is very good; it is common to measure microgram levels of material with ease.

The application of the fluorometry technique is greatly expanded by conversion of non-fluorescing compounds into fluorescent derivatives. For example, formaldehyde, a cosmetic preservative, is determined through quantitative conversion to its fluorescent lutidine derivative. Aluminum can be determined qualitatively and quantitatively in deodorants and antiperspirants through the fluorescent aluminium salt of 8-hydroxy- quinoline.

Mass Spectrometry

Submicrogram sample of pure compounds may be identified readily by mass spectrometry. A sample is introduced into a highly evacuated chamber (ca 10^{-10} atmospheres) and bombarded with a beam of electrons powerful enough to strip away one or more electrons from its molecular orbitals. These collisions produce a number of positively charged molecular fragments along with a frequently occurring positively charged species of the same molecular weight as the sample molecule. These species are separated electromagnetically by various instrumental techniques into discrete particle types represented by different relative mass-to-charge ratios. A plot of particle mass vs. relative abundance is obtained which represents the mass spectrum of the sample. Some samples may be identified by comparison with standard reference mass spectra but the structural elucidation of unknowns requires skilled interpretation. The positively charged molecular fragments form spectral peak patterns which are characteristic of certain structural features. The molecular weight of the unknown compound may be determined if its corresponding parent ion peak is present in the spectrum.

Mass spectral analysis has been used for the verification of suspected structures of derivatives of cosmetic compounds. Various alkanolamines in hair sprays must be acetylated prior to their determination by gas chromatography. Some contain several – OH groups as well as a – NH group. Mass spectral analysis determines whether or not the – NH group was acetylated and the number of – OH groups converted to acetates.

Nuclear Magnetic Resonance

Many spinning atomic nuclei, such as those of hydrogen (protons), boron, fluorine, and phosphorus, possess angular momentum and a magnetic moment. Because of the most widely studied of the nuclei are protons, the description of their nuclear magnetic resonance (NMR) behaviour is emphasised. When organic molecules containing protons are placed in a large magnetic field of known fixed strength and this field is swept with small known magnetic fields at right angles to the sample, certain of the applied frequencies (or small magnetic fields) interact with the magnetic moments of the protons, causing the protons to "flip" from their orientation with the large magnetic field to an orientation against it. Energy absorbed during this "flip" is considered to be "nuclear magnetic resonance" energy. The amount of absorbed energy required to cause a proton to flip depends upon its structural location in the molecule, because the electronic envelope surrounding a proton has a significant influence on its magnetic properties. An NMR plot of the radio frequency energy absorbed by a molecule vs. the changing magnetic field strength can yield valuable information about the various types and numbers of hydrogen atoms in the molecule. Thus ;nuclear magnetic resonance is an important tool for the structural elucidation of many complex molecules.

Nuclear magnetic resonance reference spectra are useful for verifying the identities of many compounds; however, it should be emphasised that no single spectral technique should be relied upon for proof of structure. Confirmation is best obtained by a number of mutually supportive instrumental and chemical approaches. As a case in point, the structure of $\beta 1$-cadinene (now known as α– cadinene), a sesquiterpene hydrocarbon isolated from olibanum oil, could not be varified by comparison with any available standard reference spectra (infrared or nuclear magnetic resonance). Through a process of elimination with a combination of chemical and spectral techniques, the number of possibilities was narrowed down to two alternative cadinene isomers, δ_1 and β_1 (now known as α). The NMR spectrum provided confirmatory evidence that the unknown is the $\delta 1$ isomer, based on the number of olefinic protons.

CHROMATOGRAPHIC TECHNIQUES IN COSMETIC ANALYSIS

Adsorption Column chromatography

Adsorption column chromatography is a useful technique for separating mixtures of organic compounds possessing varying degrees of polarities.

In principle, the more polar the compound the more strongly it is held by the adsorbent. In applying this technique, a solution or slurry of the sample in a solvent of relatively low polarity is introduced into a chromatography column containing a porous bed of finely divided adsorbent such as silica, alumina, Florisil (magnesium silicate), or magnesia. The components of a mixture are separated through the successive use of eluting solvent of increasing polarity. Even though a practical knowledge of the relative polar strengths of various solvents or mixtures may be gained from experience, some information on this subject has been published and may be used by the analyst in establishing an experimental design for his intended purpose.

Column Preparation, Sample Application and Elution

The preferred method for preparing the column is to prepare a wet slurry of the adsorbent using the least polar solvent of the proposed solvent system. This slurry is then added in increments to the column containing some of this least polar solvent, and each increment is "packed" into the column with the aid of 5–6 psig of air pressure. To prevent channeling, the liquid level should not be allowed to fall below the top of the adsorbent bed within the column, either during its preparation or during use.

The sample is dissolved or dispersed in a small amount of the initial eluting solvent with gentle warming if necessary to increase the solubility of the sample. This sample solution is then added to the column and a constant flow rate is maintained by gravity or by the application of air pressure. The column is then eluted successively with solvents of increasing polarity. Uniform aliquots are collected and the chromatographic procedure is continued until all components of interest have been collected.

Qualitative and Quantitative Analysis

Components in the eluted aliquots may be determined by gravimetric or volumetric analysis or such instrumental techniques as infrared (IR), ultraviolet uv, nuclear magnetic resonance, and mass spectrometry. Other helpful techniques are thin layer chromatography (TLC), refractometry, fluorometry, and polarimetry.

Variables and Efficiency

Reproducibility and efficiency of separation are dependent on certain variables, most of which can be controlled by the analyst. For example, the selection of a smaller mesh size adsorbent offers a correspondingly larger surface area for adsorption which favours improved separations. Other factors affecting accuracy, reproducibility, and efficiency of adsorption chromatographic procedures include proper selection of solvent polarity, viscosity, and compatibility of successive solvents; packing procedure; method of sample application; and flow rate. Although ambient temperature is satisfactory in most cases, the temperature of the column can affect the separation process.

Application to Cosmetic Analysis

The cosmetic analyst is frequently confronted with the problem of separating complex mixtures of cosmetic ingredients with polarities ranging from non-polar aliphatic bydrocarbons to such highly polar compounds as polyols. The selective elution of components of increasing polarities can be demonstrated by the analysis of a commercial grade of glyceryl monostearate. The order of elution is aliphatic hydrocarbons, triglycerides, fatty acids, diglycerides, monoglycerides, and finally glycerol.

Partition Column Chromatography

The partition column chromatography is generally a glass tube packed with a solid support which has been coated with a stationary or immobile phase, one of two immiscible, equilibrated liquids. The sample is introduced at the top of the column and the column is then developed by introduction of a moving or mobile phase, the other liquid of this immiscible pair of liquids. As the mobile phase, moves down the column, the sample component of interest (solute) will move in the system at a rate which depends on its relative solubilities in the two phases. This is expressed as the partition coefficient and is defined as the concentration of the solute in the mobile phase divided by its concentration in the immobile phase under equilibrium conditions. This value is constant for any given solute in a specific system. Usually, development of the column is continued until all solutes of interest have been eluted from the column. These eluates are collected in uniform aliquots and reserved for analysis by chemical or instrumental techniques.

In conventional practice, the more polar liquid of the solvent pair is used as the immobile phase. This is referred to as normal partition chromatography. In reverse phase partition chromatography the less polar solvent is the immobile phase.

Partition chromatography is generally used for the separation of chemically similar compounds that have some solubility in both liquid phases and different partition coefficients. Adsorption chromatography is primarily useful for the separation of compounds into different chemical classes.

Solid Support

The ideal solid support consists of small, uniform inert particles with high permeability and large surface areas. Of the materials commonly used as solid supports, diatomaceous earths such as Celite or Filter-Cel most closely fulfill these requirements. Other materials that have been used as solid supports include cellulose powder, potato starch, modified cellulose, polyamides, and silica gel.

Commercial grades of diatomaceous earth require sieving to the desired mesh range followed by washing with HCl, distilled water, and finally methanol or ethanol to remove impurities. After drying at 120°C, the support is suitable for preparing columns. Analytical grades of diatomaceous earth do not require further treatment. If the support is to be used for reverse phase partition chromatography, it must be silanised with a preparation such as dimethyldichlorosilane by exposing the support to vapours of the silanising reagent in a closed container or by treating the support with a toluene solution of the silanising reagent. If non-silanised support is used to prepare a reverse phase partition column, the polar mobile phase will wet the support, displace the immobile phase, and render the column useless.

Selection of the Liquid Phase

The first step in the design of an analytical partition chromatography columns is to determine the composition of the mobile and immobile liquid phases. The analyst first selects two partially immiscible solvents in which the component to be separated is soluble. Typically, this may involve a solvent pair such as hexane and methanol. Usually a third and possibly a fourth solvent is introduced into the system to modify the partitioning of the solute between the two phases. Chloroform, for example, may be introduced to increase solubility in the non-polar phase. Water can be used to increase immiscibility of the two phases as well as to change the solute solubility in the polar phase. Equal volumes of the two liquids selected as the mobile and immobile phases are added to a separatory funnel along with several milligrams of the compound to be determined. The system is then mixed thoroughly by shaking to establish equilibrium. After the liquid phases have separated, the amount of solute in each phase is determined. The partition coefficient should be approximately 0.01. If it is not, other solvents are introduced to adjust the partition coefficient to the desired value. The phase in which the solute has the highest concentration is always used as the immobile phase.

Preparation of Column

After a suitable solvent system has been selected, the appropriate amount of each component of the solvent system is added to a separatory funnel and mixed thoroughly. The equilibrated phases are then separated and stored in stoppered flasks until used. Silanised support is used for reverse phase and non-silanised support for normal partition chromatography.

For analytical columns a glass chromatographic tube approximately 2 cm id is usually used. There are several methods for packing the column. For example, the support is coated by mixing with a calculated amount of immobile phase. Until uniform, and then is added to the column in increments, with tamping, until the column beck is the desired height. Alternatively, the uncoated support is packed into the empty tube and then washed with immobile phase. Mobile phase is then added and allowed to flow through the column until no immobile phase is observed in the eluate. Other methods of column packing are variations of the above techniques. After the column has been prepared, approximately 10 mg of the sample to be analysed is added to the column in one of the following ways :

1. The sample is dissolved in the immobile phase, mixed with a small portion of the support and packed on the top of the prepared column.

2. The sample is dissolved in a minimum amount of mobile phase and added to the column.

3. When neither of the above methods is applicable, the sample is dissolved in a volatile solvent and mixed with a small amount of support. The solvent is then removed and the dried mixture is added to the column.

After the column has been prepared and the sample added, the column is developed with the mobile phase. During development, the level of mobile phase should not be allowed to fall below the level of the coated support. Ideally, the flow rate should be about 8 ml/hr/cm^2 obtained either by gravity or applied air pressure. Development is continued until the components of interest have been eluted. If the components are coloured or can be rendered visible under uv light, each resolved band is collected separately. If components are not visible, a series of uniform aliquots are collected for analysis to determine composition.

Application to Cosmetic Analysis

Many active ingredients in sunscreen preparations, such as *p*-hydroxybenzoates, cinnamates, and aminobenzoates, are successfully separated by partition chromatography and determined by uv spectrometry. Sixteen cosmetic preservatives have also been separated and determined in different cosmetic products.

Ion Exchange Chromatography

Organic or inorganic compounds containing ionic functional groups can be separated from other ionic or non-ionic compounds by ion exchange chromatography. The ion exchanger is normally a solid, finely divided, insoluble material containing ionic sites which are available for the attraction of oppositely charged ions in solution. Although naturally occurring materials such as the alkaline aluminosilicates (zeolites) have served in this capacity, synthetic organic polymers (resins) containing various functional groups are nearly always used for analytical purposes. The separation is usually carried out in a glass column containing the ion exchange resin selected to perform a specific separation. The sample is introduced onto the column in the appropriate solvent and the column is then usually washed with a solvent to elute all non-ionic compounds.

After sample introduction and removal of non-ionic components, the column is developed by displacement chromatography or elution chromatography. Displacement chromatography is carried out by forcing the sample component of interest (solute) from the resin by adding a solution (eluant) containing an excess of an ionic solute that is more strongly attached to the ionic sites on the resin than is the sample solute. In elution chromatography, the eluant contains an ionic solute that is less strongly attracted to the ionic sites on the resin. The sample solute is equilibrated between the resin and the eluant. As the eluant flows each solute moves down the column at a rate dependent upon pH and ionic concentration of the eluant and the ionic attraction between the solutes and ionic sites on the resin.

Column Preparation, Sample Addition and Elution

For most analytical purposes, a 1 x 20–25 cm chromatographic tube is filled with 10–15 ml of pretreated resin. In order to ensure column uniformity, the resin is added in increments as a thick slurry to a tube already one-third filled with liquid, which is gradually drained as the addition proceeds. Each successive addition should be made before the resin has completely settled. Ion exchange resins in acid or base form are packed in columns containing distilled water or a non-aqueous solvent, while those in the "salt" form are added to the appropriate salt or buffer solution. After the column is packed, the resin in the column is washed with the same liquid used for packing until the pH of the effluent is the same as that of the liquid added at the top. The resin in the column should always have liquid above it.

After the level of liquid in the column is adjusted to just cover the top of the ion exchange resin, the sample is added as a solution in the appropriate solvent, i.e., distilled water or organic solvent if the resin is in acid or base form, or buffer if the resin is in "salt" form. The sample solution is added slowly to the top of the column and allowed to percolate into the resin bed at the same flow rate that will be used during the chromato-graphy step. The walls should be rinsed several times with the selected solvent and the rinse solution allowed to settle into the resin bed. Uniform aliquots are collected continuously until development is complete.

The amount of sample added to the column depends on the total ion exchange capacity of the resin and the type of chromatography used. The total "sample load" in the elution procedure should not exceed 1% of the total ion exchange capacity of the resin in the column for analytical purposes or 5-10% for preparative work. Sample load in displacement chromatography may range from 25 to 50% of the total ion exchange capacity of the resin.

A flow rate of 0.005-0.05 ml of solution/ml of resin/minute is suitable in analytical determinations for particle sizes of 0.15-0.5 mm but in any case it should not exceed 0.05 ml/minute.

After eluates have been collected they can be analysed by IR or uv spectrometry or any other applicable chemical or instrumental technique.

Applications to Cosmetic Analysis

Alkanolamine salts of various acid polymers are used in some hair spray formulations. The alkanolamine can be separated from the acid polymer by a strongly acid ion exchange resin, Type I. The polymer is eluted with 75% ethanol. The amine is displaced from the resin with HCl (1 +1) and determined by gas-liquid chromatography (GLC). Triethanolamine lauryl sulphate is separated into its acidic and basic components by chromatography on the strongly basic ion exchange resin, Amberlite CG-400. The triethanolamine is eluted with water and determined by GLC.

Amberlite CG-400 is also used to remove interfering surfactants from solution prior to TLC identification of hexachlorophene. These surfactants, if not removed, frequently alter the R_f of hexachlorophene, making its identification more difficult.

Alkanolamines may interfere with the GLC determination of glycerol in cosmetic creams. Alkanolamines and glycerol remain in the aqueous phase when the sample is extracted from an acidified solution of methanol-water with $CHCl_3$ or petroleum ether. Glycerol may be separated and recovered by elution with wagter in a column which contains pretreated, strongly acidic resin. The alkanolamine is retained by the resin.

Boric acid in certain deodorant preparations can be accurately determined after removal of interfering zinc or aluminum ions with the cationic exchange resin Amberlite.

Alkanolamindes and/or soap can be separated from shampoos containing alkyl sulphates and/or sulphonates. A weakly basic anion exchange resin. Amberlite, is suitable for this separation. It must, however, be throughly pretreated by being washed with all of the same solvents to be used during the separation. Acidified ethanol elutes the alkanolamide and/or soap from the column, and the sulphate-sulphonate mixture retained by the resin is then isolated by elution with a basic (ammonium carbonate) methanol solution.

Thin Layer Chromatography

Over the past decade TLC has become an increasingly popular analytical tool for the analysis of cosmetic raw materials and products. The principles of adsorption TLC are based on those previously discussed in the section on adsorption chromatography. The principal differences are : A smaller mesh size adsorbent is supported as a thin layer with the aid of a binder, such as calcium sulphate, on a plastic sheet or a glass plate, and the mobile liquid phase (developer) separates but does not remove the sample components from the TLC adsorbent layer. Silica Gel and aluminum oxide are the adsorbents most frequently used. Although adsorption TLC is the most common type, TL C separations may also be achieved with partition or ion exchange coating materials according to the principles of ion exchange and partition chromatography discussed previously.

General Techniques

The sample is spotted on the plate near one edge (origin) and the plate is placed in an almost vertical position in an enclosed chamber containing developer previously added to a height of 1.0 cm. The origin should be above the developer after the plate is in place. As the developer rises through the adsorbent layer by capillary action, the components of the sample are separated. After the developer reaches a predesignated height (solvent front), the plate is removed from the chamber and allowed to dry. Each component may appear as a circular or elliptical spot somewhere between the origin and the solvent front. If the spot is not visible, chemical or other pretreatment may be required for its detection.

The use of several developments (multiple development) is often helpful in achieving a separation. After an initial development, the plate is removed from the chamber and allowed to dry, and one of its edges is immersed in the same or a different developer. If the same edge is immersed, the second development occurs in the same direction, but if the plate is rotated 90° it is developed perpendicular to the original direction. This technique is referred to as two-dimensional thin layer chromato- graphy.

Each separated component can be isolated by preparative TLC, performed with the use of thicker adsorbent layers (500 μm) than those used for analytical purposes (250μm). The adsorbent is lightly scored around the area containing the component. All of the material within the scored area is removed from the plate, and the component is separated from the adsorbent by extraction with a suitable solvent. Any chemical or instrumental procedure previously described may then be applied to its identification and/or determination. Components may also be determined without their removal from the plate (*in situ*) by visible, uv, or fluorometric spectral scaning with a densitometer.

Variables

Many factors influence the reproducibility of R_f values as well as separation of components. In adsorption TLC, separations are influenced by variation in the composition, purity, particle size, uniformity, layer thickness, and moisture content (activity) of the adsorbent, as well as the composition of the developing solvent, degree of vapour saturation and shape of the developing chamber, temperature, development technique, and sample composition.

Application to Cosmetic Analysis

Citral and citronellal are identified and determined in various essential oils. After their separation on Silica Gel, the plate is sprayed with a modified Schiff's reagent to produce distinctively coloured derivatives which are removed from the plate and determined spectrophotometrically.

Mixtures of naturally occurring coumarins and psoralens (furanocoumarins) in certain citrus oils are separated on Silica Gel and each compound is tentatively identified through its R_f and its fluorescent colour when viewed under uv radiation. Their isolation by the preparative TLC technique provides sufficient material for further investigations. Bergapten, a psoralen with the potential for causing a phototoxic reaction on human skin, occurs naturally in certain essential oils. It is identified in fragrance products through comparison of its fluorescent colour and spatial relationship with those of a standard. It is also determined at levels as low as 0.001% by weight by comparison with various amounts of standard. Separation is achieved by using two-dimensional multiple development with two different solvent systems.

Natural resins can sometimes be differentiated by the respective patterns of their acidic constituents on TLC plate. The components are visualised with the acid indicator spray, bromocresol green.

Thirty different hair dye intermediates used in commercial products are detected through two-dimensional development of the sample with accompanying standards in two different solvent systems. Although some of the compounds or their oxidation products are naturally coloured, others are identified only after the application of various chemical sprays. Their spatial relationship and colours are compared to those of the standards. Some of these intermediates can be detected in commercial hair dyes at levels as low as 0.02%. TLC is helpful in the identification and determination of the products formed by the oxidation of one of the above intermediates, *p*-phenylenediamine in alkaline solution.

The identification of preservatives in cosmetic products is facilitated by TLC on plates coated with Silica Gel impregnated with fluorescent additives. The uv-absorbing compounds show up as redish brown spots under short wave uv light, which is useful as a preliminary identification step.

High Pressure Liquid Chromatography

High pressure liquid chromatography (HPLC) is merely an extension of adsorption, partition, and ion exchange column chromatography. All theoretical and practical considerations that apply to these forms of chromatography apply to HPLC as well. Although efficiency and resolution can be significantly increased by reducing column diameter, support or adsobent particle size, and sample size, practical considerations limit the steps that can be taken in this direction. Instrumentation is now available which overcomes these limitations and significantly shortens analysis time. The high inlet pressure available in HPLC systems allow the use of narrow diameter columns and small uniform particles of packing materials. High efficiency chromatographic separations also require systems of low dead volume, a problem effectively handled by the use of micro detectors and capillary tubing.

HPLC systems usually employ : (a) inlet pressures of 500–5000 psig; (b) column lengths of 10–100 cm; (c) column diameters of 1–6 mm id (average, 2 mm); and (d) eluant flow rates of 10 to several hundred ml/ hour. Many HPLC systems are also equipped with gradient elution devices which can change the composition of the eluant continuously during the course of an analysis. The detectors most commonly used are uv/visible of fixed or variable wavelength. Refractive index (RI) detectors are also used. The uv detectors are sensitive but are limited to the detection of aromatic and other compounds that are strong uv-absorbers. The RI detector is universal but is relatively insensitive and different to use with gradient elution.

GAS CHROMATOGRAPHY IN COSMETIC ANALYSIS

Gas chromatography has become an increasingly important analytical tool for separating, identifying, quantifying, and isolating ingredients from a wide variety of complex cosmetic formulations. Individual components may be separated rapidly by this technique (usually in less than one hour) and in many cases identified and determined at very low levels.

Gas chromatography actually comprises two alternative separation modes, one based on adsorption (gas-solid chromatography, GSC) and the other based on partition (gas-liquid chromatography, GLC) interactions.

Gas Liquid Chromatography

In GLC, a light inert carrier gas such as helium or nitrogen serves as the "mobile phase." This mobile phase flows continuously through a copper, glass, or stainless steel column packed with a relatively non-volatile film of "stationary liquid," which is coated either on a large number of small, inert, solid particles ("solid support") contained therein or directly on the inside column walls. Such "packed column" will be emphasised because of their high frequency of use in current cosmetic analysis and their dual utility for analytical and preparative functions. Narrow bore capillary columns (0.04–0.05" id), which have the stationary liquid phase coated directly on their inner walls, are used almost exclusively for analytical purposes because of the very limited amounts of sample they can handle successfully. Either column is supported in a thermostatically controlled oven in the gas chromatograph so that is may be maintained at a preselected temperature or range of temperatures.

A sample in the solid, liquid, or gaseous state is introduced into the chromatograph via an "injection port," which is usually maintained at an elevated temperature to aid in volatilisation. (Lower injection port temperatures are sufficient for sample constituents with higher vapour pressures, such as gases and low boiling liquids.) In some cases, a chemical derivative of the sample may have to be prepared to form a product volatile enough so that it can be separated by GLC. No decomposition or destruction of components should occur at the temperatures required for volatilisation. The solid support coated with stationary phase should be readily permeable to the carrier gas flow. Vapour pressure of the stationary liquid phase should be minimal or non-existent at the operating temperature of the column.

The separation of volatilised components is influenced by a number of factors as the mixture is swept through the column by a flow of carrier gas. At the head of the column, each component of the vapourised mixture partitions itself in an equilibrium between the carrier gas and the stationary liquid phase. These multiple equilibria are continually established as the carrier gas sweeps the solutes through the column. The degree of interaction of each of the solutes with the liquid phase depends upon combinations of various electronic forces which selectively retard each component until it exists from the column as a separate entity. Separation is therefore based on the continuing competition between the liquid and gas phases for the volatilised solutes. The velocities of the solutes differ at a rate reflected mathematically by the partition coefficient, K, which is a measure of the degree that each component is retained by the liquid phase. For a given solute A,

K = Concentration of solute A in stationary phase/concentration of solute A in mobile phase.

Preparation of Packed Columns

Selection and Preparation of Tubing

Stainless steel copper, aluminum, and glass are all common materials from which tubing for columns may be manufactured. Some chemical entities in the sample or the stationary phase may be catalytically converted by the composition of these metallic tubes. Glass is the least likely material to contribute to such adverse activity, and it has the added bonus of furnishing a clever view of the progress made during the column packing procedure. However, glass tubes are fragile and expensive, and they usually must be ordered specially to fit a given gas chromatograph. Packed columns may serve in an analytical (1/8–1/4" od) or preparative (3/8–1/2" od) capacity. In order to fit in the oven, tubes must be either U-shaped or, more, often, coiled. After the tubes are coiled, they are cleaned with solvents, filled with packing material (solid support coated with stationary phase), and connected to the chromatograph with Swagelok fittings.

The tubes are cleaned with solvents prior to packing to remove industrial contaminants used in their manufacture. Usually a cacuum is applied to one end and a detergent solution and/or a series of organic solvents is introduced at the opposite end. Each successive organise solvent should have a higher polarity, the final one being the same as the solvent used for coating the liquid phase onto the solid support–eg., pentane, chloroform, acetone, and the liquid phase solvent.

Preparation of Solid Support

The support should be sieved in order to select the appropriate narrow range of particle (mesh) sizes required for efficient column performance, as previously discussed. Most of the fines should be removed; if they are created by sieving an easily fractured support, the support should instead be added to water and the fines eliminated by decantation. Many solid supports are commercially available in the required mesh range and are adequate for use as is.

Packing the Column

A well packed column should have a uniform distribution of closely packed solid particles (not crushed or fractured) to keep the pressure drop of carrier gas between the column's inlet and outlet at a minimum. One end of the clean, previously shaped tube is plugged with a gas-permeable material such as silanised glass wool or a thin metal fritted disk so that the packing material will remain in the tube. As the packing material is poured through a funnel temporarily attached to the open end, a full vacuum is applied to the plugged end while the column is tapped lightly and/or vibrated to facilitate proper settling. When no more material can be transferred into the column, it is assumed to be full and properly packed. Alternatively, 40–50 psig of inert gas or air can be applied to a specially designed reservoir (commercially available) containing the packing material. The reservoir is attached to the open end of the column, and the column is tapped or vibrated mildly until no more material is transferred into the column. Care should be taken not to disconnect any part of the apparatus until after the pressure is turned off and enough time has elapsed for the pressure to equilibrate to ambient conditions.

After the column has been packed, the open end is plugged with silanised glass wool or a fritted metal disk, and nuts and ferrules are attached to both ends (if they have not been attached previously) to provide for connection of the column to the instrument. (Special plasticised ferrules are available for glass columns).

Specialised details must be observed in packing certain types of supports. For example, only gently tapping or minimal vibration should be used for easily fractured solids; packed porous polymer beads, because of their shrinkage, should be conditioned in an oven for at least two hours at 25–50°C below the maximum recommended operating temperature with a slow carrier gas flow, followed by column removal and further packing.

Column Conditioning

After packing, all freshly prepared columns should be conditioned, primarily to eliminate various volatile impurities introduced by the coating and packing procedure or previously present in the liquid phase or solid support. Common impurities include water, unpolymerised monomeric species from which the liquid phase was synthesised, and solvents. Conditioning may also aid in achieving a more even distribution of the liquid phase throughout the packing material.

One end of the column, usually the one to which the packing was added, is attached to the inlet portion of the chromatograph while the other end is left unconnected in order not to contaminate or damage the detector.

Generally, the column, under low carrier gas flow, is heated gradually to 10–20°C above the expected operating temperature. The column is conditioned overnight at this temperature.

Certain liquid phases, require specialised treatment; for example, they may be conditioned initially for various time periods at specified temperatures with no carrier gas flow. To obtain accurate quantitative results, it is frequently necessary that certain other highly specialised and unique steps be taken. Several examples are presented below under determination.

Sample Preparation

One or more physical and/or chemical steps frequently must be taken in order to separate and isolate the components to be measured in the sample from the rest of the ingredients that may interfere with the analysis. It is also useful to concentrate the sample, especially when handling small quantities.

Reduced or ambient pressure distillation is helpful for the isolation or removal of volatile materials. The higher boiling sesquiterpene hydrocarbon portions, frequently present in small amounts in essential oils used in fragrance compositions, may be isolated along with other higher boiling compounds as the residue remaining after distillation of the more abundant, volatile terpene hydrocarbons. Such a residue is then separated further on alumina into sesquiterpene hydrocarbon fractions by liquid column chromatography. Azeotropic distillation is also useful. In this process, a liquid immiscible with the sample is added and the temperature is raised to the boiling point. The components of interest are quantitatively distilled over along with the immiscible liquid. This procedure is useful for the separation and isolation of propylene glycol from a variety of cosmetic products. In this case, iso-octane is the immiscible liquid of choice since one of the prerequisites for its selection is that only a minimum amount is required for quantitative transfer for the component of interest, propylene glycol.

Extraction with immiscible solvent systems is effective when selectivity is achieved for the ingredients of interest. Hexachlorophene is extracted from whole blood with an ether-alcohol (18 + 7) solution in a study of the extent of its penetration through mammalian skin. Glycerol is separated from most other ingredients in cosmetic creams through the addition of water (in which it is soluble) followed by extraction (and separation) of most other organic ingredients in the cream with chloroform or petroleum ether. Most cosmetic ingredients, except for highly polar water-soluble compounds such as glycerol, are soluble in these organic solvents. Glycerol is isolated from toothpastes or gums by extraction with 2-methoxyethanol, in which it is soluble. Any insoluble materials are separated by filtration of the extract.

The preparative liquid column chromatographic methods are also useful tools for separation and isolation. As indicated above, an alumina column is useful for fractionating various sesquiterpene hydrocarbon mixtures; a silica gel column is helpful for removing interfering hydrocarbons from fatty acid esters and alcohols determined in lipsticks.

The chemical reactivity of any functional group of a cosmetic ingredient may be useful for its retrieval from a mixture. The acidic (phenolic) nature of hexachlorophene, for example, facilitates its alkaline extraction from whole blood.

In headspace analysis, vapours of solutions of sufficiently volatile ingredients may be injected directly into the gas chromatograph without any need for elaborate sample clean-up or separation procedures. The sample is placed in an enclosed system so that an equilibrium of the component(s) is established between the gaseous and liquid phases. An aliquot of the vapour is then withdrawn through a septum or membrane covering and injected into the chromatograph. Cosmetics containing methanol, ethanol, or isopropanol, as well as chloroform in toothpastes, are easily handled by this technique. These ingredients can be identified and also determined by headspace analysis. A number of propellants and solvents found in aerosol hair spray formulations may also be identified.

In practice, the solute molecules not only partition between the two phases but may also be adsorbed by the so called "inert" solid support. Such an adverse effect may be significant even after the support has been "deactivated". The tendency toward adsorption on the active sites of the support is directly proportional to solute polarity, i.e., acids are adsorbed most readily, followed by phenols and amines. Adsorption, manifested in peak tailing, leads to incomplete separations and, in turn, to inaccurate qualitative and quantitative results. If such highly polar compounds are quantitatively converted to less polar derivatives not able to form hydrogen bonds with the stationary liquid phase and/or support, this problem can be minimised or eliminated. For example, phenols or alcohols are treated with acid anhydrides or azomethanes to form ester or ether derivatives, respectively. In addition, alkanoloamines, used as neutralisers for acidic polymer resins added to various aerosol hair spray formulations, are converted to their corresponding difunctional amide and acetate derivatives with acetic anhydride-pyridine $(2 + 1)$ reagent (if the amine is tertiary, only an acetate is formed).

Because high molecular weight compounds may have inordinately long retention times, it may be necessary to convert them, by chemical means, to lower molecular weight products which are more volatile and therefore more amenable to GLC. In some cases, these products may also have the potential, because of their high polarity, for being easily adsorbed on the support. Both problems are eliminated in an analysis of castor oil in lipsticks by the following technique : Castor oil, the relatively non-volatile triglyceride of ricinoleic acid, is converted by transesterification with a methanolbenzene-sulphuric acid solution (300 + 100 + 3.7) to glycerol and the methyl ester of ricinoleic acid. The amount of castor oil present is then determined by a GLC analysis for methyl ricinoleate. Multiple products from reactions such as this one also afford further confirmatory evidence for identification by the accumulation of additional retention time data. Mixtures of certain higher molecular weight isomeric fatty acid esters of fatty alcohols are difficult to separate; however, after transesterification with methanol, they become readily separable mixtures of fatty alcohols and methyl esters of fatty acids. The alcohols can be verified by acetylation. The alcohol peaks then disappear and retention times for the corresponding acetate peaks are obtained.

Detectors

In selecting a detector, points to consider are (1) sensitivity, (2) signal-to-noise ratio, (3) linearity, (4) stability, (5) specificity (range of application), and (6) destructive effect on the effluent (reactivity with the sample molecules). Thermal conductivity, flame ionisation, and electron capture detectors are used more frequently than other types in the GLC analysis of cosmetics.

Most common is the thermal conductivity detector in which a metallic filament, heated by the passage of a constant electrical potential, exhibits a given resistance which is subject to change when a corresponding change is induced in its environmental temperature. An inert carrier gas is diverted over two such heated filaments that are part of a Wheatstone bridge assembly. The heat loss from both filaments, maintained through a block set at constant temperature, is equal until a component is swept over one of them. At this point, the heat conductance away from this filament is affected, along with its temperature and resistance. The bridge circuit measures the difference in the electrical signal generated between the two filaments because of their difference in resistance and emits a signal which restores balance and indicates the presence of the solute. In order to achieve optimum sensitivity and wide linearly of response, the carrier gas should have a low molecular weight, high thermal conductivity and low viscocity. Helium is ideal in all these respects and is usually employed as the carrier gas when using a thermal conductivity detector. The thermal conductivity detector performs best with a high bridge current and low block temperature, and its performance may be adversely affected by carrier gas flow fluctuations or ambient temperature effects. This detector is less sensitive (about 1×10^{-9} g/second) than those discussed below.

In the flame ionisation detector, the organic vapour of the solute enters a flame supported by hydrogen and air, and it is converted to cationic species and free electrons. A gap between two electrodes with a difference in applied potential is oriented so as to monitor the current increase over that generated from background. This detector is destructive to the compounds measured and relatively insensitive to inorganic compounds such as water, hydrogen sulphide, carbon disulphide, and carbon dioxide; however, it is more sensitive to organic compounds (about 3×10^{-12} g/second) than the thermal conductivity detector. The presence of inorganic compounds may decrease the sensitivity of the flame ionisation detector to organic compounds. This detector has a wide linear response. Either nitrogen or belium may be used with it as a carrier gas because both (i) have small background conductivity–necessary for the detection of proportionately large currents produced by sample components; (ii) have minimal viscosity and (iii) are inert. Optimum sensitivity is dependent on carrier gas and combustion gas (hydrogen and air) flow rates.

The election capture detector is also dependent upon ionisation of the sample but, unlike the flame ionisation detector, it does not destroy the compounds measured. Certain types of vapour molecules, when bombarded with electrons, accept or "capture" them and become negatively charged. These highly energised electrons are emitted from a radioactive source, usually ^{63}Ni. The negatively charged molecules produced enter a gap between oppositely charged electrodes where a current has previously been established by ionisation of the carrier gas. When the negatively charged, slower moving components enter this gap, the current is diminished and the sample is detected accordingly. This detector is much more selective than those discussed above, since it detects only electron-accepting molecules containing halogen, sulphur, organo-metallic, phosphorus, or polyaromatic substituents. It is also the most sensitive of the three at about 3×10^{-14} g/second. Although nitrogen has been used as a carrier gas with electron capture detectors, it may foster other ionic mechanisms that may erroneously be attributed to electron capture. In order to avoid such effects, argon containing 5–10% (v/v) methane (sometimes butane) is used as carrier gas, and pulsed electrical waves are applied across the electrode gap.

Table 44.1 lists the range of operating temperatures chosen for each type of detector with corresponding injector and column temperature ranges selected from a cross-section dealing with the gas chromatographic analysis of cosmetic products and raw materials.

Table - 44.1

Operating temperature ranges (°C) for various types of detectors with accompanying injector and column temperatures[a].

	Thermal Conductivity	Flame Ionisation	Electron Capture
Detector[b]	240–320	190–300	300
Injector[b]	240–320	200–310	270–275
Column[c]	65–250	70–270	125–250

a Based on methods developed for the analysis of cosmetics and cosmetic raw materials.

b A selected isothermal temperature is chosen for any given analysis.

c Most temperatures are selected for isothermal runs within this range; some are a programmed span of temperatures from this range for a given analysis.

Identification

The time between injection of a sample onto the column and elution of a component represented by its peak on a chromatogram is known as the "retention time" of that component. Its reproduction is difficult because of many inherent variables associated with GLC. However, reproducible relative retention times may be calculated by adding a known compound, called an internal standard, to the sample and comparing the time it takes for emergence of this compound to that required for the unknown. Relative retention times are frequently expressed in terms of Kovats indices or McReynolds constants.

Many of the raw materials used in cosmetic products are complex mixtures of ingredients. A distinctive GLC peak pattern (fingerprint) may emerge based on the relative retention times of the various components. Comparison of these relative retention times with those of standard materials can be very helpful in identifying unknown constituents. For example, the sesquiterpene hydrocarbon fractions of many essential oils used in fragrance compositions contain characteristic identifiable combinations of specific sesquiterpene hydrocarbons which generate peaks that are representative of or unique for a given oil. Comparison is made of their peaks with those peaks from a similar fraction obtained from a standard oil.

Mere knowledge of the retention time of an ingredient does not provide confirmatory evidence of its identity. The pure unknown compound may be isolated by trapping as it elutes from the column and then subjected to various "wet" chemical or instrumental techniques to confirm its identity or elucidate its structure. Instrumental techniques frequently used for this purpose include ultraviolet and infrared spectrophotometry, fluorometry, nuclear magnetic resonance spectroscopy, mass spectromety, refractometry, and optical rotation (polarimetry and circular dichroism). Melting point and boiling point measurements are also useful. With mass spectrometry and, less often, infrared spectrophotometry, it is possible, and indeed common, to connect the instrument directly in series to the exit port of the GLC column via an interface which oviates trapping or handling of the compound.

Determination

The internal standard method is the preferred approach for GLC analysis of cosmetics because :

1. Errors which could arise from non-linear detector response are minimised.
2. Identical aliquots of the standard and sample solutions are not required for injection.
3. Identical concentrations of the sample and standard are not required. The standard is a volumertrically prepared solution consisting of a known concentration of a purified compound that is identical in structure to that to be determined in the sample. The internal standard is a compound different from the one being determined and should meet the following criteria : absent from the sample, miscible with the component to be determined in the chosen solvent system, pure, non-reactive with any chemical in the sample or solvent, and chemically and chemically and thermodynamically stable. The internal standard should also generate a symmetrical peak on the recorder with a retention time close to but not identical with that of the compound to be determined or any other constituent of the sample solution.

In applying the internal standard technique, a suitable volume of a known concentration of the internal standard is added to the sample solution containing all of the unknown constituent such that the peak heights generated by both in the resulting chromatogram are similar (within 10--25%). Increasing accuracy is usually assured as the ratio of peak heights approaches unity. Although each peak should be no less than 50% full scale on the recorder, 75–95% is preferred.

An identical (or similar) amount of internal standard is then added to a separate vessel into which an experimentally determined amount of the compound of interest from a standard solution containing only that compound has been added such that the peak height ratio of unknown to internal standard is similar to that in the sample solution. The total solution volume is adjusted so that it is similar to that of the sample solution containing the internal standard. The above criteria for peak heights and ratios also apply here.

Aliquots of each solution should be injected alternately at least twice so that all peak heights for the unknown in all chromatograms vary by less than ± 10%. An average value is obtained for the peak height ratios for each solution. Values which vary by more than 10% from this average should be rejected.

The percentage by weight of unknown in the sample may be calculated as follows :

% Unknown = [$R_u R_s$) x weight unknown in standard x

(weight internal standard in sample/weight internal standard in

standard)/weight of sample] x 100

Where R_s = average peak height ratio of sample solution (peak height unknown in sample/peak height internal standard in sample of several injetions), and R_s = average peak height ratio of standard solution (peak height unknown in standard/peak height internal standard in standard of several injections).

If possible, all determinations should be made on the same day in order to minimise instrumental errors resulting from carrier gas flow rate change, temperature deviations, detector response variables, etc. It is also best to work at the same attenuation and range settings of the instrument for both sample and standard solutions throughout the determination.

Two examples of potential errors that may arise in internal standard analyses are illustrated : In the headspace determination of chloroform in toothpaste, the difference in absorption by the rubber dam and smaller concentration (10%) of the 1, 1, 1-trichloroethane internal standard compared to the choloroform necessitates that all measurements be made over a short time span before peak ratios change drastically, Second, the peak response for ethanol may vary because of the dependence of this response on the time between emergence of the internal standard from the previous injection and the injection of the current ethanol sample. This phenomenon, caused by support adsorption, requires injection of all ethanol samples at a preset time differential.

ANALYSIS OF CREAMS AND LOTIONS

Three types of ingredients are essential in the formulation of cosmetic emulsions. One ingredient is water. Another is "fatty" or water-insoluble material such as beeswax, spermaceti, hydrocarbons, lanolin, fatty acids, alcohols of high molecular weight, glycerides, isopropyl myrisate, etc. The third essential ingredient is a surface active agent that emulsifies the water and "fatty" material. Some common emulsifiers are soaps, glyceryl monostearate, alkyl sulphates, lanolin, quaternary ammonium salts, and polyoxyethylene compounds.

Because these products are either water-in-oil or oil-in-water types of emulsions, they can, in most cases, be analysed in a similar manner.

GENERAL ANALYSIS

Net Contents

1. If the product is a cream, weigh the intact container at the beginning of the analysis. After the analysis is completed, remove any remaining sample and weigh the empty container. Calculate the weight of the product by difference.

2. If the product is a lotion, mark the outside of the bottle at the surface level of the liquid before beginning the analysis. Upon completing the analysis, empty the bottle and note the volume of water required to fill it to the mark.

3. For aerosol products in metallic containers, weigh the intact container, chill in a dry ice chest for 2 hours, and punch out the top of the chilled container with a cold chisel and hammer.

    (a) If contents are liquid, pour out the contents and weigh the parts of the container together. Calculate the contents by difference.

    (b) If contents are solid, place the opened can with the frozen material in a 4 L beaker and let it warm to room temperature. Decant the liquefied contents and proceed as in above.

Description of Product

Note colour, odour, and other physical characteristics of the product.

Type of Emulsion

1. Smear a thin film of the product, ca 1" square by about 1/16" thick, on a watch glass. Sprinkle small amounts of a finely ground oil-soluble dye and a water-soluble dye on separate areas of the film. Spreading of the oil-soluble dye indicates a water-in-oil emulsion; spreading of the water-soluble dye indicates an oil-in-water emulsion.

2. As an alternative procedure, determine the type of emulsion by noting whether a portion of the product readily mixes with mineral oil (w/o emulsion) or water (o/w emulsion).

3. Another procedure involves electrical conductivity, as follows :

"Equipment for this may be easily constructed by wiring in series a 30,000 ohm 1/2-watt resistor, electric contacts for the test sample, a resistorless neon lamp (1/4-watt 104 to 120 v.), and a push-button switch. The sample is placed across the test contacts and the circuit is closed. If the neon lamp glows, the emulsion is o/w; if it does not, the emulsion is w/o. There are occasions when the lamp will glow dimly or will start to glow upon continued application of the electric current. This usually indicates either a dual emulsion or a gradual inversion of the emulsion. The presence of electrolytes, particularly at high levels, may result in conductivity even though the emulsion is essentially w/o."

pH of Emulsion

1. For o/w cream emulsions, mix 1 g of cream with 9 ml of water and determine the pH of the resulting mixture with a glass electrode instrument. Report the pH (1 part cream plus 9 parts water).
2. For o/w lotion emulsions, determine the pH directly on the liquid.
3. Alternatively, determine the approximate pH of (a) and/or (b) with short range pH test paper.

Ashing at 600°C

Weigh about 5 g of the product in a flat-bottom platinum dish and heat on the steam bath under a jet of air for 1 hour. Remove the dish and add 1 g of ashless cellulose powder, then mix with a glass stirring rod. Wipe any adhering material from the stirring rod with a piece of filter paper and add the paper to the dish. Heat the dish under an infrared (IR) heating lamp until the sample is charred. Complete ashing at 600°C in a muffle oven.

Examination of Ash

1. *Borates* – Mix a portion of ash with a few drops of H_2SO_4 in a platinum dish, add several ml of methanol, stir well, place in a darkened hood; and ignite. A green flame indicates the presence of boron.
2. *Carbonates* – Mix a portion of ash with a drop of HCl. An odourless effervescence indicates the presence of carbonates.
3. *Other water-soluble salts* – Dissolve the remainder of the ash in water or dilute HNO_3, filter off any insoluble material, and test aliquots of the filtrate for chlorides with $AgNO_3$, for sulphates with $BaCl_2$, and for phosphates with ammonium molybdate. Also check for Na and K by platinum wire flame tests.
4. *Water-insoluble ash* (Commonly TiO_2, ZnO, or talc) – ignite the ash in a platinum crucible. The appearance of a yellow colour that

fades on cooling indicates the possible presence of ZnO. Dissolve the ZnO in acid and precipitate as ZnS for confirmatory test.

Solubilise TiO_2 by heating in a covered porcelain crucible with 8 ml of H_2SO_4 and 4 g of Na_2SO_4. Cool and carefully pour the solution into 50 ml of ice-cold water. Test for titanium colorimetrically with H_2O_2.

Fuse talc with a 1 + 10 mixture of Na_2CO_3 and K_2CO_3 and test for magnesium and silica.

5. *Infrared spectrum of ash* – Prepare a mineral oil mull or KBr disk of the ash and obtain its infrared spectrum. This spectrum is helpful in identifying the nature of the ash.

6. *X-ray fluorescence spectroscopy* – Elements with atomic numbers equal to or greater than that of aluminum can readily be identified by X-ray fluorescence spectroscopy.

Non-volatile Matter at 105°C

Weigh about 1 g of the product into a large weighing bottle and heat on a steam bath under a jet of air for 30 minutes. Continue heating at 105°C in an oven for 2 hours. Cool in a desiccator, weigh, and report as non-volatile matter (2 hours at 105°C).

Infrared Examinations of Non-volatile Matter

Smear a film of the non-volatile matter on a salt crystal and obtain the IR spectrum of the film. Examine this spectrum carefully for clues to the composition of the sample. The positions of the absorbance peaks indicate the identity of the ingredients present; the absorbance values indicate the relative amounts of the various components present.

In particular, look for the presence of esters, hydrocarbons, alcohol polyhydroxy compounds, polyoxyethylene compounds, amides, soaps fatty acids, and alkanolamines.

Chloroform-Extractable Matter

This extraction is applicable to soap emulsions such as the beeswax-borax, alkanolamine, glyceryl monostearate, and alkali metal types. The emulsification of the $CHCl_3$ may preclude its use with creams emulsified by other surface active agents.

1. Transfer about 3 g of sample to a separatory funnel with 50 ml of water, strongly acidify with HCl, and extract with four 35 ml portions of $CHCl_3$. Combine the $CHCl_3$ extracts wash with 10 ml of water, and add the washing to the reserved extracted aqueous solution. Filter the $CHCl_3$ extracts through a cotton plug into a tared 250 ml

beaker, evaporate the solvent on a steam bath under a jet of air, and dry the residue at 105°C in an oven for 15 minutes. Cool in a desiccator and weigh as $CHCl_3$-extractable matter.

2. Test $CHCl_3$-extractable matter for lanolin or sterols, or both, by the Liebermann-Burchard reaction:

    Dissolve a small portion of the material in 10 ml of $CHCl_3$, add 5 ml of acetic anhydride and follow with 5–10 drops of H_2SO_4. Stir well. The appearance of a characteristic green colour indicates the presence of lanolin or sterols.

3. Obtain an IR spectrum of a film of the $CHCl_3$-extractable matter and examine the spectrum to ascertain what material may be present.

Material Not Extractable by Chloroform from Acid Aqueous Solution

1. *Total non-extractable matter* – Dilute the reserved extracted aqueous solution from above to 100 ml with water in a volumetric flask. Pipet out a 40 ml aliquot into a tared 100 ml beaker and evaporate the water on a steam bath under a jet of air. Dry the residue at 105°C in an oven for 10 minutes, cool in a desiccator, and weigh as non-extractable matter.

    (a) Obtain an IR spectrum of a film of the material and note whether a polyhydroxy compound or an alkanolamine hydrochloride (usually triethanolamine) or both may be present.

    (b) As an additional test for alkanolamine, add excess *n*-propyl alcohol to the residue in a beaker, boil to a small volume, chill, scratch the sides of the beaker with a glass rod to induce crystallisation, filter off the crystals, and dry. Determine the melting point of the crystals of alkanolamine hydrochloride or obtain an IR film spectrum of a mineral oil mull of the crystals.

2. *Chemical test for glycerol* – Neutralise a 10 ml aliquot of the extracted aqueous solution, (a), to methyl red with CO_2-free $0.1N$ NaOh, making the final adjustment with $0.02N$ NaOH and leaving the solution just barely yellow. Add 30 ml of $0.02M$ KIO_4 and stir well. If the red colour of methyl red appears immediately, glycerol, is probably present.

    (c) *Additional chemical test for glycerol* – place 3 ml of the aqueous solution containing glycerol in a large test tube. Add 3 ml of freshly prepared 10% catechol solution, then 6 ml of H_2SO_4. Heat in boiling water for 30 minutes. An orange-red colour indicates the presence of glycerol.

Saponification of Chloroform-Extractable Matter

1. Reflux the $CHCl_3$-extractable matter for 2 hours with 25 ml of 95% alcohol, 1 g of KOH, and 50 ml of benzene. Transfer the saponified mixture to a separatory funnel (with Teflon or ungreased glass stopcock), add 50 ml of hot water, shake well, and draw off the aqueous layer. Continue the extraction with two additional 50 ml portions of hot benzene. Reserve the extracted aqueous solution. Combine the benzene extracts, and wash with three 30 ml portions of 30% alcohol, shaking very gently with the first washing and more vigorously with the other two. Add the washings to the reserved extracted aqueous solution. Filter the washed benzene extract through a cotton plug into a 250 ml tared beaker, evaporate the benezene on the steam bath, and dry the residue at 105°C in an oven for 15 minutes. Cool and weigh as unsaponifiable matter. Obtain its IR Spectrum.

2. Acidify the reserved aqueous solution (a) with HCl and extract with three 30 ml of portions of $CHCl_3$. Reserve the extracted aqueous solution and use it to test for combined glycerol and a polyxyethylene compound. Wash the combined $CHCl_3$ extracts with water. Filter the washed $CHCl_3$ extract through a cotton plug into a tared 250 ml beaker, evaporate the $CHCl_3$ on the steam bath under a jet of air, dry the residue at 105°C in an oven for 15 minutes, cool, and weigh as fatty acids.

Examination of the Saponifiable Matter

1. Equivalent weight of fatty acids – Dissolve saponifiable matter in 50 ml of alcohol that has been neutralised to phenolphthalein with 0.1 N alkali. Titrate with 0.1 N NaOH to a phenolphthalein end point. Calculate the equivalent weight of fatty acids.

2. Hanus iodine absorption number.

Hydrocarbons and Alcohols in Unsaponifiable Matter

Dissolve the unsaponifiable matter in 50 ml of boiling heptane and cool the solution to room·temperature with stirring.

1. If there is any precipitated matter, filter the resulting mixture through filter paper, wash the residue well with petroleum ether, and reserve the filtrate. Dissolve the residue by pouring hot $CHCl_3$ through the filter paper, and evaporate the $CHCl_3$ on the steam bath. Dry at 105°C in an oven for 10 minutes, cool in a desiccator, let stand in air 10 minutes, and weigh as alcohols insoluble in heptane-petroleum ether.

Evaporate the reserved heptane-petroleum ether solution on the steam bath and take up the residue in 50 ml of warm petroleum ether (b.p., 30–75°C). Transfer the solution, with the aid of 25 ml of petroleum ether, to a glass chromatographic tube holding a 9 x 3/4" activated alumina column (Alcoa grade F–20, 80–200 mesh), and let the solution flow through the column at a rate of 3–5 ml/minute, collecting the petroleum ether eluates in a 400 ml beaker. Follow this solution with 175 ml of petroleum ether. Reserve the petroleum ether eluate.

Remove the petroleum ether from the column by passing 50 ml of 95% alcohol through the column under air pressure. Then, again using air pressure, force 125 ml of boiling alcohol through the column at a rapid rate (4–7 minutes for 125 ml). Collect these two eluates in a tared 250 ml beaker labelled *First Hot Alcohol Fraction*. Pass another 50 ml of boiling alcohol through the column and collect it in a tared 250 ml beaker labelled *Second* Evaporate each of the hot alcohol fractions to dryness on the steam bath under a jet of air, redissolve the residue in 10 ml of $CHCl_3$, and evaporate to dryness again. Dry the residue at 105°C in an oven for 10 minutes, cool and weigh as alcohols soluble in heptane-petroleum ether.

Evaporate the reserved petroleum ether eluate to about 50 ml on the steam bath under a jet of air, transfer to a tared 250 ml of beaker with 50 ml of petroleum ether, and evaporate the solvent on the steam bath. The residue will be hydrocarbons. Dry at 105°C in an oven for 10 minutes, cool, and weigh. Obtain an IR film spectrum of the hydrocarbons.

(b) If there is no precipitated matter, evaporate the heptane solution on the steam bath and proceed as in (a), beginning "take up the residue in 50 ml of warm petroleum ether...."

Examination of Alcohols in Unsaponifiable Matter

(a) Obtain the IR spectra of the alcohols.

(b) Combine all alcohol fractions and determine the solubility of the combined fractions in cold methanol to aid in identifying the wax.

Weigh a sample not exceeding 0.5 g into a 150 ml beaker, add 80 ml of methanol, cover the beaker with a watch glass, and heat on a hot plate until solution is complete. Transfer the beaker to an ice bath and stir the solution vigorously with a thermometer until the temperature is 5°C. Pour the resulting mixture through a 4" Buchner funnel containing an 11 cm No. 595 S & S filter paper, with 1/2" of the edge turned up, wetted with methanol. Filter by gravity or gentle suction. Do not allow the material on the filter to dry or cake. Wash the residue with 20 ml of ice-chilled methanol and drain it dry with suction. Transfer the filtrate to a tared beaker with the aid of $CHCl_3$, evaporate to dryness on the steam bath, heat at 100°C in an oven for 10 minutes, cool in a desiccator, and weigh. Repeat the drying in the oven until the weight is constant to 1–2 mg. Table 44.2 gives the results obtained with beeswax alcohols.

Table 44.2
Solubility of beeswax alcohols in cold methanol[a]

Sample, g	Soluble Alcohols, g	Insoluble Alcohols, g (By Difference)
0.1	0.027	0.073
0.2	0.040	0.160
0.3	0.045	0.255
0.4	0.054	0.346
0.5	0.062	0.438

a A 0.500 g sample of spermaceti alcohols contains a maximum of 0.008 g of insoluble alcohols (10).

Composition of Chloroform-Extractable Matter

1. *Hydrocarbons* – For direct and easy identification of hydrocarbons, determine their IR spectra.

2. *Fatty acids* – If the IR spectrum of the $CHCl_3$- extractable material indicates only fatty acids, no further analysis is necessary and the IR spectrum of the non-volatile matter will probably have the characteristic absorption maximum of soap at about 6.5 μm.

    The presence of saponifiable matter but no unsaponifiable matter suggests several possibilities. The fatty acids may have originally been present as a triglyceride, a monoglyceride, the ester of some other polyhydroxy compound, or the ester of a water-soluble alcohol such as isopropyl alcohol.

3. *Waxes* – Some of the more common waxes such as spermaceti, beeswax, and lanolin contain roughly equal amounts of saponifiable and unsaponifiable matter. If the IR spectrum of the $CHCl_3$- extractable matter indicates that only esters and possibly hydrocarbons are present, and if the amounts of fatty alcohols and acids are approximately equal, it may be assumed that the waxes are equal to the sum of the alcohols and fatty acids.

Testing of Cosmetics 210

Some indications as to the types of waxes may be obtained from the IR spectra, the equivalent weight of the fatty acids, the solubility of the alcohols in methanol, and a test for lanolin.

4. *Waxes plus other materials* – If both saponifiable fatty acids and unsaponifiable alcohols are present in unequal amounts, there are several possibilities. If the alcohols greatly exceed the acids, multiply the weight of the acids by two and calculate the resulting value as waxes. Subtract the weight of acids from the weight of alcohols and calculate the remaining value as free alcohols. (It is assumed that the IR spectrum of the material before saponification indicates esters and alcohols.) Conversely, if the fatty acids exceed the alcohols, multiply the weight of alcohols by two to obtain a value for waxes. Calculate the unassigned fatty acids as free fatty acids, soap, or some fatty acid compound which has no unsaponifiable matter. (Again, reliance is placed on the IR spectra and chemical tests).

5. *Charts* – A diagrammatic summary of the analysis of mixtures of hydrocarbons, beeswax, and spermaceti is presented in Figs. 44.1, 44.2 and 44.3. With suitable modifications this scheme is applicable to the analysis of most "fatty materials" or their mixtures.

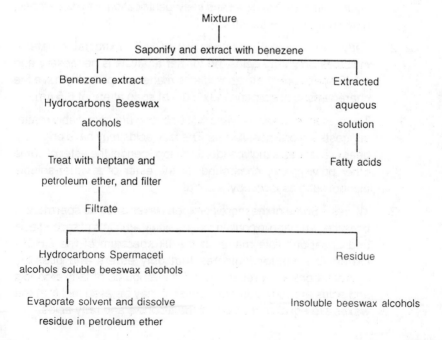

Fig. 44.1 Preparation of a mixture of hydrocarbons, beeswax, and spermaceti for chromatography.

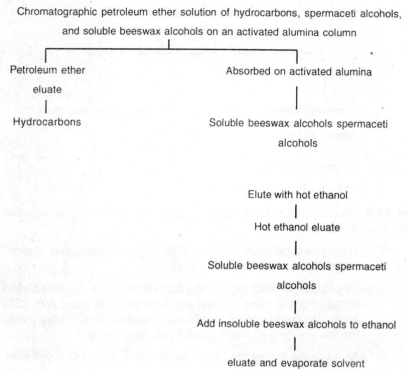

Fig. 44.2 Chromatography of hydrocarbons, spermaceti alcohols, and soluble beeswax alcohols.

Other Solvent Extraction Procedures

1. In attempting to isolate materials from products by immiscible solvent extraction, the successive use of solvents other than $CHCl_3$ is very helpful. In general, the selectivity of solvents for organic materials decreases in the following order : petroleum ether, carbon tetrachloride, benzene, ether, ethyl acetate, and $CHCl_3$. The correct adjustment of pH of the aqueous solution being extracted often ensures a successful extraction.

Testing of Cosmetics 212

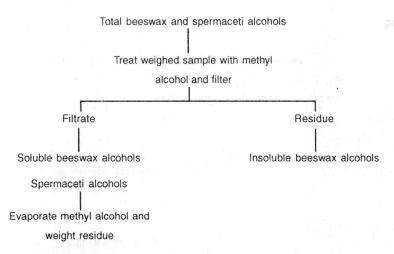

Fig. 44.3 Solubility of combined total beeswax and spermaceti alcohols in cold methyl alcohol.

2. The system petroleum ether – 80% methanol separates organic compounds on the basis of polarity.

3. Ethyl ether does not extract fatty acids from a 25% alcohol solution containing 1% KOH. In washing such ether extracts with 25% alcohol to remove alkali, shake with the dilute alcohol very gently for first washing to avoid emulsification.

4. Non-volatile matter may often be directly extracted by solvents.

5. A useful procedure is partition chromatography with a silicon-coated Celite; heptane and aqueous alcohol solutions are used as the immiscible solvents.

Adsorption Chromatography on silica Gel in Analysis of Isolated Fatty Materials

Mixtures consisting of extracted organic compounds are often best separated by adsorption chromatography on silica gel using eluants of increasing polarity. This technique, employing solvents ranging in polarity from iso-octane to methanol, is usually applicable to mixtures of materials increasing in polarity from aliphatic hydrocarbons to highly ethoxylated compounds or polyols.

1. *Preparation of silica gel column* – Insert a small glass wool plug into the bottom of a 24 x 1/2" id glass chromatographic tube, stopper the bottom of the tube with a rubber policeman, and fill with 20–30 ml of iso-octane. Slurry 10 g of silica gel with 30 ml of iso-octane, pour ca half of the slurry into the chromatographic tube, remove

the rubber policeman, and pack the column by applying 5–6 psi pressure to the tube. Do not permit the solvent to drain below the surface of the silica gel at any time during the analysis. Add the remainder of the slurry to the tube and pack as before.

2. *Sample addition* – Accurately weigh ca 200 mg of material, dissolve or disperse in 20 ml of hot iso-octane, transfer the hot solution to the chromatographic tube, and elute at the rate of 1/2 to 1 ml/minute. Regulate all flow rates by gravity or application of air pressure to the tube. Collect all eluates in 20 ml fractions in consecutively numbered, tared 50 ml beakers. Rinse sample beaker with two 10 ml portions of hot iso-octane, allowing each rinsing to elute separately at a flow rate of 2 ml/minute.

3. *Column elution* – Increase the flow rate to 3 ml/minute and continue the elution with the following solvents in the order indicated: 80 ml of iso-octane; 100 ml of ether-iso-octane (1 + 19); 100 ml of ether-iso-octane (1 + 9); 100 ml of ether-iso-octane (1 + 3); 200 ml of ether-iso-octane (1 + 1); 200 ml of ether; and 100 ml of methanol.

4. *Analysis of eluates* – Evaporate the eluates on the steam bath under a jet of air and heat the residues at 105°C for 10 minutes in a drying oven. Cool and weigh the residues.

   Plot as a bar graph the weight of the residues as the ordinate against the corresponding eluate numbers as abscissa. Indicate on the bar graph the eluant for each residue.

   The plot will consist of $\geq$ 1 peak. Choose the largest residue in each peak and obtain its infrared film spectrum. Use the IR spectra to characterise the residues.

   It is worth noting that the interpretation of the IR spectra by visual inspection could occasionally be in error. For this reason it may sometimes be necessary to compare the eluting pattern of the isolated component to that of the suspected raw material.

Determination of Water by Toluene Distillation

Transfer a 10–20 g sample to a 250 ml Erlenmeyer flask and add 50 ml of toluene and a few glass beads. Connect the flask to a Dean & Stark distilling tube receiver, and distill until no more water collects in the receiver. Cool read the volume of water under the toluene at room temperature, and from this volume calculated the percentage of water.

Examination of Aqueous Fraction from Toluene Distillation

1. *Specific gravity or density* – Determine with a small specific gravity bottle, or pipet 2 ml into a weighing bottle and weigh.

2. *Propylene glycol*

(a) Transfer 3 ml of an aqueous solution of propylene glycol to a large test tube, and add 3 ml of freshly prepared 10% catechol solution and then 6 ml of H_2SO_4. Heat in boiling water for 30 minutes. If the solution turns red and a precipitate forms, propylene glycol is present.

(b) To several ml of solution add 5 ml of $0.02M$ KIO_4. After 1 minute add an excess of 5% alkali followed by $0.1N$ I_2 solution. If a precipitate of iodoform forms immediately, propylene glycol is present.

Silicons in Creams

The IR spectra of silicons are very characteristic, but often the silicons are present in such small percentages that they are easily overlooked in the IR spectra of the product. Some selective separation is necessary. The extraction procedures used in the course of the analysis may concentrate the silicon enough so that it can be recognised. One of a number of special procedures for silicons is as follows:

Shake the emulsion with twice its volume of (1 + 1) dioxane-toluene mixture, centrifuge, and draw off the top layer, which is mostly toluene containing the silicon plus a small amount of organic material. Evaporate the toluene. Examine the IR film spectrum of the residue for the presence of a silicon.

Determination of Esters of *p*-Hydroxybenzoic Acid

Esters of *p*-hydroxybenzoic acid can be isolated from emulsion products by partition chromatography and determined by ultraviolet uv spectrophotometry. The *p*-hydroxybenzoates are quantitatively eluted by the acidified 10% alcohol eluate and are determined as combined esters of *p*-hydroxybenzoic acid.

Emulsifiers

1. *Beeswax-borax w/o cream* gives positive tests for boron and sodium in ash; it contains less than 35% water.

2. *Beeswax-borax o/w cream* gives positive tests for boron and sodium in ash; the pH of a mixture of 1 part cream plus 9 parts water is usually between 8 and 9.

3. *Soap o/w cream* has the following characteristics: the pH of a mixture of 1 part cream plus 9 parts water is usually between 8 and 9; a Na_2CO_3 **ash** is obtained; the water content is over 70%;

the IR absorption maximum of the soap may be discerned at about 6.5 µm in the spectrum of the non-volatile matter; and glycerol or other polyhydroxy compounds are probably present.

4. *Triethanolamine-soap o/w cream* yields no ash; the pH of a mixture of 1 part cream plus 9 parts water is usually between 7 and 8; the water content is over 70%; the IR absorption maximum of soap may be observed at about 6.5 µm in the spectrum of the non-volatile matter; glycerol or other polyhydroxy compounds are likely to be present; and triethanolamine will be found in the acid aqueous solution after extraction by $CHCl_3$.

5. *Glyceryl monostearate-soap o/w cream* gives a positive test for combined glycerol; more than 60% water is present; and glyceryl monostearate may be detected in the IR spectrum of the $CHCl_3$-extractable matter.

It may be possible to isolate some of the glyceryl monostearate by dissolving the $CHCl_3$- extractable matter in hot heptane and chilling the solution in an ice bath. Remove any precipitated glyceryl monostearate and identify by an IR film spectrum.

AEROSOL PRODUCTS

1. Analyse the product that emerges from the pressurised can. The propellant dissipates almost immediately and is not available for analysis.

2. To identify a halogenated propellant, spray a small amount of product into a suction flask and immediately stopper the top of the flask. Allow the gases emerging from the side arm of the flask to flow into a cell suitable for determination of spectra of gases. Obtain the IR spectrum of propellant, and identify. If the concentration of propellant in the gas cell is too great, remove the excess with a pipet fitted with a rubber bulb.

(If too much of the product is released into the suction flask, the flask becomes chilled, and only the more volatile constituent of the propellant vapourises).

ANALYSIS OF LIPSTICKS

A lipstick generally consists of a moulded, solid fatty base containing dissolved coal-tar dyes and suspended pigments. The base is usually composed of waxes, oils, and fatty material; typical ingredients might include carnauba wax, candelilla wax, beeswax, hydrocarbons, castor oil oleyl alcohol, butyl stearate, polyethylene glycols, Propylene glycol, lanolin, and cocoa butter.

Testing of Cosmetics

The characteristics and quantity of the waxes present in the lipstick determine the gloss and hardness of the product. The oils are selected primarily on the basis of their solvent effects on the fluorescein dyes. Oils may account for more than half the total weight of the lipstick. The fatty material gives the lipstick film more body, softens the skin of the lips, and promotes the dispersion of insoluble pigments.

Dyes, including the fluoresceins, are used predominantly to stain the lips; lakes and other pigments are used for their brightening and covering effects. A typical product may contain as much as 10% lakes and other pigments and only 2-3% pure dyes in a fatty base. The use of colour additives in lipsticks is regulated by the Food and Drug Administration.

Because of the tendency of all oil-fat-wax mixtures to decompose rapidly, antioxidants and preservatives are added to lipsticks to prevent rancidity and deterioration. Flavours are also added to camouflage any unpleasant fatty taste and odours of the base.

General Analysis

Determine net content, non-volatile matter, ash and infrared spectra as described earlier. Note: colour, odour and other physical characteristics of the lipstick.

Lakes and Fillers

Accurately weigh 0.25-0.30 g of lipstick into a 100 ml beaker. Add 10 ml of trichloroethylene, cover with a watch glass, and heat on the steam bath to dissolve hydrocarbons, waxes etc. Filter the warm mixture under vacuum into a 250 ml suction flask through a tared. Gooch crucible containing double glass fibre filter disks for extra fine precipitates. To prevent contamination of the solvent by rubber fittings, wrap the Gooch crucible with a piece of Al foil so that the foil projects slightly below the bottom of the crucible. Wash the beaker and Gooch crucible with five 5 ml portions of trichloroethylene, followed by 5 ml portions of acetone until the washings are colourless or nearly colourless. Reserve the filtrate for determination by 5.7. Dry the crucible in an oven at 105°C for 2 hours, cool in a desiccator, let stand in air for 10 minutes, and weigh as lakes and fillers.

Trichloroethylene-Acetone Solubles

Transfer the reserved filtrate in the suction flask from above into a tared 100 ml beaker, using two 5 ml portions of trichloroethylene and two 5 ml portions of acetone. Evaporate the solvents on the steam bath under a gentle jet of air. Add 10-15 ml of $CHCl_3$ to the beaker, cover with a watch glass, and reflux on the steam bath until the sides of the beaker are free of any adhering material. Remove the watch glass and evaporate to dryness on the steam bath under a gentle jet of air. Dry the beaker in an oven at 105°C for 15 minutes, cool in a desiccator, let stand in air for 10 minutes, and weigh as trichloroethylene-acetone solubles. This fraction contains all of the ingredient of the lipstick except lakes, fillers, and volatile materials. Reserve for determination of trichloro ethylene - acetene soluble and lenolin or sterols.

Chromatographic Analysis of Trichloroethylene-Acetone Solubles

Prepare silica gel column, introduce the sample and carry out elution as per the process described earlier.

Treatment of eluates—Evaporate the eluates on the steam bath under a jet of air and heat the residues in an oven at 105°C for 10 minutes. Cool in a desiccator and weigh the residues. Obtain an IR spectrum of each residue, using the smallest amount possible to obtain the spectrum. Use the spectra to characterise the residues as containing aliphatic hydrocarbons, liquid or solid alcohols, castor oil, and esters, including isopropyl esters, acetates, etc. Reserve the residues.

Gas-Liquid Chromatographic (GLC) Determination of Castor Oil

1. *Apparatus*

    (a) Gas chromatograph—with hydrogen flame detector. Operating conditions: temperatures (°C) – detector 235, injection port 300, column 235; helium carrier gas flow rate, 85 ml/minute.

    (b) GLC column –6' x 4 mm id glass tube backed with 100-120 mesh Chromosorb W HP coated with 5% SP- 2100. Coated the support with the liquid phase by the funnel coating procedure. Condition the column overnight at 250°C with a helium flow rate of ca 10 ml/minute.

    (c) Refluxing apparatus – All glass, with T24/40 joints, consisting of 100 ml round-bottom flask and water-cooled refluxing condenser, heated with an electric heating mantle.

2. *Reagents*

    (a) Transesterification mixture – Menthol-benzene-sulphuric acid (3+1+0.037). Prepare fresh every 2 or 3 days.

    (b) Dicyclohexyl phthalate internal standard solution–20 mg/ml. Accurately weigh ca 1 g of dicyclohexyl phthalate in a 50 ml volumetric flask, and dilute to volume with toluene.

    (c) Methyl ricinoleate standard solution – 209 mg/ml. Purify ether-extractable methyl ricionleate by adsorption chromatography as follows: Tamp a small glass wool plug into the bottom of a 24 x 1/4" id glass chromatographic tube. Fill the tube with ca 100 ml of $CHCl_3$. Slurry 40g of silica gel in 100 ml of $CHCl_3$ and pack half of the slurry in the tube under 5-6 psi of air pressure. In this and subsequent steps, do not let the solvent drain below the surface of the silica gel. Pack the remainder of the slurry as before. Dissolve the ether extract of the methyl ricinoleate in 40 ml of hot $CHCl_3$ and add to the chromatographic column. Rinse the beaker with two 20 ml portions of hot $CHCl_3$ and add to the column after eluting the initial solution. Continue eluting the column with 120 ml of $CHCl_3$ and 200 ml of $CHCl_3$-ether (9+1). Discard the $CHCl_3$ eluate and collect the $CHCl_3$-ether (9+1) eluate in 25 ml portions in tared 50 ml beakers. Evaporate the eluates on the steam bath under a gentle jet of air, and dry the residues in an oven at 105°C for 5 minutes. Cool and weigh the residues. Combine the 4 largest residues and rechromatography as before. Again combine the 4 largest residues and reserve. Accurately weigh ca 1 g of residue in a 50 ml volumetric flask, and dilute to volume with toluene.

3. *Transesterification* – Accurately weigh a 200-300 mg lipstick sample into a tared 100 ml round-bottom boiling flask. Add 20 ml of transesterification mixture and 3 glass beads to the flask. Connect the flask to water-jacketed reflux condenser with a 24/40 male joint. Attach a heating mantle and adjust the voltage on the power source so that the solution in the flask boils gently. Reflux the solution for 2½ hours. Cool the condenser and rinse with 10 ml of water. Transfer the transesterification mixture and rinse into a 125 ml separatory funnel. Rinse the condenser and boiling flask with an additional 10 ml of water and add to the seperatory funnel. Rinse the condenser and flask with 25 ml of ether, transfer the rinsing to the funnel, and shake well. Draw off the lower aqueous layer into a second 125 ml separatory funnel and extract with 20 ml of ether. Discard the water layer. Combine the two ether extracts, rinse the second 125 ml separatory funnel with a small amount of ether, and add to the ether extracts. Wash the combined ether extracts with three 5 ml portions of water and discard the wash each time. Filter the ether extracts through a cotton plug washed with 20 ml of ether into a 125 ml Erlenmeyer flask. Rinse the separator with two 5 ml portions of ether, and filter the rinsings through the cotton plug. Wash the plug with 20 ml of ether. Reduce the volume of ether to 30-40 ml by evaporating under a gentle jet of air, and reserve the remainder for (4)

4. *Determination* – Add 1 ml of dicyclohexyl phthalate internal standard solution to the reserved ether extract from (c). Inject 2-5 µl of sample

solution into the gas chromatograph. Adjust the operating conditions to elute the methyl ricinoleate peak in ca 8-10 minutes. Compare the peak heights of the sample and internal standard, and, if necessary, add 1.0 ml aliquots of dicyclohexyl phthalate internal standard solution until the ratio of sample peak height most nearly approaches 1.

Prepare a standard solution containing 6.0 ml of dicyclohexyl phthalate internal standard solution and 4.0 ml of methyl ricinoleate standard solution, and inject 2-5 µl into the gas chromatograph. Compare the peak heights and, if necessary, add 1.0 ml aliquots of standard solution or internal standard solution so that the ratio of peak heights most nearly approaches that obtained before for the sample (ca 1).

Inject a 2-5 µl aliquot of standard solution and adjust the range and attenuation to keep the peaks from 60 to 95% of full scale. Under the conditions determined previously, alternately inject 2-5 µl aliquots of the standard and sample solutions, making a minimum of 2 injections of each.

Calculate the peak height rations at follows :

R_u = peak height of sample methyl ricinoleate/peak height of dicyclohexyl phthalate

R_s = peak height of standard methyl ricinoleate/peak height of dicyclohexyl phthalate

Neither R_u nor R_s values from each set of injections should differ by > 5%. Determine average values of R_u and R_s, and calculate the amount of methyl ricinoleate in the sample as follows :

Methyl ricinoleate, mg

$= (R_u/R_s) \times M \times (I_s/I')$,

Where M= mg methyl ricinoleate in standard, I_s = mg internal standard in sample, and I' = mg internal standard in standard.

The castor oil content of the lipstick can be estimated by dividing the methyl ricinoleate content by a factor of 0.9.

ANALYSIS OF SHAMPOOS

Every shampoo contains one or more surface active agents. In commercial preparations the two most widely used surfactants are soaps and alkyl sulphates. They may be salts of either alkali metals or alkanolamines. The vehicle for the surface active agent is ordinarily water. Many other materials are used in conjunction with the surfactant to sequester cations, control the viscosity of a liquid product, and alter the characteristics of the foam; or to serve as hair conditioners, bacteriostats, opacifiers, etc.

Some of these materials are lanolin, the Versenes, water-soluble gums, hexachlorophene, fatty acid-alkanolamine condensates, polyoxyethylene compounds, alcohols of high molecular weight, hydrocarbons, and inorganic salts.

General Analysis

Net Contents

1. At the begining of the examination, mark the outside of bottle at the surface level of the liquid. At the end of the examination, empty the bottle and note the volume of water required to fill it to the mark.

2. Determine net content, pH, ash at 600°C, distillation examination of ash, non-volatile matter and water by toluene using the procedure described earlier.

Description of Shampoo

Infrared Examination of Non-volatile Matter

1. Obtain an infrared (IR) film spectrum of the non-volatile matter on a salt crystal.

It may be necessary to prepare the sample by slurrying the non-volatile matter with alcohol, placing a film of the mixture on a salt crystal, and drying at 105°C in an oven for 5 minutes.

2. Examine the spectrum for the possible presence of soap, alkyl sulphates, alkanolamines, fatty acid-alkanolamine condensates, polyoxyethylene compounds, polyhydroxy compounds, and quaternary ammonium compounds.

Test for Ammonia

1. Make a portion of the shampoo strongly alkaline with 30% NaOH, and note whether the odour of ammonia can be detected.

2. Alternatively, hold a piece of moistened red litmus paper over the shampoo which has been made strongly alkaline. If the paper turns blue, ammonia is present.

Test for Basic Nitrogen Compounds Including Ammonia

Mix about 1 g of shampoo with 8 g of anhydrous Na_2CO_3 in a large Pyrex test tube, cover with another 2 g of Na_2CO_3, and heat the mixture strongly over a gas flame. If a moistened red litmus paper turns blue when it is held in the vapours, ammonia or some other basic nitrogen compound is present.

Lanolin and/or Sterols

The extract from any method of extraction that removes the fatty material will contain the lanolin and/or sterols. Test a portion of such an extract by the Liebesrmann-Burchard colorimetric test.

Water-soluble Gums

1. *Preparation of water-repellent glass plate on which film is formed* – Wash a 4" square of window pane glass thoroughly with soap and water, and dry it with a towel. Dip a solid glass stirring rod in a bottle of Desicote and streak and adhering liquid across the top of the plate. Repeat the streaking process several times. Rub the plate with lens paper to distribute the Desicote evenly, and then rub it with clean lens paper to remove any excess Desicote. The plate is now ready for use. The coated plate may be used for two or three films provided it is washed with cold water and dried with a towel after each use. The plate can be recoated by repeating the described procedure.

2. *Preparation of gum solution* – Precipitate any water-soluble gums by adding alcohol to the shampoo. Centrifuge to concentrate the gum, decant, and discard the supernatant liquid. Redisperse the gum in a minimum amount of water, reprecipitate with alcohol, centrifuge, and decant as before. Dissolve the residue in 10 - 25 ml of water.

3. *Preparation and identification of gum film* – Place the water-repellent glass plate over an open 2" aperture in the steam bath. Pour the aqueous gum solution on the plate so that a circle of liquid about 2" in diameter is formed (about 10 ml is required). Heat the plate on the steam bath until all the liquid has evaporated. Remove the film with forceps (if the film is stuck to the plate it can usually be removed by scraping with a razor blade). Transfer the film to a beaker and dry at 105°C for an hour. Place a piece of dried film between two salt plates and obtain the IR spectrum. To identify the gum, compare the spectrum with spectra of known gums.

ANALYSIS OF NAIL LACQUERS

Most nail lacquers are solutions of nitrocellulsoe, Plasticisers, and resins in mixed volatile organic solvents. Colour and opacity are produced by pigments suspended in the lacquer.

In nail lacquers, n-butyl phthalate, camphor, and tricresyl phosphate are common platicisers; an aryl sulphonamide-formaldehyde polymer is a frequently used resin, and the pigments are likely to be organic lakes, guanine, and titanium dioxide. The solvents are usually mixtures of toluene, butyl acetate, ethyl acetate, ethanol, isopropanol, and butanol, and occasionally include acetone, xylenes, or methyl ethyl ketone.

A typical nail lacquer might contain 12% nitrocellulose, 5% n-butyl phthalate, 5% aryl sulphonamides-formaldehyde resin, 1-3% camphor, and 1-2% pigment. The solvent may approximate 35% toluene, 40% butyl acetate, 15% ethyl acetate, and 10% ethanol. Ethanol is sometimes present as the packing solvent for the nitrocellulose.

General Analysis

Net Contents

Remove the brush and cap from the bottle and mark the height of the liquid on the outside of the bottle. When analysis has been completed, empty the bottle, rinse it with acetone, and fill it with water to the previously inscribed mark; then empty the water into a graduated cylinder and record the volume of liquid.

Description of Nail Lacquer

Note colour, odour, opacity, and other physical characteristics of the nail lacquer.

Infrared Film Spectrum of the Nail Lacquer

1. Prepare a sample by coating a salt crystal with a thin film of the lacquer and drying at 105°C in an oven for 5 minutes.

2. Observe whether the infrared (IR) spectrum can be interpreted as a mixture of nitrocellulose, n-butyl phthalate, and aryl sulphonamide-formaldehyde resin.

Non-volatile Matter at 105°C

After discarding the brush from the bottle top, weigh the closed bottle of nail lacquer. Pour ca 1.0-1.2 g into a tared weighing bottle 65 mm high and 45 mm in diameter, and weigh the nail lacquer bottle again. The difference in weight is the sample weight. With the top removed, manipulate the weighing bottle so that the lacquer covers the entire inside surface of the bottle as a thin film. Then heat the lacquer at 105°C in an oven for 2 hours. Cool and weigh the residue as non-volatic matter.

Determination of Non-volatile Constituents

The overwhelming majority of commercial nail lacquers contain these non-volatile components: nitrocellulose, organic lakes, inorganic pigments such as TiO2, n-butyl phthalate, and an aryl sulphonamide-formaldehyde resin. The following is a method of analysis (Fig. 44.4) for these nail lacquer ingredients :

(a) Dilute a 4-6 g sample with 5 ml of acetone, add 20 ml of benzene, and pour slowly with stirring into a 400 ml beaker containing 150 ml of hot benzene. Rinse the sample container with 5 ml of acetone and add the rinsings to the benzene. Evaporate the benzene on the steam bath under a gentle jet of air to about 80 ml, dilute with 90 ml of benzene, and cool to room temperature. Pour the mixture into a 250 ml centrifuge tube, rinse the precipitation beaker with 10 ml of benzene, and add the rinsings to the centrifuge tube. Reserve the precipitation beaker and any precipitate that adhered to the sides. After centrifuging, decant the supernatant liquid into a 250 ml beaker labelled no. 1 and set it aside.

(b) Dissolve the residue in the precipitation beaker and the centrifuge tube from (a) with 15, 10, and 10 ml portions of acetone, and pour the combined acetone solutions into a 100 ml beaker. Evaporate the acetone on the steam bath, redissolve the residue in 10 ml of acetone, add 20 ml of benzene, and repeat the precipitation and centrifuging procedure described in (a) Decant the supernatant liquid into a beaker labelled no. 2. Reserve the precipitation beaker and the centrifuge tube containing the residues.

(c) Filter the decanted liquids in beakers No. 1, (a) and No.2 (b) through the same 12.5 cm filter paper into two tared beakers labelled I and II. Reserve the filter paper and beakers Nos. 1 and 2.

(d) Evaporate the filtrates in beakers I and II, (c) on the steam bath under jets of air, and dry the residues in an oven at 105°C for 10 minutes. Cool and weigh I and II as combined resin and plasticiser.

(e) Rinse the reserved beakers Nos. 1 and 2 (c) with two 30 ml portions of hot methyl ethyl ketone and pour the rinsings through the reserved filter paper, (c) into a tared beaker. Discard the filter paper, evaporate the filtrate on the steam bath under a jet of air, dry the residue in an oven at 105°C for 20 minutes, cool, and weigh as a mixture consisting essentially of nitrocellulose and pigments.

Obtain an IR film spectrum of the residue from a film prepared in the following manner : Dissolve a little of the material in acetone, pour some of the solution on a salt crystal, let the acetone evaporate in air, dry the film on the crystal in an oven at 105°C for 5 minutes, and cool to room temperature.

(f) Dissolve the residues in the reserved precipitation beaker and the centrifuge tube, (b) in acetone and transfer the acetone solutions to a tared 250 ml beaker. Evaporate the acetone on the steam bath, redissolve the residue in 5 ml of acetone, and add 75 ml of alcohol-ether solution (1+2) followed by 10 ml of water. Evaporate the solvent on the steam bath under a gentle jet of air and dry the residue in an oven at 105°C for 1 1/2 hours. Cool, and weigh as nitrocellulose plus pigments.

Obtain an IR film spectrum of the residue as described in (e)

(g) Use 32 ml of methanol to dissolve and transfer the resin and plasticiser residues in beakers I and II (d) into a 250 ml separatory funnel. Add 8 ml of water and extract with four 40 ml portions of petroleum ether. Reserve the extracted methanol solution. Set the separatory funnels aside for rinsing later.

(h) Filter the combined petroleum ether extracts (g) through a 12.5 cm filter paper into a tared 250 ml beaker. Follow with an additional 40 ml of petroleum ether wash through the filter paper. Reserve the filter paper. Evaporate the filtrate on the steam bath under a jet of air, dry the residue in an oven at 105°C for 10 minutes, cool and weigh as butyl phthalate.

Obtain an IR film spectrum of the material from a liquid film spread on a salt crystal. Also obtain the ultraviolet uv spectrum of an alcohol solution of the phthalate.

(i) Transfer the reserved extracted methanol solution, (g) to a 500 ml separatory funnel, add 50 ml of $CHCl_3$, dilute with 200 ml of water, and acidify with a little HCl. Shake the mixture well and draw off the $CHCl_3$ layer. Continue the extraction with additional 50, 50 and 30 ml portions of $CHCl_3$. Reserve the extracted aqueous solution. Set the separatory funnel aside for rinsing later.

(j) Filter the combined $CHCl_3$ extracts, (i), through the reserved filter paper, (h), and follow with an additional 40 ml wash with $CHCl_3$. Reserve the filter paper. Evaporate the filtrate on the steam bath under a jet of air, dry the residue in an oven at 105°C for 10 minutes, cool, and weigh as aryl sulphonamide- formaldehyde resin.

Obtain an IR film spectrum of the resin as described in (e) Also obtain a uv spectrum of an alcohol solution of the material.

(k) Filter the extracted aqueous solution, (i), through the reserved filter paper, (j), Discard the filtrate. Rinse all the separatory funnels used in the extractions, (g) and (i), with two 30 ml portions of acetone, and filter the acetone solutions through the filter paper into a tared 250 ml beaker. Discard the filter paper. Evaporate the filtrate on the steam bath, dry the residue in an oven at 105°C for 10 minutes, cool, and weigh as a mixture of resin and nitrocellulose.

Obtain an IR film spectrum of the material as in (e).

Separation of Nitrocellulose from Pigments

1. *Guanine* – The mother-of-pearl appearance of some nail lacquers arises from the presence of guanine. To analyse such a product, dilute a weighed sample with acetone, centrifuge, and decant the acetone. Identify the guanine residue from the infrared spectrum of a mineral oil mull or from a film prepared by rubbing the guanine between two salt crystals with a drop of acetone. Separate the crystals and evaporate the acetone at 105°C in an oven.

2. *Opaque coloured nail lacquers* – The opaque coloured effect is achieved through the dispersion of finely divided organic lakes and inorganic pigments such as TiO_2. The nitrocellulose may be separated from the colouring agents by the following procedure (3):

Dissolve, disperse, and transfer the residues of precipitated nitrocellulose and pigments, from steps of the non-volatile estimation process into a 50 ml heavy-duty centrifuge tube with the aid of 25 ml of hot methyl ethyl ketone. Add 4 drops of water and 50 mg of silicic acid (Mallinckrodt's chromatographic grade) to the solutions. Centrifuge at high speed for one hour and decant the supernatant liquid into a 250 ml separator. Treat the residue in the centrifuge tube with successive 15 and 10 ml portions of methyl ethyl ketone, centrifuging 15 minutes each time and decanting as before into the separator. Discard the residue in the centrifuge tube.

Add 1 ml of HCl to the separator, shake 2-3 minutes, and extract with 50 ml of water saturated with methyl ethyl ketone. Discard the extract. Make the methyl ethyl ketone solution slightly basic with ammonia, and extract with 50 ml of an aqueous solution which is weakly ammonical and saturated with the ketone and which contains 0.5% ammonium chloride. Continue the alkaline extracts until no further colour is extracted (three extractions usually suffice). Discard the extracts, re-acidify the ketone solution with HCl, and wash with two 25 ml portions of water that is weakly acid with HCl and saturated with the ketone. Discard the washings.

Filter the extracted methyl ethyl ketone solution through an 11 cm filter paper into a 250 ml tared beaker. Wash the separator and the filter paper with two 25 ml portions of hot methyl ethyl ketone, collecting the washings in the tared beaker.

Evaporate the volatile solvent on the steam bath under a gentle jet of air Redissolve the residue in 5 ml of acetone and add 75 ml of alcohol-ether solution (1+2) followed by 10 ml of water. Again evaporate the solvent on the steam bath under a gentle jet of air and dry at 105°C in an oven for 1 1/2 hours. Cool, and weigh as nitrocellulose.

In separating the nitrocellulose and the pigments from the nail lacquers, traces of pigment may adhere to the sides of the glassware or on the filter paper. These traces can be dissolved by alcohol strongly acidified with HCl.

Tricresyl Phosphate in Nail Lacquers

When tricresyl phosphate is used with n-butyl phthalate as the plasticiser, the two substances are isolated together. The IR spectra of these two materials differ sufficiently so that each can be identified in the presence of the other. If it is necessary to determine the amount of each component, the uv spectra differ enough so that the methods for the analysis of two-component mixtures can be applied.

Acrylonitrile-Butadiene Polymer

An acrylonitrile-butadiene polymer may be detected in the infrared spectrum of the non-volatile matter. The CN absorbance peak is at 4.45 μm.

When the polymer is present as an additional ingredient in a nail lacquer, it is isolated by precipitation with methanol. The methanol solution may be used for the usual nail lacquer analysis.

Base Coats

1. Base coats are preparations which are applied prior to the nail lacquer. They are usually solutions of polymeric substances. The polymers are most readily recognised by examination of the IR spectrum of the non-volatile matter. Ultra-violet spectra, sometimes of films on a quartz surface, are also helpful if the polymers have aromatic constituents. When a base coat contains two or more polymers, it is good practice to separate them, e.g., by extraction.
2. Acrylonitrile-butadiene and phenol-formaldehyde-polymers are among those used in base coats.

Infrared Spectrophotometric Analysis

Description and Interpretation of Spectra

A commercial colourless nail lacquer, known to contain nitrocelllulose, n-butyl phthalate and aryl sulphonamide-formaldehyde resin as non-volatile ingredients, was analysed. The IR spectra of the following fractions were examined.

1. *Non-volatile matter*
   (a) The presence of nitrocellulose is immediately apparent from the absorption maximum just beyond 6 μm and the one at 12 μm.
   (b) Although there is no positive identification for n-butyl phthalate, the indication of carbonyl absorption at 5.85 μm suggests that it might very well be a constituent of the product. Likewise the absorption at 8.6 μm may arise from an aryl sulphonamide-formaldehyde resin.

2. *Nitrocellulose*
   (a) The principal absorption maxima at 6.05 and 7.8 μm are characteristic of the covalent nitrate groups. The strong absorption at 11.9 μm is also associated with the nitrate group and that at 9.4 μm with the cellulose ring. Note the broad but weak OH bond absorption just before 3 μm and the weak C–H absorption just before 3.5 μm. The minor absorption maxima also aid in identifying nitrocellulose.
   (b) In the analysis of coloured opaque nail lacquers containing suspended pigments, the precipitation of the nitrocellulose entrains the pigments. However, it is difficult to differentiate the infrared film spectrum of the contaminated nitrocellulose from that of pure nitrocellulose. In part this is due to the small amount of pigment, 1-2%, ordinarily present in nail lacquers.

3. *n-Butyl phthalate*
   (a) The characteristic strong absorption maxima of phthalats are the carbonyl ester absorption at 5.8 μm and the maxima at 7.8, 8.9, and 9.3 μm. The weak doublet centred around 6.3 μm always appears in phthalates. The other absorption peaks are also helpful for identification.
   (b) The intensity of the C–H absorption in the 3.5 μm region is indicative of the length of the alkyl carbon chain of the ester.

4. *Aryl sulphonamide-formaldehyde resin* – is the spectrum of a commercial sample of the resin.
   (a) The major absorption maxima attributable to sulphonamides appear at 7.5 and 8.6 μm. The weak C-H bond absorption in the 3.5 μm region as well as the relatively strong absorption between 12 and 15 μm indicates the aromatic nature of the material. The weak but sharp absorption peak just before 3 μm suggests N - H linkages. The absorption at other wave lenghts aids in uniquely identifying the resin.

Testing of Cosmetics

(b) There is some difference in absorption between the commercial and isolated resins in the 13.5 μm region. The resin may be slightly altered chemically, in the course of the analysis, or else some component of the resin may be lost in the extraction procedure.

Infrared Spectra of Guanine and Tricresyl Phosphate

1. *Guanine from commercial Nail Lacquer* - Spectra of known sample of guanine obtained by heating the hydrochloride to 200°C. Guanine has many identifying absorption maxima. Two readily recognisable linkages are the N-H absorption between 2.9 and 3.5 μm and carbonyl absorption below 6 μm.

2. *Tricresyl phosphate* - Technical grade (80% para and 20% meta isomers). The spectrum of an n-butyl phthalate-trcresyl phosphate mixture spectrum can easily be interpreted as a composite of the widely differing individual spectra of the phthalate and phosphate.

The weak C-H absorption maximum at 3.5 μm, the absorption between 6 and 7 μm and that beyond 12 μm strongly suggest the aromatic character of tricresyl phosphate. The strongest absorption maximum, however, occurs between 10 and 11 μm and is attributed to the phosphate radical.

Gas-Liquid Chromatorgraphy

Gas-Liquid Chromatographic (GLC) Determination of Solvent and Camphor (Plasticiser)

1. *Apparatus and Reagents* - (1) Gas chromatograph - F& M Model 810, or equivalent, equipped with a thermal conductivity detector capable of operating in a rapid program mode after an initial isothermal period. Operating temperatures (°C) : injection port 260; detector 250; column initially 118 until solvents elute (ca 20 minutes), then programmed to 240 at 60/minute, held isothermal until camphor elutes (ca 7 minutes), and returned to the starting temperature, Helium carrier gas flow rate: 80ml/minute.

    (a) *GLC column* - Copper tubing, 20' x 1/4" outer diameter packed with 70-80 mesh Gas-Chrom R coated with 10% PEG 20M.

    (b) *Stock solutions* - Accurately weigh ca 5 g each of isopropanol, ethyl acetate, toluene, butyl acetate, butanol, camphor (dl), and propyl acetate (internal standard) into separate 25 ml volumetric flasks and dilute each to volume with iso-octane (distilled in glass).

2. *Preparations of samples* - Accurately weigh ca 1·g of nail lacquer into a tared 25 ml glass-stoppered Erlenmeyer flask. Slowly add, with stirring, 10-15 ml of iso-octane. Pulverise the resulting precipitate with

a stirring rod. Add 1.0 ml of n-propyl acetate internal standard solution. Stir the mixture and let it settle for 4-5 minutes before analysis.

3. *Preparation of standard solution* – Prepare a standard solution containing the following amounts of the stock solutions from (a): 2.0 ml of ethyl acetate (ca 400 mg), 3.0 ml of propyl acetate internal standard (ca 600 mg), 4.0 ml of toluene (ca 1200 mg), 4.0 ml of butyl acetate (ca 800 mg), 6.0 ml of butanol (ca 1200 mg), and 2.0 ml of camphor (ca 400 mg).

4. *GLC determination* – Inject 10-15 µl of sample onto the column, using the operating temperatures given in (a). Adjust the sample volume and / or attenuation to bring each peak to ca 50-90% of full scale deflection (do not adjust the iso-octane peak). The sample volume should not exceed 15 µl. In a similar manner, inject the standard solution and a determine the correct injection volume and attenuations. Identify the solvents in the sample by comparing their retention times with those of the components of the standard solution. After determining the correct operating conditions, alternatively inject the sample and standard ≥ 3 times each.

5. *Calculations* - Calculate the amount of each solvent or plasticiser in the sample as follows :

% Solvent or plasticiser = $(R_u / R_s) \times K_s \times (IS_u/IS_s) \times (100/W)$,

Where R_u = peak height of solvent in sample x attenuation /peak height of internal standard in sample x attenuation, R_s = peak height of standard solvent in standard solution x attenuation/peak height of internal standard in standard solution x attenuation , K_s = mg of standard solvent in standard solution, IS_u = mg of internal standard in sample solution IS_s = mg of internal standard in standard solution, and W = mg of sample.

Gas-Liquid Chromatographic Determination of Acetone, Xylene, and Methyl Ethyl Ketone

Acetone, xylene, and methyl ethyl ketone may also be determined by GLC with a minor temperature adjustment (1-2°C) for methyl ethyl ketone and a longer initial isothermal operating period for xylene. If either ethanol or isopropanol is present by itself, the alcohol can be identified by its retention time. Mixtures of these alcohols cannot be resolved under the conditions described. The shape of the curve indicates the presence of a mixture and some estimate can be made of the relative amounts of each. It should be noted that mixtures of alcohols may also be determined by headspace analysis.

ANALYSIS OF SUNSCREEN PRODUCTS

Sunscreens are incorporated into cosmetic preparations for the selective absorption of potentially harmful burning radiation between 290 and 320 nm while permitting the transmission of longer wavelenghts that permit tanning. A variety of chemical compounds, mostly aromatic, are available for incorporation into creams, lotions and solutions as sunscreens. These preparations can be roughly classified according to the vehicle or base in which the sunscreen is incorporated, e.g., hydrocarbons, vegetable oils, alcohols and oil-in-water or water-in-oil emulsions.

Determine net contents, description of product, non-volatile matter at 105°C, ash content and pH as per the procedure described earlier.

Infrared Examination of Non-volatile Matter

Examine the infrared (IR) spectrum for possible identification of sunscreens as well as other materials.

Determination of Sunscreen

1. *In an alcohol base* – Dilute a known amount of the product to a definite volume with alcohol Identify and determine the sunscreen from the ultra-violet uv spectrum of the resulting solution. Make dilutions as necessary.

2. *In an emulsion base* – It is generally necessary to isolate the sunscreen from the emulsion before its determination. The method for the isolation and determination of amyl p-dimethylaminobenzoate described in Official Methods of Analysis, (AOAC), with some modifications, is also applicable to the determination of certain other sunscreens. For example, elute 2-ethoxyethyl *p*-methoxycinnamate with acidified 50% alcohol and homomenthylsalicylate with acidified 70% alcohol. Before eluting with eluants of high alcohol concentration, wash the eluant with 2-3 ml of the immobile solvent, *n*-heptane-CCl_4 (1+1). Determine these sunscreens in acid solution by uv spectrophot- ometry.

3. *In a hydrocarbon or vegetable oil base*

    (a) Dilute the preparation with spectrophotometric grade iso-octane. Identify the determine the sunscreen from the uv spectrum of the isooctane solution.

    (b) Alternatively, it may be necessary to isolate the sunscreen from the hydrocarbon or vegetable oil base by partition chromato-graphy before the determinative step. If so, chromatography the preparation directly without prior solvent extraction, and then proceed as in (2).

Analysis of Sunscreen Vehicle

1. *Alcohol base* - See determination of sunscreen.

2. *Hydrocarbon or vegetable oil base* - An examination of the IR spectrum of the non-volatile matter should be sufficient for the characterisation of these base ingredients.

3. *Emulsions* - These preparations are normally mixtures of several ingredients. The base ingredients can generally be determined by methods used for creams and lotions. (Fig. 44.4),

SKIN SENSITISATION AND SENSITIVITY TESTING

A variety of substances are used in the manufacture of cosmetics. Therefore, finished cosmetics when used on human body have potential for several type of adverse reactions. The adverse effects that may be caused include skin irritation and allergic sensitisation, contact urticaria, stinging, phototoxicity and photoallergy. Skin irritation and allergic sensitisation is the most frequently encountered adverse effect. With growing consumer awareness and enforcement of consumer protection act, it is necessary for cosmetic manufacturer to assess the potential of adverse effects of his product. Safety considerations are not only relevant to consumers but also to factory workers who handle cosmetic raw materials in large quantities.

The substances that induce inflammation are known as irritants. Inflammation may be caused by use either immediately or through prolonged use or on repeated use. Irritants may be classified as primary irritants and secondary irritants. Primary irritants cause inflammation on the first contact (the duration of contact may be of several hours). Secondary irritants are harmless on first contact but cause inflammation on repeated contact and inflammation becomes more severe with progressive contacts.

In view of the potential of the of the cosmetic for harmful effects mentioned above, some tests have been designed to predict the potential of substances to induce irritation or sensitisation.

Sensitivity Testing

For detection of potential primary irritation, Draize test or its slight modification is used. In this test, Albino rabbits are clipped and the substance to be tested is applied to : intact skin, abraded skin, or lightly scarified skin.

All of them are covered with a patch for 24 hours. The sites of applications are examined at intervals and changes are assessed and recorded. The skin of rabbit is more susceptible than man. However, this method of testing can lead to false positive and false negative. It is advisable to compare results of test substance with the result of known harmless substance. Bureau of India Standards 4011 - 1982 (6.1 - Test for Irritant Potential) recommends that if there is no reaction in any of the animals, the

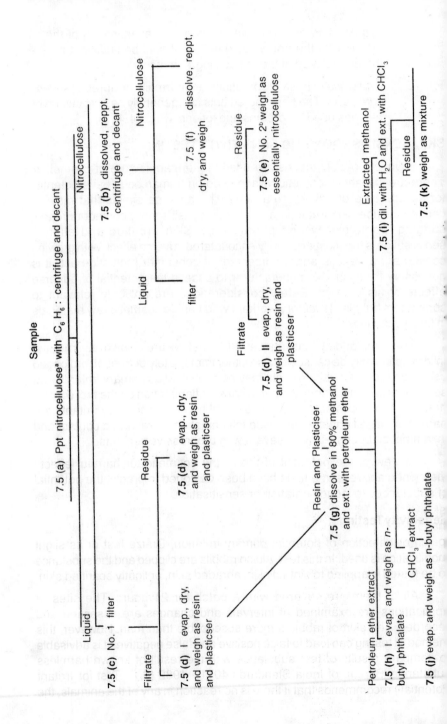

same test should be performed on 10 human volunteers applying the substance on the skin of the forearm.

Patch Test

On humans, sensitivity testing of cosmetics may be performed either as a diagnostic or as a prophetic test. By diagnostic test if is intended to discover whether the cosmetic used has caused dermitis and if cosmetic is known, the ingredient which has caused it. It is known as diagnostic patch test. Prophetic test is done to assess whether a new cosmetic should be placed on the market or not. This test is known as prophetic patch test. General procedure of patch test is given below.

Place about 0.1-0.3 gm of cosmetic to be tested on a piece of cotton fabric or flannel (2-3 sq.cm. in size) and apply this to the skin of arms, thighs or back. This patch is covered with a patch of cellophane (about 5 sq.cm.) and sealed with adhesive plaster (about 40 sq.cm.). Apply several patches at one time. Out of these several patches some of them should be of similar cosmetic of other brand available in the market and known not to cause any harm to the skin. Other similar cosmetics act as controls. These patches are allowed to remain on the skin for 24-72 hours. If there are no reactions, the same patch may be reapplied to the same place or a fresh patch of the same material may be made and applied. This may be continued till :

1. Either a reaction is produced under one or more patches, or
2. Investigator is confirmed that no reaction will occur.

Reading and grading of patches is best done by an experienced dermatologist. Sites of patches should be examined after 30 minutes of removal or patch. Observation can be made a little earlier but not earlier than 15 minutes. Usually the skin under adhesive tape gets inflammed, the skin under cellophane tape remains clear, the skin under test patch may not have reaction or may have reactions like erythema, erythema with papules, papulo-vascular reaction or ulceration or neurosis. Patch test reactions, usually, are graded as under :

Description of Observation	Symbol
No reaction	–
Erythema only	+
Erythema with papules	++
Papulovascular	+++
Ulceration of Neurosis	++++

Open Patch Test

In case of cosmetics containing higher percentage of potential irritants like hair dyes, shampoos, hair tonics, patches should not be sealed. These should be used as open patches. Open patch test is performed on sensitive part of skin, e.g., bend of elbow, popliteal space of the skin behind the ears. The site of patch is inspected after 24 hours. If there is no reaction, the test is repeated once more on the same site. If still no reaction is there, the test is repeated a third time. If no reaction is observed on third application, the person may be taken as not hypersensitive.

Prophetic Patch Test

Before a programme of prophetic skin test is undertaken, the investigator should perform test on himself to as certain that the material is not primary irritant. After satisfying himself, the investigator can select ten subjects. He should get signed from each of the subjects a waiver for any damage. The amount of money to be paid should also be got agreed upon. If the results of the test are favourable, the investigator may use more subjects. For full scale prophetic patch test, 200 normal subjects are used. The cosmetic to be used is placed on the skin of the subjects for one to five days depending upon the nature of the cosmetic and judgement of investigator. The purpose of this application is inducing or establishing sensitivity and also detecting the presence of any primary irritant the patch sites are examined and observations are made. Subjects are observed for three more days for development of any late reactions. After 7-10 days patches are again applied to the same area of those subjects who did not show reaction to the test. One or more similar cosmetics known to have been used for years without complaints are used as controls. If there are no reactions or one or two reactions out of 200, new product can be placed on trial sale in small community of about 10,000 persons.

Prophetic patch test may be covered or open. Many a time, question is asked what is percentage of hypersensitive persons that is allowable. Schwartz suggests that incidence more than one in 10,000 may not result in safe cosmetics.

Repeated Insult Test

The prophetic patch test has certain shortcomings, to name :

1. Quick absorption of potential skin irritant through skin.
2. Rapid evaporation of volatile skin irritant from the patch.
3. Small amount of cosmetic in patch in comparison to large amount in actual use.

4. Small area of skin used in comparison with skin surface area used in actual use of cosmetic.

5. Short exposure of skin to cosmetic than the exposure actual in use.

To overcome some of the shortcomings of prophetic patch test, its modification in the form of repeated insult technique has been suggested. Draize described this technique as under.

The repeated insult technique consists in applying the finished cosmetic, or if the test substance is an ingredient of the cosmetic, it is applied in the same concentration as is found in the finished formulation incorporated in a bland base. The bland base must necessarily vary according to the nature and solubility of the test substance. Therefore, the diluting bland base may vary from physiologic saline to such nonirritating, nonsensitising organic solvent as dimethyl phthalate. Ordinarily 0.5 gram or 0.5 ml. of the test sample is applied by usual patch test procedure. The skin of the back or upper arm is used, such areas as are ordinarily covered by wearing apparel. The test material is maintained in situ for 24 hours. Allowing 15 to 20 minutes after the removal of the patches, readings are made and the reactions recorded. The test subject is allowed 24 hours of rest and the second test patch is applied to a different test site, otherwise the procedure is identical to that of the first application. Each individual is thus subjected to a series of 10 such consecutive exposures, exclusive of Sundays and nonwork days. Following the 10 individual exposures the subject is given 10 to 14 days rest after which item a "retest application" is made similar to one of the original 10 applications. A comparison of the reaction following "retest" with the average reading of the 10 original applications permits an appraisal of the sensitising propensities of the test substance Preferably the test subjects should be equally divided as to sex and cover as wide an age range as practicable.

To be comprehensive, a panel of 200 test subjects should be employed. Two hundred subjects represent an auspicious number and smaller groups possibly should be used at first, gradually building up to 200 subjects. It would be unwise to use a large number if it were possible to demonstrate on a smaller panel, 25 or 50 individuals that the substance is a potent sensitiser and unfit for its intended use.

Another modification of patch test for volatile substances has been described in BIS : 4011 in section 5.3.1 reader may refer to the same.

In BIS: 4011 - 1982 it has been suggested that this test should first be performed on 10 laboratory animals and if there is no reaction in any of the animals, it should be performed on 10 human volunteers.

Photopatch Test

Certain substances are not harmful by themselves but they become harmful when exposed to sunlight. It has also been mentioned earlier that substances that absorb light wave lengths between 300-800 nm have potential of phototoxicity. In case, a substance is considered phototoxic, photopatch test may be performed. To perform this test, the substance to be tested is applied in duplicate patches in the same manner as for standard patch test. After 24 hours, one of the patches in the pair is exposed to sunlight for 30 minutes. Alternatively the patch can also be exposed to ultraviolet light. The light exposed patch is covered again. One additional site in the adjoining area of the skin is exposed to sunlight or ultraviolet light as has been done in case of one patch of the pair. The time of exposure is also same as for the exposed patch. This site acts as control. After further 24 hours the patches are opened and examined. If the patch not exposed to light and the skin area exposed to light do not show reaction but the patch site which has been exposed to light shows reaction, the test indicates that substance is phototoxic. If no reactions are observed on patch sites and control skin site, the substance may be taken as non-phototoxic.

Test for Sensitising Potential

An individual is not likely to be allergic to a substance, if he is exposed to it for the first time. In immunological terms, it can be said that lymphocytes of that individual acquire capability to recognise and elicit immunological response. Thus next exposure of that individual to the substance has chance of sensitising him. With the number of exposure his chances of developing hyper-sensitivity increase.

Test for sensitising potential has been described in BIS : 4011. It has been recommended that standard patch tests with same chemical or cosmetic are repeated in the same 200 volunteers after an interval of 10-14 days. The number of persons who will show positive reaction will represent the sensitising potential of the substance or cosmetic which has been tested.

Provocative Patch Test

Weak sensitising agents, generally, do not sensitise a person with first exposure. Repeated exposures, however, to even weak sensitising agent may make a person hyper-sensitive. This can be indicated by provocative patch test. In this test, 10-15 applications of a substance or cosmetic are made on alternative days on the same spot of skin in 10 volunteers. Standard patch test is perfomed after 10 days of the last application. The test will show, how many persons have been sensitised. It has also been recommended in the Indian Standard that in case of unknown chemicals, the test should be first performed on animals like guineapigs or rabbits.

Use Test

In use test, the cosmetic to be tested is actually used and its adverse effects, if any, are observed. BIS : 4011 suggests that 15 volunteers should be asked to use the cosmetic and they should make 15 applications of it. If there is no adverse reaction, cosmetic can be released for trial.

Skin Testing with some Specific Cosmetics

Creams

Dermatitis, usually with cleansing and emollient type creams, is not frequent. Dermatitis may occur with creams containing substances like mercurials, salicylic acid, deodorant creams containing salts of aluminium, bleaching creams containing oxidising agents and vanishing creams (because of alkalinity). Another important ingredients in creams is perfume which may cause dermatitis. Allergy has also been reported because of lanolin. Hydroxy fatty acids in lanolin are said to be allergic in nature.

To carry out diagnostic test, rub cream into an unaffected suitable part of the body (e.g., forearm) for five days. However, if positive reaction occurs before five days, rubbing of cream may not be continued. While carrying out prophetic patch test, the patch may be covered. A similar cream available in market for long time without any adverse effects may be chosen as control. The best test remains the user test.

Deodorants and Antiperspirants

Dermatitis from deodorants is infrequent. However, some phenolic antimicrobials can cause dermatitis. Perfumes of deodorants can cause dermatitis in hyper-sensitive persons.

Deodorants in powder and cream form can be tested using diagnostic patch test. In these forms the patches can be covered. But perfumes in solution should not be sealed in patch test. Perfume should be sprayed on the skin and the skin should be kept open.

On the other hand, dermatitis from antiperspirant is not uncommon. Aluminium chloride in antiperspirant is more irritant that aluminium sulphate. Often modern antiperspirant preparations are buffered to minimise irritation. Both diagnostic and prophetic patch tests can be employed for these cosmetics.

Depilatories

Depilatories (chemical) contain sulphides of alkali (e.g., NaS), alkaline earth (BaS) or thio-glycolic acid. These substance are reducing agents and disrupt cystine linkages of hair protein and thereby act as depilatories. These are capable of acting a primary irritants. Often some degree of erytherma is associated with depilatories. Intensity will depend upon concentration, pH and time of exposure. Therefore losed patch tests for diagnostic purposes are not recommended.

In case of testing of new depilatory, actual user test should be employed with well established depilatory in market as control. However, before undertaking actual user test, irritant properties of new depilatory may be assessed by carrying out prophetic test on 10 subjects with well established depilatory as control. The following procedure could be followed for the prophetic patch test.

Prepare inactive base of depilatory. Prepare dilutions given below of the well established depilatory and depilatory to be tested:

>one part depilatory + one part base
>
>one part depilatory + two parts base
>
>one part depilatory + three parts base
>
>one part depilatory + four parts base
>
>+
>
>One part depilatory + n part base

Place patches of well established depilatory dilutions on one thigh and patches of depilatory dilutions to be tested on other thigh of the subject. Examine the patches on two thighs after appropriate time. This time could be 24-48 hours.

Hair Dyes

If prophetic patch test is to be carried out on new hair dye, its composition should be ascertained. Because it may contain primary irritant, e.g., ammonia (more than 1% ammonia is primary irritant). Prophetic patch should not be closed, if the dye contains primary irritant.

Normally hair dye is applied to grey hair and is allowed to remain in contact with hair for about 1-1 1/2 hour. Excess of unconsumed hair dye is washed with shampoo. Hair dye is applied every four to six weeks to colour emerging roots of hair. In view of this open prophetic patch test should be used in case of hair dyes. The test could be carried out as follows :

Prepare hair dye for application and paint one square inch skin on the forearm or behind the ear. Repeat it every day for three days (application should not be washed off during this period). On the other forearm run a control with well established hair dye available in market. Repeat the procedure after seven to fourteen days. Reaction of the dye to be tested should not be more than the reaction with control dye.

If the new hair dye passes this test, it should be tried on 1000 subjects twice. When found satisfactory on trial, it may be placed on the market.

Cold Wave Lotion

Thioglycollates are used in permanent waving lotions. Thioglycollates in higher pH on long exposure can cause dermatitis. However, dermatitis from cold wave lotions is not frequent. Closed prophetic patch test can be performed with long established cold wave lotion. The following procedure could be followed :

Place 0.2 ml of new preparation on a piece of flannel (3 sq.cm. in are). Place this patch on forearm, cover it with uncoated cellophane (about 9 sq.cm. in area) and cover this with adhesive plaster (about 18 sq. cm. in area). A similar patch of control waving lotion is placed on the other forearm. Remove the patches after 24 hours and examine the patch sites after 15 - 30 minutes of removal of patches. Reaction should not be more than the reaction with control. The test is repeated after 7-10 days for finding out sensitisation potential. This test should be perfomed on 100 female subjects. This Test is more stringent than actual user test as in practice cold wave lotion does not come in contact with scalp and even if it comes in contact, the contact time is not more than 3 hours. Another factor for stringency is that in practice, cold wave lotion treatment is given once in a few months while the second patch test is followed with in 7 -10 days.

Lipsticks

Before introduction of indelible type lipstick cheilitis was rare. Cheilitis occurred frequently with the use of bromofluorescein type dyes in lipstick formula. This adverse effect was caused by photosensitising effect of fluorescent dyes. However, the fluorescent dyes being used in modern cosmetics are less photo-sensitive than earlier ones. Addition of pigment lakes which act opacifiers reduce photo-sensitisation.

Closed prophetic test can be performed on lipsticks. After removing the patch, the patch site should be exposed to bright sunlight for several hours to observe the tendency of the lipstick to photosensitisation A well-established lipstick in market should be used as control. At least 200 subjects should be taken for this test. Along with patch test, they should also use the lipstick under test and should continue to use for at least one month. If results of patch test and actual user test are favourable, an extensive user test on additional 800 subjects should be carried out before the lipstick is put on the market.

Nail Polish

With use of nail polish fingers have been rarely affected. However,

Testing of Cosmetics

dermatitis may be caused at those places which are frequently and habitually touched, stroked or scratched by finger nails. Solvents of nail Polish evaporate quickly. As such, causative factors could be resins, colour and pigments.

Earlier actual loss of nail occurred due to phenolic type of resin and synthetic rubber. Their use has been discontinued since then. Splitting of nails on long usage of nail polish has been observed.

In case of nail polishes, open prophetic patch test is carried out. The following procedure could be used :

Apply new nail polish about 1 sq. inch in area on forearm. A well-known and established nail polish should similarly be applied to the other forearm. Do not cover the patch. Apply test nail polish on nails of hand which has patch of test nail polish. Similarly apply control nail polish on the nails of forearm which has patch of control nail polish. Remove patches after 48 hours and after 7 - 10 days repeat the test on same subjects. Continue the use of nail polishes for two months. In performing this test take 200 subjects. Compare the results of test nail polish and control nail polish. Reactions with test nail polish should not be greater than the control nail polish. If new nail polish passes this test, user test on additional 800 subjects should be carried out before nail polish is put on the market.

Testing of hair & bath preparations for eye irritation properties

Eyes can be accidentally exposed to shampoos, other hair preparations and bath preparations. Draize and Kelly designed test on eye mucosa of albino rabbit. Such tests can be conducted as follows :

Instill 0.1 ml of test substance in conjunctival sac of one eye nine albino rabbits (the other eye works as control). Divide rabbits in three groups comprising of three rabbits each.

Group - 1   Leave the eyes of this group unwashed.

Group - 2   Wash the treated eyes with 20 ml of lukewarm water after 2 seconds of instillation of test substance.

Group - 3   Wash the treated eyes after 4 seconds of instillation of test substance with 20 ml of lukewarm water.

Read the occular reactions with hand slit lamp for seven days or till any residual injury persists.

Any preparation, which leaves corneal or iris lesions for more than 7 days, is considered severe eye irritant. Eye irritant effect of combination of synthetic detergents is greater than produced singly by them. All synthetic detergents preparations used on hair or during bath should be assessed for their eye irritating effect.

Efficacy Testing

The majority of skin-care products are sold to improve the appearance and feel of the skin, and are broadly classified as moisturisers. The condition and appearance of the skin is a function of its softness and flexibility, which is adversely affected by loss of water. Tests for moisture content and moisture transmission, as well as the viscoelastic response, ultrasound techniques, and electrical properties of skin have been the subject of much study, with the development of increasingly sophisticated instrumentation to show the condition of the skin and its water content. Most of these new methods have evolved to help evaluate the potential performance of products, and are very useful in screening formulations, levels of ingredients and other stepwise formula variables.

Cell Turnover Testing

A very useful test to determine cell turnover rate utilises the dansyl chloride test, in which dansyl chloride, which fluoresces under a long-wave uv or woods lamp, is applied to the skin. This material penetrates the stratum corneum to a uniform depth. The cell turnover rate, or transit time, is determined by disappearance of the stain compared to a non-treatment site.

Instrumental Tests

The instrumental test is proving to be of great value is profilometry, which is especially useful in the assessment of the changes to the skin's surface caused by the anti-ageing effect of retinoid therapy on sun damaged skin. Two primary methods are used inprofilometry. One method employs replicas and the other uses photographs. Fully hydrated skin has altered surface characteristics, as measured by both lower peaks and greater distance between peaks. This is also the case with skin that has fewer lines and wrinkles due to effects other than hydration. In evaluation with a replica, an instrument with a stylus produces a tracing of the topography of the skin, based on a replica produced by dental impression material. With two-dimensional photographs, computerised image analysis techniques are used to review the image.

The gas-bearing electrodynamometer (GBE), has been widely used to evaluate the viscoelastic properties of the stratum corneum, both in vivo and in vitro. More recently computer handling of data generated by this device has improved its utility. The Twistometre device measures resistance to torsion of the skin, as applied by a rotating disc inside an external ring, which acts as a stator. This device is used to evaluate the skin's softness and suppleness. There has been a long history of the measurement of not only the water content of skin, but also the flow of moisture from the skin, which is known as the moisture vapour transmission rate (MVTR) or the moisture/water loss or transepidermal moisture loss (TEML). MVTR is a technique that has shown continual refinement. Progress has continued to the more recent development of a well-accepted instrument, the Servo-Med evaporimeter. Most of the work on the direct measurement of water content in skin has utilised an infrared (IR) spectrophotometer.

Testing For Moisturisers

The tests consist of the flow of moisture through a barrier, which is often a synthetic film with a transmission rate similar to that of skin. This technique (MVTR) combined with a water-holding technique to measure hydration or the ability of the formulate or test material to maintain humectancy is very useful in evaluating or predicting potential in vivo results.

Test methods other than MVTR and water-holding capacity include scanning colourimetric techniques, scanning electron microscopy (SEM) and biomechanical properties of skin under various in vitro conditions. *In vitro* test methods can be instructive when their correlation to in vivo performance has been established. In the author's experience, a battery of tests and an excellent history of correlation are necessary for the test to be of predictive clinical value. The problem is that, when *in vitro* tests are used with excised skin or a synthetic membrane, unlike the human skin, there is a lack of the biological underpinnings of the epidermis, which is anything but an inert, static or dead layer.

Test For Sebum

This device (Sebutape) is a film that visualises and traps sebum. The tape can then be analysed, and total relative sebum amount computed using image analysis. If quantification is not the only requirement, the sebum can be solvent-extracted, gravimetrically analysed and broken down into component parts. This can be a very useful technique for assessing the instant removal of sebum by cleansers, or the effect on sebum production of various treatments.

Test for Cleanser Mildness

A wide variety of cleansers are available on the market and will be covered within this chapter. Tests for cleansers have focused primarily on testing soap or detergent formulations for mildness. In this test, dilute solutions of soaps or test solutions are maintained in a cup held against the skin of human volunteers. The skin is then evaluated for redness, scaling, and fissuring, often against high irritancy (non-fatted soap bar) and low irritancy (fatted sodium cocoisethionate bar) controls. A more recent modification of this method calls for a shorter test, and measures the increase in MVTR by a Servo-Med evaporimeter. This has shown close correlation with the longer duration visual assessment technique. These methods differs from the Soap Chamber Test in that the Forearm Test adjusts frequency for humidity, while the Flex Test is reported to be unaffected by humidity. For evaluation of facial cleansers of all types for mildness and drying potential, the method outlined by Frosch utilisers half-face testing with realistic use conditions. In order to obtain suitable dryness scores, this test is best run during periods of low relative humidity. Cleanser tests for efficacy, evaluating soil and make-up removal, as well as esthetic properties and after-cleansing skin-feel must also be done to obtain a complete picture.

A combination of all these test methods, together with adequate clinical and consumer trial and observation, should enable one to have a great insight not only into the performance of products but, more importantly, as to how and why products work, and how variations in formula affect performance. The is necessary for the enlightened formulator.

Stability Testing

Stability testing is done to ensure that a developed product will be fit for use during its expected life. Stability testing should be done early in the development cycle to remedy any problems before final testing. A well-run stability trial can provide much information about a product in a relatively short period of time. Prototype products in packaging representing the ultimate trade package material, can be placed at ambient, and elevated (e.g., 37°C and 45°C) temperatures, refrigerated and cycled through freeze/thaw cycles and placed in high humidity chambers. During these trials, testing should focus on attributes most important to the products performance, or on the integrity of any active ingredients. In addition, there should be physical testing, for example pH and viscosity, chemical content of active ingredients, water content, etc. The formulator must not overlook attributes relating to consumer perception, such as fragrance, colour, rub-in characteristics and appearance. Two or three months of successful elevated temperature testing and three of four freeze/thaw cycles will usually indicate that products will have an adequate shelf-life. It is important, however, to continue testing for longer periods at ambient temperature, to obtain an understanding of the product's ultimate shelf-life. Further testing whenever changes are made to the supply of raw materials or to the formulation is essential.

Chapter - 15

NATURAL PERFUMES

Natural perfumes are still in considerable demand inspite of easy availability of synthetic perfumes as substitutes of Natural Perfumes. The natural essence are extracted from odoriferious, plants, herbs, grasses and wide variety of wild flavour grown in abundance in our forests and valleys.

The perfumes made rom true flower oils have a charm and fragrance of their on which is appreciated by people who are accustomed to using "perfume-parexcellence", and which fact is strongly reflected to those who do the blending of scnets for powders, toilet requisites and kerchief perfumery.

There are mainly two classes of natural perfumes based upon its origins.

1. Vegetable origin perfumes

2. Animal origin perfumes

Vegetable Origin Perfumes

The most common example of an aromatic substance of vegetable origin is the flower which is unsurpassed in the freshness of the perfume due to the minute traces of essential oil present in its petals. Besides flower, perfumes are capable of extraction from various herbs, roots, barks, leaves, stems, fuits and other parts of vegetable plants. For instance, perfumes can be obtained from the flowers of cloves, etc; leaves and stems of patchouli, cinnamon, etc. barks of cassia, cinnamon etc., woods of cedar, sandal, etc., roots of sassafras, vetiver etc., rhizomes of ginger, orris, etc; fruits of lemon, etc., seeds of bitter almonds, anise, etc., gums or resinous exudations from myrrh, olibanum etc.,

It is thus apparent that the fragrance is not confined to full-blown flowers only but may be suitably derived from all organs of the plants. Mention may also be made here that some plants also are capable of yielding more than one odour quite distinct and characteristic in nature. The most commonly noted example is no doubt the orange tree from which three distinct perfumes may be secured, one from the leaves, one from the fruits and one from the rind of the fruit.

2. Animal Origin Perfumes

Perfumes are also obtained from animal origin. These occur almost exclusively as glandular secretions and enter into commerce in their natural state. The chief among them are musk, ambergris, castor and civet.

Animal perfumes are specially distinguished for their property of giving permanence to the odour of other bodies with which these are mixed. The odour they possess is also characterised by wide diffusion hardly surpassed by anything else. They are held in very high esteem and are, therefore, liable to indiscriminate adulteration.

Four main perfumes derived from animal origin are Musk, Ambergris, Civet and Castor described as under :-

Musk

Musk, to cite an example, is obtaned from musk deer and possesses an inimitable odour. Its presence even in small doses is capable of detection by perfumers. But this being a rare object and valuable, it undergoes considerable adulteration.

Genuine musk often becomes nearly inodorous by keeping, but recovers its smell on being exposed to the vapour of ammonia, or by being moistened with ammonia water.

Amergris

Ambergris is found in the intestines of spermaceti whales and is much prized in perfumery. Its presence even in minute traces is perceptible and permeates the whale with exalting odour. Its tincture is hence sometimes made the basis in the preparation of ottos, essences, etc.

Ambergris is solid, opaque, ash-coloured, streaked or variegated, fatty, inflammable, remarkably light and highly odorous. It has a pleasant musk-like odour, which is supposed to be derived from the squid (Sepia moschata) on which the animal feeds, the horny beaks of which are often found embedded in the masses. the odour is peculiar and not easily described or imitated, of a very diffusive and penetrating character, and perceptible in minute quantities. Ambergris is rugged on the surfaced does not effervesce with acids; melts at 140^0-150^0F into a yellowish resin-like mass; at 212^0 F sublimes as a white vapour very soluble in alcohol, ether, and the volatile and fixed oils. it appears to be abody analogous to cholesterine. Its specific gravity is 0.780 to 0.926.

Civet

Civet is another animal perfume having very strong smell and hence should only be used in a diluted state in manufacturing perfumery. If added in excess, the smell is unbearable and even nauseous. But when added in measured doses, it imparts a most pleasant fragrance to the preparation and makes it lasting.

Castor

Castor, an unctuous substance derived from the heaver, is also incorporated in small quanttities only in making perfumery.

It gives a black tincture, which added in big qunatities would discolour the whole preparation. Its odour specially improves on keeping.

Essences from natural herbal sources

The important herbs used as perfumes are mentioned below alongwith its properties.

1. Sandalwood oil

- Contains 89-96% santalol which is antiseptic.

2. Rosemary oil

- Fine tonic for scalp
- Skin deodorant
- For preventing baldness, dandruff and clears scurf.

3. Lavender Oil

- as calmative
- antiphlogistic

Floral extracts are used in the manufacture of handkerchief perfumes, scents, essences, etc. The process of preparation is essentially the same in every case. Fresh scented flowers are selected, freed from green stalks and cleaned from dirt and dust. the picked flowers are then digested in spirit. After a time the liquid is filtered and the scent carefully botttled. Some of the important essences are described as under :-

Bakul

Procedure : Take Bakul flowers 8 oz., clean and free from dust; put them in a stoppered phial and pour in 20 oz. Cologne spirit. Close the mouth. Leave aside fro 3 days and filter. Again soak 12 oz. fresh flowers in the filtered spirit and leave aside undisturbed for 48 hours. Finally filter and put in a stoppered phial.

Henna

Procedure : Mehndi flowers 8 oz., proof spirit 16 oz. Put these two ingredients together in a stoppered phial for 15 days. Wring out the flowers and throw them away. Put 12 oz. fresh flowers in this spirit and filter after 7 days. Store in a stoppered bottle.

Bela

Procedure: Take 16 oz. Bela flowers free from stalks and 20 oz. Cologne spirit. Put these two ingredients in a wide-mouthed stoppered phial for 48 hours. Wring out the flowers and put in 8 oz. fresh flowers. Set aside for 24 hours and then filter through filter paper. Store carefully in a stoppered phial.

Champaka

Procedure: Procure 100 Chmpaka flowers and then put in a stoppered phial. Pour 24 oz. spirit of wine into it and leave for 48 hours. Strain the liquid and throw away the exhausted flowers.

Put in 200 fresh flower and leave for 24 hours. Finally filter through filter paper and bottle.

Rose

Procedure: Procedure 16 oz. dried buds of Rose (any scented variety) and 20 oz. spirit of wine. Put the two together into a wide-mouthed stoppered phial for 20 days. Filter through filter paper and store in a stoppered phial.

Chameli

Procedure: Take 12 oz. Chameli flowers free from stalks, put in a wide-mouthed stoppered phial and pur in 16 oz. Cologne spirit. Leave for 48 hours, strain and throw away the flowers. Put in 8 oz. fresh flowers, leave for 24 hours, then filter and store in a stoppered phial.

Jasmine

Procedure: Procure 16 oz. single asmine free from stalks and 12 oz. spirit. Put these two together into a wide-mouthed stoppered phial for 24 hours. Strain and throw away the exhausted flowers. Put in 8 oz. fresh flowers, close up the mouth tightly and leave for 24 hours. Fianlly filter through filter paper and store in a stoppered phial.

Khus

Procedure: Procure 12 oz. Khus root; pick them and free them from dirt. Pound them finely. Soak the roots in 16 oz. spirits of wine and put the two together into a wide-mouthed stoppered phial. After a month filter through filter paper and put in a stoppered phial.

Orange

Procedure: Procure 8 oz. dries peels of Orange and mince them fine. Soak them in 12 oz. spirit in a wide-mouthed stoppered phial. Close up its mouth and set aside for 1 month. Finally filter through filter paper and store tin a stoppered phial.

Lavender

Procedure : Take fresh Lavender flowers 20 oz. and spirit 32 oz. Put the two together into a stoppered phial. Close the mouth and leave for 1 month. Filter through filter paper and store in a stoppered phial.

Bergamot

Procedure : Oil of Bergamot 4 oz. and spirit of wine 30 oz. are taken in a stoppered bottle and kept for 7 days. Finally filter and then pack.

Sandalwood

Procedure : mix together 4 oz. of Sandalwood dust and 8 oz. of white chalk and digest in 12 oz. of spirit and set aside in a stoppered bottle for a week. Then strain through filter paper and to the filtrate add 1 oz. of sandal oil. Store in a bottle for 2 weeks before phialing.

OTHER USEFUL PUBLICATIONS

★ HANDBOOK OF SYNTHETIC & HERBAL COSMETICS
★ COSMETICS PROCESSES & FORMULATIONS HANDBOOK
★ HAND BOOK OF PERFUEMS WITH FORMULATIONS
★ ESSENTIAL OILS PROCESSES & FORMULATIONS HAND BOOK
★ HAND BOOK OF ESSENTIAL OILS MFG. & AROMATIC PLANTS
★ HANDBOOK OF PERFUMES & FLAVOURS
★ HAND BOOK OF HERBS, MEDICINAL & AROMATIC PLANTS CULTIVATION

AVAILABLE AT :

ENGINEERS INDIA RESEARCH INSTITUTE

Regd. Off. : 4449, Nai Sarak (S1), Main Road, Delhi-6 (India)
Ph. : 3918117, 3916431, 3960797, 3920361 Fax : 91-11-3916431
E-mail : eirisidi@bol.net.in Website : startindustry.com

Chapter - 16

HERBAL EXTRACTION

Herbal extracts are the products obtained by extracting herbs through suitable process and extraction mediums. A process flow sheet for herbal extractions is as under :-

Process flowsheet for herbal extraction

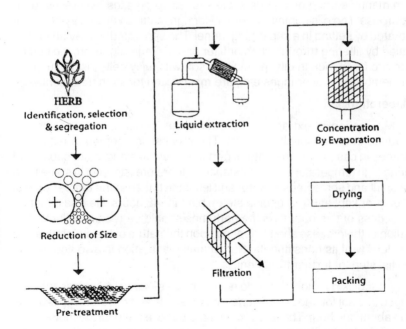

Extraction of Perfumes & Essences

For extraction of perfumes & essences there are basically following methods.

1. Expression
2. Maceration
3. Digestion
4. Infusion
5. Absorption or Enflaourage
6. Distillation
7. Solvent Extration

1. Expression

The raw materials are packed in a strong cloth bag and the oils are expressed in a press by strong pressure. The bodies are sometimes squeezed with great force in a small squeezer and the extract is collected from below. When manufacturing on a large scale squeezing presses may be used for the purpose. The oils contain water and foreign matters which may be easily separated by setting in a separating funnel. The separated oil may be further clarified by filtering through cloth or filter paper. Generally, aromatic bodies which are fresh, rich in oils, plump and soft with juicy cells inside such as, citrus lemon, peel of oranges etc., are most suited for such treatment.

2. Maceration

Maceration is extracting the odoriferous principle by steeping the substance in some suitable solvent. The process is adopted in extracting perfumes in case when the natural perfume is volatile and is not capable of bearing high temperature. The substance is, therefore, steeped in some fixed oil or spirit and sometimes in water and left undisturbed in the temperature of the room or kept at 65^0 C upon a steam bath for 48 hours. Be it said that for the success of this operation the perfumes should be readily solluble. The duration of the process should depend upon the nature of the substance and the solubility of its constituents. Sometimes maceration is also adopted as an initial step for further treatment.

After picking, most floers do not generate essential oil unless they are plunged into hot fat. the hot fat penetrates the cells and absorbs the essential oils in about one hour. The used flowers are removed and further flowers are immersed in the fat. This is repeated about eight to fourteen time. The essential oils are recovered in the manner described in the previous paragraph.

A perfume is composed of various constituent which are called notes. A scale of-100 is used, based on an assessment of the volatility of the substances. This is done by noting the time taken for a substance to evaporate completely from a slip of paper.

A certain period of ageing is required before an alcoholic perfume can be bottled and ready for use. When the perfume is maturing it acquires a balanced odour. Any fats or was particles originating from natural extracts are precipitated. this ageing takes two months. Maturation of the perfume is due to a chemical reaction between the components, together with the maturation of the spirits.

Alcoholic perfumes can only mature in glass bottles. Air and light must be excluded. They must be cooled for at least twenty-four hours in a refrigerator before they can be filtered, and should be kept as cold as possible before filtering.

3. Digestion

Digestion consists of extracting the fragrant element by the aid of warm liquids, which are not allowed to attain boiling temperatures. One usually submits to digestion only those substances which are very slow to yield up their perfume and for which are very slow to yield up their perfume and for which employment of heat to some extent is indispensable. To shorten the process, may be raised keeping the mixture well stirred.

4. Infusion

Non-volatile bodies may be subjected for extraction of their perfumes to the process of infusion which consists in steeping the substances in some boiling liquid in a closed vessel to prevent evaporation of the perfumed substances if any. The period of infusion varies according to the greater or less solubility in the solvent of the body to be extracted.

5. Absorption of Enfleurage

This method uses cold fat, as fat will absorb essential oil. A thin layer of fat is spread on a sheet of glass which is held in a wooden frame. Freshly picked flowers are spread over the fat and left for twenty hours. After this time the flowers have given up their oil to the fat and begin to wither. The frame is then turned over and the flower fall off. The remainder of the flowers are depending on the type of flower. In due course that fat absorbs the flower perfume and it is then known as pomade. This is washed in alcohol until all the perfume and it is then known as pomade. This is washed in alcohol until all the perfume is transferred to the alcohol, which is then evaporated under vacuum pressure in a cold still. leaving the concentrated flower oil.

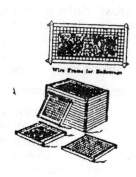

6. Distillation

This is the oldest method and is applied to plants whose odour will not be destroyed by stream. The materials are either placed in a still filled with water, or steam is passed directly into them from a boiler. The boiling water or steam penetrates the plants, breaks down the cell walls and reaches the tiny droplets of essential oil secreted in the vege ole matter, causing them to vaporise. 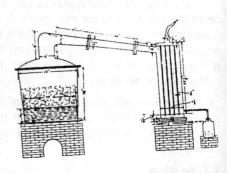 These two vapours, that is the water vapour and the essential oil vapour, are then passed into a condensing chamber whose sides are kept cool by a current of cold water. Inside the chamber, the mixed vapours liquefy and the mixture flows into a separating flash where the water and oil automatically separate.

7. Solvent extraction:

In this method, fresh plant material is placed in a container which is sealed down and is flooded with the liquid solvent (such as ether or petroleum). This evaporates at a low temperature. The solvent then penetrates the plant tissue and dissolves out the essence together with some colouring matter and waxes. The solution is then pumped out and the solvent is removed by evaporation under reduced pressure. The substance left behind consists of waxes m ed with he floral essences. The wax is separated, leaving a liquid which is concentrated essential oil.

Solvent extraction of perfume

The material is placed in the left-hand container and a spirit solvent is added. The solvent together with a mixture of wax and essential oil runs into the lower half of the still. Gentle heat from an electric heater is applied and the solvent is distilled off, leaving behind in the still a mixture, of "concrete", of wax and oil which is drained off later. The solvent is condensed through the colling tube and collected in two receivers, one of which is closed while the other is being emptied.

Repening of perfumes

For making the extracted perfume, tenacious and of agreeable character is is allowed to keep undisturbed in closely sealed vessel in a place not too warm and unexposed to the direct action of sunlight. This greatly ripens the preparation, improves its quality and makes it clearer by the deposition of sediments in soulution. To make the fixation complete the volatile portions of the perfumes are to be fixed by less evanescent bodies. The alcohol, when in use, poroduces a disagreeable smell which is also to be remedied.

Chapter - 17

PRESERVATION OF COSMETICS

The cosmetics in general contain oils, fats, moisture which are subject to deterioration due to number fo factors such as oxidation of fats, microbial growth. Cosmetic preparations which contain oils and fats are required to be protected against the growth of molds and from becoming rancid. By the effect of rancidity the cosmetics get discoloured and qauire undesirable odours. For preventing the cosmetics to get deteriorated, preservatives are required to be added in the cosmetic preparations.

A preservative is a substance which prevents the decomposition of the cosmetic preparation by discouraging the growth of bacteria and fungus, thereby preserving its original colour, odour and qualities.

For the growth of molds, access of the air to the cosmetics is required as these are aerobic. to prevent his a piece of waxes paper or foil is placed on the surface and the lid of the jar is screwed as well.

The materials used for preserving the cosmetics from spoilage by microorganisms are having function to prevent the multiplication of bacteria and fungi throughout the period of its use.

Antioxidants

Antioxidant are used to prevent the oxidation of certain materials in cosmetic preparation. These materials which are subject to oxidation are castor oil, corn oil, almond oil, olive oil sesame oil etc.

The antioxidants hould have following properties:-

1. It should have no odour of its own.
2. The cosmetic preparation should not deteriorate if kept for some time.
3. It should not be toxic.
4. It should be colourless.

For dissolving the antioxidant in the oil phase, it should be warmed up to $60°$-$70°$ centigrade.

Factors for Deterioration of Cosmetics

1. Presence of Molds

The molds are fungi with a filamentous type of growth; they usually reproduce by means of spores. These spores falling on a moist surface germinate and produce branching filaments or hyphae. Later fruiting bodies are formed with masses of colorless or pigmented spores.

The following are probably the most frequent molds encountered in cosmetics.

Penicillum is an extremely widespread genus of fungi, most often seen as a green, velvety growth on decaying vegetables and fruits. its vegetative growth of mycelium is a network of fine, branching tubular threads with cross walls marking off cell limits. Some of the branches are characterized by a tuft of fingerlike branches at the tip, at the end of which long chains of microscopic single celled spores occur. This fungus is able to decompose proteins, fats and carbohydrates.

Aspergilus is similar to the preceding in many ways and is also seen frequently on decaying fruits and vegetables. Its colors are varied: green, yellow, brown and black. The spores are also borne in chains but in this case the tip of the mycelial branch bearing them is club shaped. The species of Aspergilus trend to grow under rather warmer conditions than Penicillium and on media containing a higher concentration of nutrients.

Rhizopur and **Mucor** belong to a group of fungi differing from the preceding genral their mycelia show no cross walss and spores are produced inside a globe or sporagium. These fungi also produce thick walled resting cells (Zygopores) by a rudimentary sexual process.

Rhizopus nigricons occurs commonly as the balck bread mold."its large balck sporangla can be distinguished with the naked eye on the surface of a fluffy white network of mycelium. It is highly proflific species causing black rot of weet potatoes and storage rots of many other vegetables.

Mucor Mucdo grows as a silvery gray turf of mycelium. Its sporangia are grayish, and are borne on single long cheards branching off the main mycelium. It too, is widespread and may be found on a great variety of decaying organic matter. Both of these genera require more moist conditions than the Penicilia or Aspergilli.

Botrytis cincrea is commonly found on decaying organic material and is commonly associated with plant disease. one of its relatives is the cause of a destructive rot of onion. Vegetative growth if fluffy gray-white to dark, with small single celled spores borne on crowded fine swellings along the rounded tips of oright branches, somewhat in the manner of bunches of grapes. It has been found in creams where it subsists on the fatty acid residues of soap substances.

Species of Alternaria are found both as saprohytes and as parasites.

Alternaria is usually dark in colour, greenish-black with creeping vegetative mycelium which sends up short unbranched threads at the ends of which chains of large many celled dark spores are formed. Alternaria has been found by Holt and Carroll to contaminate creams and lotions the sealers of the caps providing the inoculum.

Stemphylium resembles Alternaria is occurring as a dark spreading mycelium with club-shaped muriform spores. However these spores are borne singly at the tips of short upright branches rather than in chains.

Cladosporium is a soil fungus withdark greenish-black mycelium. its spores are usually olive green and they appear in chains which branch in a treelike fashion on upright mycelial threads. This fungus is found frequently among soil isolates.

Yeasts also occur as common contaminants; they are classified along with mold as fungi. The yeast are generally nonfilamentous spherical or ellipsoidal cells which reproduce by budding. They are found in soil and air and are common contaminants of culture media. Their greatest commercial uses are in the manufacture of bread and in the production aof alcohol and alcoholic beverages.

The **bacteria** are smaller than yeasts and reproduce aby fission or in some cases by formation or spores. Saprophytic forms occur widely in nature. Little informations present on the bacteria contaminating cosmetics; however, bacillus subtills, B mycoides, Aerobacter aerogenes, and Pseudomonas sp commonly present in air and soil and capable of vigorous growth may be taken as representatives.

2. Factors Influencing the Growth of Microorganisms :

As a group, the microorganisms are the most omnivours of living things since they are capable of supporting their metabolic processes by utilisation of the most diverse food sources. According to Lamanna and Mallette, it may be speculated that there is probably not a single naturally occuring compound for which a persistent search would not reveal on or more kinds of bacteria capable of utilizing it as a nutrient. it is remarkable that there are bacteria which can utilize organic compound having no known existence outside the laboratory of the organic chemist.

On the other hand, many microorganisms show a remarkable specificity as to sources of food. This is true of a number of parasitic microorganisms as well as those organisms which cause decay.

The following may serve as substrates for microganisms found in cosmetics:

1. Carbohydrates and glycosides : Natural gums and mucilages, pectinase, starches, dextrins and sugars.
2. Alcohol : glycerol, mannitol and fatty alcohols.
3. Fatty acids and their esters; animal and vegetable fats, oil and waxes.
4. Steroids; Cholesterol, ergosterol and lanolin.
5. Proteins, peptones and main acids.
6. Vitamins

In addtion to a carbon source an adequate, suitable nitrogen source is necessary. This may be organic and serve also as a source of carbon such as protein, or it may be inorganic such as ammonia. The latter is readilly utilized by most molds.

3. Growth Factors :

Growth factors have been defined as those organic compounds required for growth which need to be present in only minute amounts. As a rule these compounds are assumed to be functioning metabolites necessary for the chemical reactions occuring in the cell. Growth factors are considered essential if growth cannot take place without them.

4. Moisture Content

Microorganisms can grow only when they have a sufficient water supply, since normally growing metabolizing cells of all kinds must be bathed in an aqueous phase. In addition to acting as an inert medium for vital systems, water also is a reactant in numerous essential reactions of the cell. It is of further interest that the amount of moisture present has a strong influence on the type of organisms which will grow in a particular product.

the bacteria in general require a high water content in their immediate environment tha do fungi; there is an intermediate range in which yeasts may become the dominant organisms.

5. PH

The PH Has a marked effect upon the number and types of microorganisms which can grow in a given substrate. Fungi are capable of growing over fiarly wide range of pH, although the rate of growth is usually; best at a PH of 4 to 6. Some acid-producing fungi can grow best in more neutral media (pH 6 to 8). In slightly acid conditions the yeast and lectic bacteria are favoured. No organism seems to be able to grow appreciably above a pH of about 9.

6. Temperature

There is a true optimum temperature for the growth of each organisms and the range of temperature ever which any particular organisms can grow is usally faily narrow. The optima for the great majority of common saprophytic bacteria, yeasts and fungi (including most types naturally occurring in air, water and soil) appear to lie in the range of 20 to 30^0 C. Since this is the temperature range at which most cosmetics are stored and used, this favourable temperature obviously plays and important part in providing optimum conditions for growth of contaminants.

7. Oxygen

The presence of oxygen or more fundamentally the oxidation reduction potential, has an includence on the type of organism which will grow in a given substrate. Those organisms which cannot develop without oxygen are called obligate aerobes. Those organisms which cannot grow in the 5 presence of oxygen are called obligate anaerobes. Those which prefer a limited access of oxygen are called microaerophiles such as the lactic acid bacteria. Finally there is a large group called facultative anaerobes which grow best in the presence of air but can gow in its absence if the medium is able to supply the missing oxygen.

Most molds are strongly aerobic and apparently none are obligate anaerobes; yeasts too, grow best in the presence of air, although they ferment material without it. The bacteria as indicated above, avry greatly in their oxygen requirements. However most of the organisam of concern in the preservative of cosmetics appear to be aerobic.

8. Other Ingrdients :

Other ingredients of the compostion even through they do not serve as sources of food for microorganism may influence their growth. In this category are preservative themselves. Also in this group are substances such as alcohols and glycols which in lower concentration serve as sources of carbon and energy for microorganism but in high concentration may inhibit their growth. Salts of various types may become inhibitory in higher concentrations.

Cosmetics preservatives may be regarded as agents which extend the storage and shilf life of cosmetics by retarding or preventing deterioration. This generally implies retardation or prevention of microbial growth, or of oxidation of fats and oils or both. To eliminate any ambiguity that might arise from this definition, the word preservative is used to refer to any compound capable of preventing growth of microorganism; antioxidant to any agent which retards oxidative deterioration in fats and oils. The term preservative is by no means synonymous with either antiseptic or germicide, although they are sometimes confused and a preservative does not necessarily fit into the category of antiseptics or germicides.

The problem of the preservation of cosmetic preparation is a complex one. The complexity is increased by the vast number of different problesm and formulations with each product and formulations presenting its own particular probles, depending on a number of factors. Some of the more important of these facts are :

1. The physical form of the preparation - liquid, emulsion, ointment, powder, etc.
2. Factors influencing growth of microorganism-nutritional factors, mositure, PH temparture etc.
3. Factors affecting the action of the preservative-concentration, nature of and amount of inoculum incompatiable substances etc.
4. Presence of compounds which are inherently bacteriostatic orfungistatic.
5. Purity and cleanliness of raw materials and maintenance of sanitary oeprations in formulating and packing and finished product.

From the foregoing, it is quite evident that deterioration may arise from several causes-physical, chemical, microbial and enzymatic. Evidence of deterioration which can be detected visually or organoleptically (changes in odor, color and texture) is of particular importance, as these changes are easily notices by the consumer. Odor changes are due to the production of volatile substances, such as aldehydes, ketones, acids, amines, sulfieds, mercaptans to color changes may be due to growth of pigmented or pigment-producing organisms to oxidative reactions, and to other chemical reaction. Changes in texture may be due to hydrolysis of starches, solubilization of proteinaceious mateiral and microbial overgrowth. In addition destruction of active ingredients such as vitamins, hormones and the like may occur.

Most cosmetic preparations are subject to deterioration. Almost all cosmetics containing water are susceptible to microbial action. Even substantially anhydrous preparations such as lipsticks may require preservatives. Mucilages, fatty acids, lipids, albumins, hormones and vitamin in mention just a few are materials that are susceptible to microbial deterioration.

All preparations containing fats and oils are subject to oxidative as well as to microbial deterioration. Microorganisms are extremely adaptable to unfavourable conditions. To be on the safe side, a preservative should be added to each cosmetic preparation, unless it can be shown that the cosmetic is inherently resistant to the growth of microorganisms.

The selection of a preservative poses itself a problem. An "ideal"antimicrobial agent or antioxidant must have the following attributes :

1. It must be effective under the conditions of use; this means that it must have few incompatibilities (physical of chemical), must retain

its effectiveness over a wide pH range, and must not alter the pH of the preparation.
2. It must be soluble to an extent commensurate with its effective concentration.
3. It must be stable and capable of sustained action.
4. It must be colorless and odorless or nearly so.
5. It must be easily and economically formulated into the product.
6. It must be nontoxic and must not produce irritation or sensitization in the concentrations employed.

This last attribute is of great consequence, because every effort is made to eliminate from cosmetic preparations any possibility of irritation of sensitization even with long continued use; also any possibility of toxicity caused by inadvertent ingestion. Fortunately compounds now exist on which as considerable amount of data has been amassed to show their safety under a wide range of conditions.

Although there is no antimicrobial agent which meets all the requirements of the ideal, some progress has been made in the field.

Preservatives such as formaldehyde, alcohol, boric acid and salicylic acid and its derivatives which were once widely used, are now known to be useful only under limited circumstances and at concentration which make them less desirable than other compounds presently available. Numerous investigators share the opinion that of the preservatives in general use today, the esters of p-hydroxybenzoic acid are the preservatives of choice since they approach the requirements of the :ideal preservatives: most closely.

Since much of the information on the use of preservatives is empirical it is necessary to consider available information on factors affecting the growth of microorganisms in cosmetics and to inqurie into the effectiveness of the preservatives from the microbiological and biochemical point of view, in order to place the choice of a preservative on a rotational basis, and to decrease the chances of unexplained and costly failures.

Chapter - 18

PACKAGING OF COSMETICS PRODUCTS

INTRODUCTION

The packaging of any product and cosmetics have same principle. However, in case of cosmetics for successful marketing more importance is given to package design and development.

Packaging utilises a wide variety of materials such as plastics, glass, paper, board, metal and wood combined with wide range of technologies including printing, machinery design and tool making.

Packaging has been defined as the means of ensuring the safe delivery of a product to the ultimate consumer, in sound condition at the minimum overall cost. Other definitions are :

1. Packaging is the art or science of, and the operations involved in, the preparations of articles or commodities for carriage, storage and delivery to the customer.
2. Packaging sells what it protects and protects what it sells.

PRINCIPLES OF PACKAGING

Packaging must contain the product, restrain the product, protect the product, identify the product, sell the product and give information about the product, and do this within a cost related to the marketing, profit, margin, selling price and image of the product.

Marketing and Packaging

The package projects the style and image, not only of the product, but often of the company which markets the brand. The pack must therefore project the image that it has been designed for, not only to the customer through advertising and point of sale but also to the retailer and wholesaler chain.

Packaging is particularly important in the self-service retail trade. The package designer has a responsibility to ensure not only that the pack has the type of appeal that will make the customer pick it up and be encouraged to purchase on impulse, but also to ensure that the pack will stack on self-service shelves and give the retailer the maximum profit per linear unit of shelf space.

Advertising has ensured that the package is now more widely seen than ever before. With the predominance of colour in advertising – in television, cinema and press advertisements and on posters – the package must be made of materials that have good aesthetic appeal and which will take the hold colour.

TECHNOLOGY AND COMPONENTS

Plastics

The use of plastics for producing primary components and point-of-sale material now dominates packaging technology. Two main groups are used–thermoplastic resins and thermosetting resins. Thermoplastics can be extruded at their melt temperature and then blow moulded or injection moulded. After cooling, the resin can be remelted by heating to the limits of thermal fatigue and oxidation. Thermosetting resins, by contrast, are moulded using an irreversible chemical reaction and the resins tend to be rigid, hard, insoluble and unaffected by heat up to decomposition temperature.

Metals

Metals are suited in cosmetics packaging are aerosol containers, powder dispensers, shallow tins and collapsible tubes. Tin plate is the most commonly used metal for the rigid packs, although aluminium also finds widespread use. The impervious nature of the metal gives me collapsible tube the great advantages of reduced risk of contamination of the product and reduced losses of volatile materials from the contents.

Laminates

The various requirements of packages for cosmetics and toiletries (such as attractive appearance; impermeability to water and volatile oils) are not always available from a single material. In such case the use of composite material in laminar form can be made. Laminates have found particular application in the production of sachets and of collapsible tubes as alternatives to pure metal tubes for toothpastes.

Laminates are used for *flat sachets* that are heat sealed around the periphery (as distinct from the fatter *pillow sachets* which are made from PVC tube and sealed ultrasonically). The laminate must be able to withstand the pressure of the contained product and provide leak-proof seals.

Glass

Glass containers are still used widely in the toiletries industry by virtue of the basic packaging characteristics of glass. Glass is chemically very inert and generally will not react with or contaminate high quality cosmetic and perfume products. Glass is manufactured in many different formulations but the most common in packaging is soda lime glass.

Paper and Board

Practically every cosmetic and toiletry products uses paper or paperboard in some form. Many grades of paper and board are available. Uses of paper and board in cosmetics packaging include labels, leaflets, corrugated cases, printed cartons and soap wraps.

Printing and Decoration

All packaging components can be printed to give a wide range of decorative effects. Different processes are used depending on the application. The five main processes used in the printing of packaging components are screen printing, letter press, flexographics, offset lithography and gravure printing.

Package Development And Design

Package development has the aim of increased sales and profit through the correct design of the package. Packaging must be considered as early as possible in the development of a new product to allow time to ensure that pack and product are compatible. The development process begins with a detailed analysis of the product so that a pack can be designed to give protection. Finally, in the development of the package the environmental aspects of the pack should be considered in terms of disposability and litter. It should also consider the re-use of scarce raw materials.

Technical Aspects of Design

The packaging material must be sufficiently strong to survive any treatment that it is liable to receive from the time to first delivery at a factory, through to filling, distribution, sale and actual use. It is essential that failure rate due to accident must be very low. Hence very strict testing and quality control of packs is essential in a factory producing toiletries or cosmetics.

A pack must be attractive to the consumer and contain the product in an efficient manner and render the product available as soon as the consumer desires to use it.

Closures

Unless it has an efficient closure, container has no value. Ideally the closure should be easy to remove and replace. However, it should give a seal that prevents the diffusion of gases and vapours and the seepage of liquids. Many bottle and tube closures consist of a screw cap containing a compressible wad. But wadless closures–achieved by new designs of thermoplastics screw and snap–on–are now extensively used for liquid products such as shampoos and hair conditioners.

PACKAGE TESTING AND COMPATIBILITY

Testing

The testing of packaging material and finished pack is required :

1. For effective material selection;
2. For assessing performance of material; and
3. For checking quality.

The packaging industry examines the properties like, mechanical, physical chemical and compatibility.

Mechanical properties for example, compression, tensile, flexural and impact strengths. *Physical properties* for example, water absorption, moisture vapour transmission rates, accelerated aging, flammability and thermal conductivity. *Chemical properties* for example, resistance to the product or the chemical environment, and corrosion testing. *Compatibility testing* is performed when the final product formulation and packaging system have been decided. Samples of the product should ideally be taken from trial batches, and the complete packaging system should be assembled using actual samples or pilot tooling samples representing the final component.

The general compatibility of the pack and product needs to be checked by storage testing which will enable an assessment to be made of the effect of the pack on the product as well as that of the product on the pack. It is important to remember that the effect of spillage on the outside of the pack is important, and should certainly be included in any testing schedule.

Shelf-life testing is also necessary in order to determine the rate at which volatiles may be lost and this includes not only water or alcohol but the perfume. The assessment of loss of perfume can only sensibly be done by nose, although weighing will obviously allow determination to be made of the loss of solvents.

Finally, the convenience of any cosmetics pack must be tested by in-use tests as well as by laboratory tests and for this purpose it is necessary to take into account both the local customs and the climate of the country in which the product is to be marketed : for instance, bathrooms in the UK tend to be cold, and tests for pourability should reflect this; similarly, products for tropical countries should be tested in conditions of high temperature and humidity.

Chapter - 19

PACKAGING OF HERBAL COSMETICS

Cosmetic products are in use for hundreds of years. Well before the commencement manufacture of these products by the organized sector, many naturally occurring of homemade articles were being used. Examples of these are shikakai and Soap-nuts for hair care, milk, cream with turmeric and gram flour for the face, and Oil (massage) for softening of skin. Most of these items were found in the kitchen or purchased in bulk and hence needed no special packaging. Thus, although these products were being used in the country for hundreds of years, systematic development and importance of packaging in true sense started only after the establishment of organized industry for cosmetic products.

With the start of cosmetics/toiletries industry in the country, homemade products slowly got replaced by products manufactured in factories e.g. creams and lotions replaced milk-cream-flour mix etc.

With the use of factory-made cosmetic products, need for the development of their effective packaging was felt. Initially most primary packages consisted of glass bottles usually of simple round shape and metal containers. Packaging at this stage was mostly from utility angle.

Most of the manufactures of cosmetic products in the initial stages were multinational companies or their licensing. They wanted their products of Indian origin to appear the same as those manufactured by the originating companies. This gave boost to the modernization in packaging of cosmetics products.

Another very important reason for the need for modernization in packaging is rapid industrialization of our society. with more and more people in our country getting educated and working women sharing equal responsibilities with men, demand for cosmetic products has steadily increased over the last few decades. Manufacturers have now fully realized the indulgence of attractive and efficient packaging system in conveying quality and brand image to the consumer.

The main factors that one must consider before deciding on the package design and packaging component(s) for packaging of cosmetics are as under :-

Determining Factors for Packaging

Determining factors may be classified under three broad considerations, viz. Technical, aesthetic and cost.

Technical Factors

Under technical consideration, the factors to be examined are chemicals and physical compatibility (of the product with the packaging material).

Aesthetic Factors

Presentability/appearance, technicalities and practicabilities for packaging design.

Cost Factors

Cost-effectiveness of a package is an important consideration.

Each of these important factors are analyzed in greater detail in following lines.

Technical Factors

Chemical Compatibility

The primary container (package) and the auxiliaries coming in contact with the product (e.g., plug, wad, liner, etc.) should not react with the product or any of its ingredients. The material from with the container is made should be impermeable to the product. If the product is liable to deterioration in sunlight, then the container must have the U.V. absorbers. To meet this requirement, one has to be very familiar with the chemical properties of the products as well as the chemical properties of packaging material components.

Chemical compatibility may be ascertained by checking product stability. Stability of the product over the period for which it is expected to lie on on the shelf is done by conducting accelerated ageing studies (at 38^0 temperature and 90% R.H). Stability study will also confirm whether the colour of the container (in case of coloured packaging materials) leaches out and affects the colour of the products or vice-a-versa.

Some plastic materials impart their own smell or modify the perfume. The perfume notes have to be checked after ageing the product in the container in the case of perfumed products.

Physical compatibility

(i) Retention of volatiles

Many health care products have a high percentage of volatiles such as water or alcohol, loss of volatiles would affect the quality of the product, perfume is usually more volatile should neither escape in vapour from the closure system nor permeate through container walls.

(ii) Leak Proof Caps

No container, however perfect, is of any value unless it has an efficient closure system. Ideally the closure should be easy to remove and replace, but should give a sea that prevents the diffusion of gases and vapours and the seepage of liquids. Most bottle and tube closures consist of a screw cap containing compressible wad, although wadless caps are coming into wider use of late. Leakproof property of the cap along with the container must be checked with the intended product and not with water. As water may not leak our through many closure systems but products like shampoo, oil can find a way to come out as each of them has got peculiar characteristics.

There is increasing trend for making the closure not only leakproof, but also tamper-indicating. This is a very desirable development.

(iii) Tamper-proof Seal

Most of the consumer products in the category of cosmetics/toiletries attract very high duties which make them expensive. A customer who is willing to pay a high price for such a product will naturally expect an intact product. A product having tamper proof seal will automatically assure its intactness to the customer. Most manufacturers are in the process of developing pilfer-proof seal for their products wherever it is not there. A few examples are : Many plastic containers now are seen with PVC heat-shrinkable pilfer proof sleeves; Glass and plastic bottles with ROPP caps; Cartons are either closed with cellotapes or glued, if not, the product inside is packed in a sealed poly bag. Aluminium collapsible tubes have metallic membrane seas on the nozzles.

(iv) Transport Hazards

Teritary packaging materials (shippers) are designed to take care of product damage during transit. If the shipper is made up of corrugated box, then grammage, type of paper, flute, number of primary packs to be packed are considered. Even the type of glue to be used while manufacturing corrugated box has to be specified. Cushioning material also plays important role in taking care of this factor.

Aesthetic Factors

(i) Presentability/Appearance

The aesthetic side of package design is basically a marketing responsibility, but a very close liaison between marketing and packaging experts is essential to ensure that a design is aesthetically functional and technically feasible. This applies not only to the container itself but also to the labelling and printing, and to the design of the display holders too.

In packaging of cosmetic products probably the package is ten time more important than the product. Esoteric shapes of crystal clear glass bottles, fancy spray systems, oversize decorative caps, glossy sophisticated labels and eye catching cartons made from laminated boards combine to make a pack of cosmetic product a piece of art. Its designing requires the imagination of a creative artist rather than scientific knowledge of a package engineer.

An attractive pack appeals to the consumer and contributes substantially to the initial sales of the product. An average product with appealing package can succeed. On the other hand even an excellent product with defective packaging is bound to fail. Good packaging is therefore very important for the success of a product.

(ii) Packaging Design - Technicalities

As far as technicalities of the package design are concerned, in general, the final pack must be sufficiently strong to survive the normal treatment it is liable to receive during manufacturing process, distribution, sale and actual use at customers' end. there is bound to be a certain failure of packs, largely due to accidents, but it is essential that this failure rate is very low, if the product has to be a commercial success. Typical possible problems we look for in package design are :

(a) Thin areas in containers-glass or plastic;

(b) Highly stressed areas-when polyolefins are used;

(c) Very small radius convex areas on the outside of clear packs that can act as effective lenses for focussing U.V. radiation, and so concentrate its harmful effects on to small areas of a product;

(d) Stability of the container-especially plastic containers with unstable bases can give rise to troubles on a mechanical filling line.

Apart from all the technical and aesthetic parameters of a pack. it must also dispense the product easily and be convenient for the consumer to handle. There is nothing more infuriating to a customer than a lotion that will not come of a container because the orifice of the nozzle is too small, or a deodorant squeeze pack that squirts a direct jet of liquid rather than the expected fine spray. problem of a badly judged orifice size in the first example and incorrect orifice dimensions and design in the second examples can stop the growth of the respective products. These two problems can easily be overlooked if proper attention is not paid while designing the pack. One of the solutions to avoid these problems is to do technical survey of similar packs used for similar products. Any shortcomings in the competitor's a pack can be a lesson to overcome similar problems while designing the pack.

(iii) Packaging Design-Practicability

The practicability includes easy availability of the material, presence of alternative suppliers, supplier's capacity, limitations as far as their machines are concerned and cost considerations.

Whenever any new packaging material has to be introduced its available must be checked. we must check the expertise, technical know how and capabilities of the existing supplier. It is always advisable to go for indigenously available packaging material where availability is not a problem. Packaging expert must visit the supplier's premises and check under what conditions the supplier is going to manufacture the material. Its also better to check whether more than one supplier are available. Manufacturing capacity must also be critically evaluated.

(iv) Packaging Design-Standard Weights and Measures for Packaged Commodities Act and Rules (SWAMPA Rules)

It is necessary to be aware of SWAMPAC Rule. Among other things, these rules specify product quantity that can be packed and sold, e.g, all creams except dental and shaving must be packed in 25, 30, 35, 40, 45, 50, 60, 70, 80, 90, 100, 120, 140, 160, 180, 200 and thereafter in multiples of hundreds grammes. Hence, while designing a pack, we have to inform Marketing that the product could be packed in certain quantities only.

Second important SWAMPAC requirement is the relation between letter height on the label and area of principal display panel of the pack.

Cost Factors

The last but not the last factor to be considered is cost. Selection of design, material shape, weight, etc. must be appropriate. Every paise saved in packaging is the real profit.

Secondly, cost economy can be achieved by mincing the handling of the packing material, e.g. corrugated boxes can be delivered to the plastic container manufacturer who in turn will pack them in the desired manner and despatch them to the factory. In this process we can avoid loading unloading, opening closing of the shippers. Moreover containers packed uniformly will help on-line operations (i.e. stamping., conveying easier.

Another example we can take is that of printing. One can go for four colour offset printing or settle with two colours. As three colour offset printing machines are to available in our country. Either we can print on four colour machine or print twice on two colour machine.

It is true that cost holds the balance between aesthetic and functional considerations. When this equilibrium is attained, the we can say the pack is cost-effective.

Packaging Materials commonly Used for Cosmetics

(a) Cartons : Coated boards, varnished, laminated embossed, E-fluted boards

(b) Flexibles : Paper, cellophene, LDPE, HDPE, BOPP, PP, PET, aluminium foil, nylon, HIP shrink and stretch films and laminates of various combinations.

(C) Rigid Plastic containers (jars, bottles etc.) Blo moulded, injection blow moulded, stretch blow moulded, injection moulded and rotatinal blow moulded.

(D) From fill & seal pouches from multilayer films.

(e) Corrugated boxes : Virgin, semi-virgin, B-grade kraft papers, A.B.C.E.-fluted.

(f) Collapsible Tubes : Aluminium and multilayer (lami tubes)-coextruded plastic tubes or soft squeeze tubes.

(g) Aerosol systems : Aluminium tin

(h) Glass Bottles ; Plain transparent, amber coloured

(i) Cushioning Material : Corrugated material, expanded LDPE and PS.

(j) Labels, Stickers, shrink sleeves; papers, PVC material, etc.

Out of all the above mentioned packaging materials, plastic materials have the major share and it is growing at a very fast rate. There has been many new developments in plastic packaging like development of multilayer pouches, multilayer co-extruded tubes (lami tubes), Stretch blow moulded pet container of various sizes and shpes besides the development of sophsiticated and fast packaging machinery & equipment. a suitable packaging system and packaging machinery is adopted depending upon the cosmetic product to be packed and various factors detailed earlier.

Chapter - 20

HERBAL COSMETICS FOR BEAUTY PARLOURS

With the growing craze for Herbal Cosmetics various big and small companies have started producing Herbal Cosmetics. To enhance the shelf life of these cosmetics, some preservatives are also added, which may have adverse side effect on our body in long run. If such preservatives are not added the chances are that the bottled cosmetic may get fungus after a while during storage.

To overcome this problem, the best way is to produce such Herbal Cosmetics free from synthetic preservatives in Beauty Parlours where these cosmetics get consumed very fast.

In the following pages some of the Herbal Cosmetics are described which can be easily and safely produced and consumed in Beauty Parlours and homes.

These Herbal Cosmetics described in details cover skin lotions, creams, face scrub, face packs, astringent lotions. Moisturisers shampoo's and Hair conditioners. These Herbal Cosmetics can be produced in Beauty Parlours and homes so that they can be consumed very fast without getting any chance to deteriorate.

Skin Lotions

Complexion lotions/sunscreen lotions for all skin types.

Complexion lotions not only improve the colour of your skin but also protect it from the harmful effects of the sun by providing a screen between skin and the sunrays. Therefore they are generally known as sunscreen lotions. We have below a few complexion lotions you can make yourself at home.

Lime Complexion Lotion

Lime flowers	25 gm
Distilled water	250 ml
Sodium benzoate	1/4 tsp

Procedure : Put the lime flowers in boiling water for an hour. Strain and let the mixture cool. Add sodium benzoatge to it. This is a very good complexion lotion and for better results add equal part of rose water to it. Keep it under refrigeration and use it with the help of cotton buds.

Lavender Complexion Lotion

Borax powder	1 tsp
Rose water	1 cup
Olive oil	2 tbsp
Lavender extract	1/2 cup

Procedure : Mix borax powder in rose water and add boiling oil to the mixture. Keep stirring, when cool add lavender extract too. It can be kept under refrigeration for more than 2 months.

Almond Complexion Lotion

Almond oil	1 tbsp
Cucumber/carrot juice	1 tsp
Glycerine	2 tsp
Liquid paraffin	1 tsp
Extract of cornflower	1 tsp

Procedure : Heat the almond oil and paraffin together and add all the other ingredients to it. Shake it well, apply it and let it remain till it dries. Rinse off with cold water preceded by lukewarm water wash. It leaves the skin looking fairer and smoother.

Sesame Complexion Lotion

Sesame oil	40 ml
Olive oil	10 ml
Almond oil	10 ml

Procedure : Mix all the oils together and apply it on the face and neck. It is an exclusive tonic to protect the skin from scorching heat of sun or is a very effective measure to get rid of sun tanning.

Brook Lime Complexion Lotion

Leaves/stems of brook lime	50 gm
Distilled water	500 ml
Sodium benzoate	1/2 tsp

Procedure : Boil the water an put the brook lime leaves/stems in it.

Leave it for an hour. Strain and let it cool. Now mix sodium benzoate in it. Apply it on the face and neck with cotton. It removes the spots and blackheads. It can be kept under refrigeration for more than 2 months.

Witch Hazel Complexion Lotion

Borax powder	15 gm
Distilled water	500 ml
Alcohol	1 cup
Witch hazel extract	1/2 cup

Procedure : Dissolve the borax powder in water over a low flame. Let it cool, the stir with rest of the ingredients. Pour the mixture into an airtight bottle and keep under regrigeration.

Pimple Removing Lotions

Pimple removing tomato lotion	1/2 tsp
Tomato juice	1 tsp
Honey	1 tsp

Procedure : Mix all the ingredients well and apply the paste on the face. Leave it on for 15 minutes. Then wash off with lukewarm water followed by a cold water rinse. It is also very good for removing spots caused by pimples.

Pimple removing garlic lotion

Multani mitti powder	1 tbsp
Honey	1 tsp
Carrot juice	1 tsp
Garlic (paste)	1/2 tsp

Procedure : Blend all these together and apply this mask on the face for 20 minutes After that wash off with lukewarm water. Never forget to give a cold water rinse becuase the pores which get opened by lukewarm water wash, get contracted if you rinse off with cold water.

Pimple removing camphor lotion

Glycerine	1 tsp
Borax Powder	1/2 tsp
Distilled water	1 cup
Camphor lotion	1/2 tsp

Procedure : Mix all these ingredients well and make a mixture of it. Apply this on the face and leave it to dry. When it is dry wash off with lukewarm water. Finally rinse off with cold water. Extra paste can be kept safe under regrigeration for further use.

Astringent Lotions for All Skin Types

Astringent lotions are antiseptic in nature and therefore these should be used by the people having skin problem-for example acne prone skin. Apply either of the followings :

Lemon Astringent Lotion

Lemon juice	2 large lemons
distilled water	16 tbsp
Tincture of benzoin	1 tbsp

Procedure : Mix all the ingredients together and use with a cotton pad.

Cornflower Astringent Lotion

Distilled water	250 ml
Cornflower	100 gm
Witch hazel	1 tsp

Procedure : Boil the water and soak the cornflower in it. Strain the mixture and mix witch hazel. You get a wonderful astringent lotion. You can use it by soaking the cotton pad in this mixture and then applying it on the desired places.

Rose Astringent Lotion

Rose petals/roots	500 gm
Disilled water	1.50 litres
Sodium benzoate	0.5 tsp

Procedure : Boil the water and soak the rose petals in it. Then mix sodium benzoate in the mixture. Apply it with cotton pads. It is very good for tightening the skin and removing the wrinkles.

Lilly Astringent Lotion

Distilled water	2 litres
Lilly flower	500 gm
Sodium benzoate	0.5 tsp

Procedure : Soak the lilly flower in boiling water for an hour. Then strain and mix sodium benzoate in it. Soak cotton buds in the mixture and apply it on the face. It leaves the skin fair and soft.

Nutmeg Astringent Lotion

Honey	1 tbsp
Nutmeg powder	1 tbsp
Clove powder	1/2 tbsp
Grate lemon peels	2 tbsp
Brandy	4 tbsp
Rose water	2 tbsp
Orange flower extract	2 tbsp
Tincture of benzoin	1/8 tsp

Procedure : Mix hem thoroughly. Let it stand for 7 days. Then use it. You can keep it for more than 2 months if kept under refrigeration.

Peppermint Astringent Lotion

Calomine lotion	4 tbsp
Witch hazel extract	4 tbsp
Peepermint extract	2 tbsp
Vinegar (cider)	1 tsp
Tincture of benzoin	1 tbsp

Procedure : Mix them thoroughly and apply on the face for deep cleansing and opening of pores. Keep the remaining under refrigeration for further applications.

Sandalwood Astringent Lotion

Sandalwood oil	8 tbsp
Sodium bicarbonate	5 gm
Almond oil	2 tsp
Rose water	4 tbsp
Orange flower extract	4 tbsp
Honey	1 tbsp

Procedure : Mix all these ingredients well. Keep it under refrigeration so that you can preserve it for months.

Rosemary Astringent Lotion

Sodium benzoate	1/2 tsp
Rosermary powder	2 tbsp

Orange peels	1 tbsp
Lemon Peels	2 tbsp
Mint leaves	30 leaves
Brandy	1/4 cup
Rose water	1 cup

Procedure : Soak orange peels, lemon peels and mint leaves in boiling rose water. Leave it so for an hour. Then strain and mix all th other ingredients to the mixture. Mix them thoroughly and keep under rerigeration.

Witch Hazel Astringent Lotion

Rose water	1 cup
Witch hazel extract	2 tbsp
Tincture of benzoin	1 tbsp

Procedure : Mix them thoroughly. Apply on the fac and neck at night and keep the rest under refrigeration for further applications.

Skin Toning Lotions

Grapefruit Skin Toning Lotion

Grapefruit (ripe)	100 gm
Yoghurt	250 gm
Sodium benzoate	0.5 tsp

Procedure : Remove the skin of the grapefruit and cut it into small pieces. Put the pieces through the blender them mix with yoghurt to make a paste. Refrigerate for an hour and add sodium benzoate, then smear over the face and neck. Leave for 30 minutes until you feel your pores tightening. Wash off with lukewarm water. It is very good for oily and sensitive skin.

Sunflower Skin Toning Lotion

Lanolin	1 cup
Sunflower oil	1 cup
Wheat germ oil	1 tsp
Witch hazel extract	1/2 cup
Sodium benzoate	1 tsp

Procedure : Melt lanolin in a pan over a low flame and stir in sunflower oil. Remove from th heat and stir in wheat germ oil and witch hazel with sodium benzoate. Bottle and refrigerate and then massage a little into the face and neck at bed time. It is an effective tonic for dry skin.

- Wheat germ oil or vitarnin E oil is very effective for dry skin. Apply it by dipping cotton bud in the oil
- Rub a piece of potato over the face and neck and leave the juice for 15 minutes to dry on and then wash off. It is very effective for oily skin and can also be used for dry skin with a moisturiser.

Skin Soothing Preparations

Cucumber Skin Soothing Preparation

Cucumber	1 medium
Lemon	1/2

Procedure : Peel and chop the cucumber and place the slices in a bowl. Squeeze the lemon over cucumber and let them stand for an hour. Then rub the cucumber slices over the face avoiding the area encircling the yes. Leave it so for 30 minutes and wash off with cold water. It is an extra luxurious preparation for oily skin.

Yoghurt Skin Soothing Preparation

Cucumber	1 small
Yoghurt	100 gm

Procedure : Put the cucumber through a blender and mix it with the yoghurt. Apply the past on the face and neck. leave to dry and then wash off with cold water. This is a good preparation for normal and sensitive skin.

Witch Hazel Skin Soothing Preparation

Cucumber	1 small
Honey	1 tsp
Witch hazel extract	1 tsp

Procedure : Grind the cucumber and mix honey and witch hazel to the pulp of cucumbe. Apply on the face and neck, and leave it on for 20 minutes. when dry, wash off with cold water. This gives a luxurious touch to the dry skin.

Cleansing Creams /Cold Creams

The following cleaning creams can be applied during winter as cold creams becuase in winter you need some creamy substance to protect your skin from the drying effects of cold wind. And cold creams do the same.

Almond Cleansing Cream (1)

White beewax	120 gm
Almond oil	500 ml

| Rose water | 1 cup |
| Borax powder | 1 tsp |

Procedure : Heat the beewax in a saucepan, when it is melt add almond oil, rose water and borax powder. Mix them thoroughly and keep stirring till the mixture cools. It can be kept under refrigeration for a long time.

Almond Cleansing Cream (2)

Sweet almond oil	1 cup
Bitter almond oil	1 cup
Sodium benzoate	1 tsp
Honey dew soap	30 gm

Procedure : Mix all the ingredients except sodium benzoate over a low flame. When the mixture cools down, add sodium benzoate. Keep it in a bottle under refrigeration.

Almond Cleansing Cream (3)

Sweet almond oil	1 cup
Ground almond	120 gm
Egg yolk	of 4 eggs
Honey	250 gm
Sodium benzoate	1 tsp

Procedure : Beat egg yolk and honey. Mix almond oil and powder making them into a paste. Now blend the beaten egg and honey to the paste of almond oil and add sodium benzoate too. You can keep this cream under refrigeration for 1-2 months.

Cucumber Cleansing Cream

Beeswax	30 gm
Spermaceti	30 gm
Olive oil	500 ml
Cocumber juice	1/2 cup
Sodium benzoate	1 tsp

Procedure : Put a bowl in an open pot filled with boiling water. Pour spermaceti and beewax in the bowl. After they have melted remove the bowl from the pot. Pour olive oil and cucumber juice. Keep stirring while the mixture is still warm add sodium benzoate.

Oatmeal Cleansing Cream

Buttermilk (Mattha)	1/2 cup
Oatmeal	50 gm
Sodium benzoate	1 tsp

Procedure : Mix sodium benzoate in the buttermilk and add oatmeal to the mixture. Make a fine paste and your cleansing cream is ready.

Chamomile Cleansing Cream

Chamomile flowers	50 gm
Distilled water	500 ml
Lemon juice	1 tsp
Sodium benzoate	1/2 tsp

Procedure : Put chamomile flowers and water in a saucepan over a low flame for 10-15 minutes. Strain and let it cool. Add lemon juice and sodium benzoate. Bottle it and keep under refrigeration.

Night Creams

Garlic Night Cream

Garlic cloves	20 gm
Vegetable lard	500 gm
Beewax	15 gm

Procedure : Put the garlic cloves in a saucepan with vegetable lard and keep it over a low flame for 30 minutes. Turn off the flame, cover the pan and leave it so for 5-6 hours. After that remove the garlic cloves and pour the mixture into screw top jars to solidify. It is very good for sensitive skin,

Apple Night Cream

Apple	500 gm
Vegetable lard	500 gm
Tincture of benzoin	1 tbsp
Rose water	1 cup

Procedure : Put the apples through the blender and add the juice and pulp to vegetable lard. Warm the mixture in a pan over a low flame. Simmer and stir until they get well mixed. Remove from the flame and add tincture of benzoin and rose water. Keep stirring all the time. Strain into a screw-top jar and use as night cream massaging it well into the face and neck. It works well for all types of skin.

Avocado Night Cream

Almond oil	1 cup
Avocado	1 medium
White beeswax	10 gm
Sodium benzoate	0.5 tsp

Procedure : Grate the avocado, put it in a piece of muslin cloth and squeeze it to get its juice. Mix the juice with the almond oil. Keep stirring until it is thoroughly mixed. Add white beeswax to make it set while still warm and pour into a screw top pot. Massage a little on the face and neck at bed time. Wash it in the morning with lukewarm water. It is very useful for dry skin.

Nourishing Creams / Daytime Creams

Nourishing creams provide nourishment to the skin. These creams can also be used as a daytime cream for they are also needed to nourish the skin. Daytime creams differ from night creams because the latter are heavy creams while the former are light creams. Being lighter in nature daytime creams do not attract dirt, hence, they can be used during the day.

Cucumber Nourishing Cream

Cucumber juice	4 tsp
Tincture of benzoin	1 tsp
Distilled water	25 ml

Procedure : Mix all the ingredients well. Place in the refrigerator for 5-6 hours before applying on the face and neck. Leave it for 20 minutes and then wash it off. Good for all types of skin.

Oatmeal Nourishing Cream

Egg yolk	2 eggs
Honey	1 tbsp
Lanolin	1 cup
Oatmeal	1 cup
Lemon juice	1 tbsp
Tincture of benzoin	1/2 tsp

Procedure : Mix together beaten yolk of egg, honey, lanolin, lemon juice and oatmeal. Stir in the tincture of benzoin. Massage on the face, neck and forehead with a circular movement and leave it on for 15 minutes. Then wash off with lukewarm water. It is very good and effective for dry skin.

Almond Nourishing Cream

Sweet almond meal	2 tbsp
Yoghurt	100 gm

Procedure : Mix almond meal with yoghurt. apply on the face and neck and leave it on for an hour. Rinse off with lukewarm water. It is good for a dry and blemished skin.

Almond Nourishing Cream

Almond oil cream	40 gm
Honey	1 tsp
Sweet almond meal	30 gm

Procedure : To almond oil, mox honey and almond meal. Massage into the skin for 15 minutes. Leave it on for 10 minutes and wash off with lukewarm water. It will take away any greasiness and leave the skin soft and smooth. It is very good for all types of skin.

Marigold Nourishing Cream

Marigold flower	500 gm
Spirit of wine	500 ml
Vegetable lard	500 gm
Essence	q.s.
Tincture of benzoin	1 tsp

Procedure : Place marigold flowers in a large glass jar and cover them with spirit of wine. Leave it in the sun for a week's time. Shake the jar every day. Heat vegetable lard and when melted stir in essence. Add tincture of benzoin to preserve it. As it starts cooling pour into a jar slowly and mix thoroughly. Good for oily skin.

Olive Nourishing Cream

Olive oil	2 tbsp
Egg yolk	2 eggs
Tincture of benzoin	1/2 tsp
Lemon juice	1 tsp

Procedure : Beat yolk of egg and mix olive oil, lemon juice and tincture of benzoin. It does wonders for dry skin.

Red Elm Nourishing Cream

Marshmallow leaves	60 gm
Distilled water	1 litre
Vegetable lard	500 gm
Beeswax	90 gm
Red elm	60 gm

Procedure : Melt refined vegetable lard and beewax in a saucepan over a low flame and then stir in slowly the extract of red elm and marshmallow until they are completely mixed. Pour into screw top jars before the mixture cools and sets. Use a little to massage into the face and neck at bed time. Suitably for oily, sensitive and patchy skin.

Anti-Wrinkle Creams

Anti-Wrinkle Carrot Cream

Carrot	250 gm
Almond/olive oil	1 tsp

Procedure : Take the carrot and put through the blender. Add olive/almond oil and mix well. Place it in a refrigerator for 1 to 2 hours then apply around the eyes and cheeks, leave it on for 30 minutes. Then lie down with eyes closed. Finally wipe off with lukewarm water. It is good for all types of skin.

Anti-Wrinkle Cucumber Cream

Cucumber (grated)	3 tbsp
Lemon juice	1/2 tsp
Brandy	1 tsp
Egg white	1 egg
Tincture of benzoin	1/2 tsp

Procedure : Mix all the ingredients and blend the mixture well. Keep it in a refrigerator for 2 hours. Massage on the face and neck in circular motions with fingertips and leave it on for 30 minutes. Then wash off with lukewarm water in which a few drops of lemon juice have been added. Good for all types of skin.

Anti-Wrinkle Egg Cream

Cucumber Juice	2 tbsp
Egg White	1 egg

Lemon Juice	1 tsp
Rum/brandy	1 tsp
Sodium benzoate/	
Tincture of benzoin	0.5 tsp

Procedure : Beat egg white and mix all the ingredients in it. Keep the mixtue under refrigeration. Apply it as required.

Anti-Wrinkle Apricot (Khubani) Cream

Almond oil	2 tbsp
Beewax	2 tbsp
Apricot extract	4 tbsp
Lemon Juice	1/2 tsp

Procedure : Take almond oil and melt it in a saucepan over low flame. Then mix apricot extract and lemon juice thoroughly. Keep it in a refrigerator for 1 to 2 hours. Massage on the cheeks and neck in circular motions with fingertips. Suitable for all types of skin.

Hand Creams
Almond Hand Cream

| Almond oil | 2 tsp |
| Honey | 1 tsp |

Procedure : Mix honey with almond oil and massage on the hands. Put on a pair of old cotton gloves and sleep in them. Wash off the hands in warm soapy water in the morning. The hands will be soft. Repeat it the following night if necessary.

Vanilla Hand Cream

Vegetable lard	250 gm
Vanilla essence	50 gm
Spermaceti	120 gm
Gum benzoin	120 gm
Almond oil	2 large cups
Tincture of benzoin	1 tsp

Procedure : Put a porcelain bowl partly submerged in a saucepan of boiling water and pour spermaceti, gum benzoin and almond oil in it. Keep the mixture so for 5-6 Hours. Then mix vanilla essence and vegetable lard to the mixture and pour it into a screw-tip jar while it is still warm. Let it set and then use.

Witch Hazel hand Cream

Brewer's yeast	2 tsp
Witch hazel extract	5 tbsp
Tincture of benzoin	0.25 tsp

Procedure : Mix together all the ingredients to make a smooth paste, refrigerate for 20 minutes and then smear over the hands. Leave it on for 30 minutes and wash off with lukewarm water.

Moisturizers for All Skin Types

Lemon Moisturizer

Gelatine	100 gm
Distilled water	1 cup
Lemon juice	2 tsp

Procedure : Pour gelatine in a bowl to make a past by adding water. Add juice of lemon and place it in the refrigerator for 20 minutes to set. Apply on the face and forehead. Leave on for 20 minutes and wash off with lukewarm water.

Watermelon Moisturizer

Watermelon	1 slice
Lemon jice	1 tsp

Procedure : Cut a watermelon is slices and place them over the face and neck while lying for 30 minutes. It will be still more effective if the juice of half a lemon is squeezed over it and it has been refrigerated for 20 minutes. It will reduce the body temperature, tighten the skin and remoisturise it.

Avocado Moisturizer

Avocado	1 medium
Honey	1 tsp
Lemon juice	1 tsp
Yoghurt	200 gm

Procedure : Put an avocado through the blender and mix honey to it. Add lemon juice and yoghurt to make it a stiff cream. Refrigerate for 30 minutes. Then massage it on the face and neck until the cream has disappeared and leave it on for overnight. It adds luster to the skin by making up the moisture deficiency.

Face Scrub

Face packs which have the quality of rubbing or scrubbing the skin are called face scrub or 'Ubtan'. By scrubbing, they bring the blood to the surface of the skin, remove dead cells, smooth and clean the skin. Face scrub do the wonders to the spotty and sluggish looking skin. The best way to use the face scrub is to spread it over the face with fingertips, when it is slightly dry remove it by scrubbing. Afterwards wash off with lukewarm water. Use one of the following face scrubs suiting to your skin type.

Face Scrubs for Normal Skin

Orange Face Scrub

Dried orange peel (powder)	2 tbsp
Oatmeal	2 tsp
Cold cream	2 tbsp

Procedure : Mix all the ingredients to get a paste and apply on the face. When it slightly dries up. Remove by scrubbing. Finally wash off with lukewarm water. But remember to rinse you face with cold water at the end.

Barley Face Scrub

Barley powder	1 tsp
Lemon juice	2 tsp
Milk	1 tsp

Procedure : Mixx all the ingredients well until you get a very smooth paste. Apply this on the face, leave it for 15 minutes and then remove by scrubbing. Wash off with lukewarm water.

Oatmeal Face scrub

Oatmeal	1 tbsp
Almond oil	1 tsp

Procedure : Mix the above two ingredients and apply it on the face for 15 minutes. Then remove it by scrubbing. finally wash it off with lukewarm water.

Face Scrubs for dry skin

Oatmeal Face Scrub

Buttermilk	3-4 tbsp
Oatmeal	2 tbsp

Procedure : Mix them together and apply it on let it dry and then wash off with lukewarm water after removing it by scrubbing.

Almond Face Scrub

Almond oil	1 tbsp
Nourishing Cream	2 tbsp

Procedure : Beat the two ingredients well to make a paste. Apply this paste liberally on your face. Let it dry slightly then wash off with lukewarm water giving the final rinse with cold water. Wash off only after removing it by scrubbing.

Face Scrubs for Oily Skin

Carrot Face Scrub

Yeast powder/brewer's yeast	1 tbsp
Yoghurt	1.5 tsp
Lemon juice	1 tsp
Carrot juice	1 tsp
Olive/almond oil	1 tsp

Procedure : Mix all the ingredients and blend well together. Apply this on the face for 15 minutes. Then wash off with lukewarm water. If the skin is v y oily omit the oil and if dry and more oil to it. Do not use this on the skin having pimples because it may cuase infection.

Shaljam Face Scrub

Carrot	50 gm
Shaljam	50 gm
Milk	25 ml

Procedure : Boil carrot and shaljam, mash-them well. Add milk to it and apply this on the face. First remove it by scrubbing and then wash off with lukewarm water.

Pea Face Scrub

Pea powder	4-6 tbsp
Lemon juice	1/4 tbsp
Rose water	2 tbsp

Procedure : Soak the pea powder in rose water and lemon juice for half an hour. Then beat it will. When beaten apply this face scrub for 15 minutes. Then wash off with lukewarm water.

Face scrubs for Combination Skin

For the treatment of combination skin with the help of face scrub, use the face scrubs recommended for dry and oily skin types on different parts of the face having respective type of skins. For example use oily skin face scrub on to juction (nose, forehead, chin) and dry skin face scrub on the cheeks.

Face Scrubs for Patchy Skin

Oatmeal Face Scrub

Milk powder	1 tbsp
Oatmeal	1 tbsp
Lemon juice	2 tbsp

Procedure : Mix all the ingredients well and apply this scrub on the face. When dry remove it by scrubbing. Then wash off with lukewarm water. give a cold water rinse too.

Banana Face Scrub

Egg yolk	2 eggs
Almond/olive oil	1 cup
Banana large	1 No.

Procedure : beat egg yolk and almond or olive oil until thoroughly mixed. Then mash a ripe banana and mix it in the mixture of egg yolk and oil. Smear over the face and neck. Leave it for 30 minutes in which a little lemon juice has been added. Also rinse off with cold water. It is very effective in removing blemishes.

Peach Face Scrub

Powdered milk	2 tsp
Honey	1 tsp
Peach/Apricot (Khubani) pulp	2 tbsp
Lemon juice	1 tsp

Procedure : Mix powdered milk with honey and peach or apricot. Smear on the face and neck. leave it on for 15 minutes before washing off in lukewarm water containing lemon juice. Also give a cold water rinse to the face.

Sunflower Face Scrub

Egg yolk	1 egg
Sunflower oil	1 tsp

Brewer's yeast	1 tsp

Procedure : Beat the egg, add yeast and oil in it. Mix well and apply it on the face. When it is dry, wash off with lukewarm water. Do not forget to give a cold water rinse.

Almond Face Scrub

Almond meal	250 gm
Milk/water	100 ml.

Procedure : Mix almond meal with milk or water to make a smooth paste and smear over the face and neck. Leave for 30 minutes and then wash off with lukewarm water and massage a little almond oil into the skin. It will remove the spots and leave the skin soft and smooth.

Strawberry Face Scrub

Strawberries	100 gm
Powdered milk	2 tsp
Lemon juice	1 tsp

Procedure : mash strawberries with powdered milk and lemon juice. Smear over the face and neck and leave it on for 15 minutes before scrubbing it, Wash off with lukewarm water containing juice of half a lemon. Give a final rinse with cold water.

Face Scrubs for All Skin Types

Oatmeal Face Scrub

Dries Orange peel (powder)	2 tbsp
Oatmeal	2 tsp
Cold Cream	2 tbsp

Procedure : Mix orange peel powder and oatmeal together, When well mixed add the cold cream. Beat well and apply the past on the face. Fianlly wash off with lukewarm water when it is slightly dry. Do not forget to give a cold water rinse.

Egg Face Scrub

Egg yolk	1 egg
Almond oil	2 tsp
Dry skimmed milk	2 tbsp
Camphor Lotion	5 drops

Procedure : beat the egg yolk and add the oil to it. Then beat again and add the milk and camphor lotion in it. Mix all the ingredients well and get a fine paste. Apply the paste on the face and leave it to dry. When it is slightly dry wash off with lukewarm water followed by a cold water rinse.

Face Packs or Face Masks

These are requuired to supplement the primary phase of skin care, i.e. cleansing. Masks stimulate the blood circulation, tone the muscles and maintain the elasticity of the skin. Also they draw out the impurities from the pores. While applying the face pack use your fingertips to spread the pack gently over the face. Remember you should not apply the face pack around your eyes and mouth, thus leaving three circles on the face. You can put the cotton pads soaked in cucumber/potato juice to provide relief to your eyes. It will be better if you can lie down while your face pack dries. Because this way you will not be stretching your skin which is being treated right then. Following are some of the face packs which you can try suiting to your convenience. There is no harm in switching from one face pack to the other depending on its availability. But these shifts should be within the variety of face packs suggested for your skin type.

Face Packs for Normal Skin

Milk Face Pack

Procedure : Damp the cotton pad and rub on the face.

Apricot Face Pack

Honey	2 tsp
Apricot extract	2 tsp
Almond oil	1/2 tsp
Lemon juice	1/2 tsp

Mix all the ingredients and apply this paste on the face. Leave it on for 15 minutes then wash off. This is very good for the firming of the skin.

Bail Fruit Face Pack

Bail fruit powder	2 tsp
Date extract	2 tbsp
Honey	1 tbsp

Procedure : All the ingredients are mixed into a paste and applied on the face for 10-15 minutes and then wash off. It yields amazing results, beyond your expections. It is very rewarding for the sagging skin because it firms the skin.

Face Packs for Dry Skin

Mint Face Pack

Youghurt	1 tbsp
Multani mitti powder	1 tbsp
Mint powder	1 tsp

Procedure : Soak multani mitti and mint powder in youghurt for half an hour. The mix them well by beating. Apply in on the face for 15 minutes and leave it to dry. When dried, wash off with lukewarm water followed by a cold water rinse.

Egg Face Pack

Honey	1/2 tsp
Egg yolk	1 egg
Milk powder	1 tsp

Procedure : Beat the egg yolk, mix the milk powder and honey in it. Beat again. When you get a paste of medium to thick consitency apply it on the ace. When it is dry, wash off with lukewarm water.

Face Packs for Oily Skin

Potato Face Pack

Potato juice	1 tsp
Multani Mitti	1 tsp

Procedure : Blend both the ingredients together and apply it on the face, leave so until it rises. Then wash off with lukewarm water. Rinse your face finally with cold water.

Cucumber Face Pack

Cucumber juice	1 tbsp
Peppermint extract	1/2 tsp
Mint juice	1 tsbsp

Procedure : Mix all the ingredients together and apply this on the face. Leave it to dry. Then wash off with lukewarm water. This face pack is very effective for the oily skin.

Papaya Face Pack

Apply 2 tbsp of papaya pulp on your face and when it is dry wash off with lukewarm water. you can also mix lemon juice in it.

Egg Face Pack

Egg white	1 egg
Multani mitti powder	1 tsp
Peppermint extract	1/2 tsp
Water	1/2 tbsp

Procedure : Soak multani mitti powder in the water for half an hour. Beat the egg and blend in all the ingredients together. Also mix the soaked multani mitti powder in the mixture. Apply this on the face for 15 minutes then wash off with lukewarm water.

Face Paks for Combination Skin

People having the combination skin are advised to apply the mask for oily and dry skins on the respective areas of their face. For example the area like T-zone troubles with oily skin should be trated with the mask which is recommended for the oily skin; and the areas which are characterized by dry skin should be given the treatment of face packs which are recommended for the people having dry skin.

Face Packs for Patchy Skin

Mint Face Pack

Youghurt	1 tbsp
Multani mitti powder	1 tbsp
Mint powder	1 tsp

Procedure : Soak multani mitti powder in youghurt for half an hour, then mix mint in it. Mix all the ingredients well. Apply the paste on the face. Leave it to dry and wash off with lukewarm water followed by a cold water rinse.

Coconut Face Pack

Sea-kale powder	1 tsp
Coconut oil	2 tsp

Procedure : Mix together sea-kale powder and coconut oil in a basin. Massage it on the face, neck and forehead for 10 to 15 minutes. Leave it on for 30 minutes and then wash off with lukewarm water in which a few drops of lemon juice have been added. Do not forget to rinse off with cold water. It will remove the blemishes and leave the skin soft and smooth.

Peppermint Face Pack

Brewer's yeast	125 gm
Witch hazel extract	1 tsp
Peppermint extract	1 tsp
Lemon juice	1 tsp

Procedure : Mix all the ingredients together. Apply to the face and forehead and lie down with the eye closed. Leave on for 30 minutes. Then wash off with lukewarm water containing a little lemon juice. It is a soothing pack for effective blood circulation.

Red Elm Face Pack

Red elm bark powder	1 tsp
Yoghurt	100 gm
Honey	1 tsp
Peppermint extract	1/2 tsp
Sodium bicarbonate	1/4 tsp

Procedure : Mix red elm with youghurt. Add honey, peppermint and bicarbonate of soda, mix them thoroughly. Aply on the face and neck and leave on for 30 minutes. Rinse off with cold water preceded by a lukewarm water wash. It will remove all greasiness from the skin. You can keep this face pack for 2-3 weeks under refrigeration.

Face Packs for All Skin Types

Milk Face Pack

Yeast powder	2 tsp
Sugar	1 tsp
Toned milk (warm)	1 cup

Procedure : Mix all the ingredients well and keep the mixture for five minutes to ferment. When fermented, apply it for 20-30 minutes. Wash off with lukewarm water giving a cold water rinse finally.

Honey Face Pack

Egg white	1 egg
Honey	1 tsp
Yoghurt	2 tsp

Procedure : Beat the egg and add yoghurt and honey to it. Mix well and apply this paste on the face. When it is dry, wash off with lukewarm water giving a cold water rinse.

Egg Face Pack

Honey	1 tsp
Egg white	1 egg

Procedure : Beat the egg and mix honey in it. Mix well and apply this on the face. Leave it to dry. When dry, wash off with lukewarm water followed by the cold water rinse.

Water Based Face Packs

Water based face packs are needed to firm the skin after cleansing, tightening, balancing and toning. These water based packs help in removing th wrinkling feeling of the skin.

Tomato Face Pack

Tomato juice	2-3 tbsp
Yoghurt	125 gm
Oatmeal	50 gm
Distilled water	100 ml

Procedure : Mix tomator juice with yoghurt. Boil the mixture of oatmeal and water for 20 minutes. Now mix both the mixture together to make a smooth paste and allow it to cool. Lie down and apply it thickly on the face and neck and leave it so for 30 minutes. Relax with eyes closed. Rinse off with cold water. It will leave the skin soft and clear of blackheads and pimples and will take away the greasy film from the skin.

Orange Face Pack

Honey	1 tbsp
Orange juice	1 tsp
Multani mitti powder	1 tsp
Rose water	2 tsp

Procedure : Soak multani mitti powder in rose water for half an hour, When soaked well and all the other ingredients and mix them sell. You get a fine paste now. Apply this on the face and when it is dry wash off with lukewarm water followed by a cold water rinse.

Honey Face Pack

Honey	1/2 tbsp
Lemon juice	1 tsp

Multani mitti powder	2 tsp
Water	2 tsp

Procedure : Soak multani mitti powder in the water for half an hour. Add honey and lemon juice to it and apply the mixture on the face. After 15 minutes wash off with lukewarm water followed by a cold water rinse.

Olive Face Pack

Almond oil	1 tbsp
Olive oil	1 tsp
Water	2 tbsp
Cornflakes powder	1 tbsp

Procedure : Mix the two oils together. Mix cornflakes powder with water. Add the oil mixture to this paste a little by little. Keep beating the paste. When the paste is ready apply it on he face and leave it to dry. Then wash off with lukewarm water followed by a cold water rinse.

Strawberry Face Pack

Strawberries	3 pieces
Rose water	1 tbsp

Procedure : Mash strawberries and add rose water to the pulp. Apply this mask on the face for 20-25 minutes. Finally rinse off with cold water preceded by a lukewarm water wash.

Shampoos for All Hair Types

Lime Shampoo

Amla	100 gm
Shikakai	200 gm
Char	100 gm
Charilla	100 gm
Khus	100 gm
Reetha	200 gm
Water	2.5 lites
Glycerine	8 tsp
Lime juice	4 tsp
Sodium benzoate	1.5

Procedure : Boil the first five ingredients in the water till the mixture becomes half of the quantity. Strain it and add rest of the ingredients. Rinse the hair and apply the shampoo for 2-3 minutes and wash off with lukewarm water.

Lavender Shampoo

Amla	100 gm
Shikakai	200 gm
henna	100 gm
Khus	100 gm
Char	100 gm
Charilla	100 gm
Reetha	200 gm
Sodium benzoate	0.5 tsp
Lavender oil	8 tsp
Water	2.5 litres

Procedure : Soak amla, shikakai, henna, khus, char, charilla and reetha for one night. In the morning boil them till the mixture remains half. Now strain the mixture and add lavender oil and sodium benzoate. You can preserve the shampoo for very long.

Methi-Shikakai Shampoo

Methi	250 gm
Shikakai	1 kg
Orange/lemon peels	handful

Procedure : Crush all these ingredients into a powdery form and use this powder shampoo as you do others. But remember to soak this powder a 1/2 cup of water 2 hours before using it to your hair.

Sandalwood Shampoo

Shikakai	200 gm
Khus	100 gm
Char	100 gm
Charilla	100 gm
Amla	100 gm
Reetha	200 gm
Sodium benzoate	0.5 tsp

Water	2.5 litres
Sandalwood oil	8 tsp

Pocedure : Except sodium benzoate and sadalwood oil, soak all the other ingredients for a night's period. Boil this in the morning till half of the quantity remains. Strain it and add sodium benzoate and sandalwood oil. Use this shampoo in the same manner as others are used. This shampoo is especially recommended for oily hair.

Neem Shampoo

Gram flour	1 kg
Sandalwood powder	250 gm
Neem leaves powder	4-5 cups
Shikakai powder	1kg

Procedure : Mix these thoroughly by sieving. Keep it in an airtight bottle. When needed for washing soak 2 tbsp of it in a cup of water then apply. Quantity can be increased or lessen as required. Good for all types of hair.

Dissolve the gum is alcohol. Stir it over a very low flame and add castor oil and glycerine to it. Keep stirring and add water. Cool and bottle it. If desired a few drops of fragrance can be added before it cools down.

Lime Hari Setting Preparation

Gelatine	1 cup
Hot water	2 cups
Lemon juice	1 tsp

Procedure : Mix all the ingredients and use it for setting your hair. The mixture is specially recommended for oily hair.

Hari Conditioners for All Hari Types

Avocado Hair Conditioner

Avocado paste	1 cup
Egg yolk	2 eggs

Procedure : Beat the egg and mix avocado to get a mixture. Apply this for 30 minutes and then wash off with lukewam water.

Sunflower Hair Conditioner

Wheat germ oil	1 cup
Sunflower	1 cup

Procedure : Mix the to oils and warm the mixture. Massage it into the head and wash off with lukewarm water in which 1 tablespoon of lemon juice has been added.

Wheat Hair Conditioner

Wheat germ oil	1 tsp
Milk	1 tbsp
Egg yolk	1 egg
Water	1 cup
Lemon juice	1 tsp
Glycerine	1 tbsp

Procedure : beat the egg and mix all the other ingredients. Massage into the head. Rinse off with lukearm water which is mixed with lemon juice.

Hair Rinses

Rinses are required to give a shiny and satiny look to the hair. They are really good to provide a shield to your hair against the hazads of pollution and sun.

Apple Hair Rinse

Malt Vinegar	200 ml
Hot water	1 litre

Procedure : Mix the two and apply on the hair. Complete the drying in a warm room. The hair will take and attractive gloss and golden tint. It is good for oily hair.

Barley Hair Rinse

Malt vinegar	1 cup
Hot water	1 cup

Procedure : Malt vinegar, when mixed with warm water and applied on the hair, leaves the hair soft and glossy and brings out the colour. Then with barley boiled water (4 parts water and one part barley) wash the hair and let it dry after the required setting being done. (It is a very efficient setting lotion for oily hair.

Chamomile Hair Rinse

Chamomile flower (powder)	1 cup
Kaolin powder	1 cup

Procedure : Take chamomile crushed flowers and kaolin powder. Make a paste of the two. Massage well into the hair and leave it on for 30 minutes. Rinse it off with lukewarm water containing juice of one lemon. Your hair will become attractive. This rinse can be used for all types of hair.

Rosemary-Chamomile Hair Rinse

Chamomile flower (powder)	2 handful
Rosemary tops (powder)	1 handful
Water	500 ml

Procedure : Take chamomile flowers and rosemary tops, place these in a saucepan. Pour boiling water over them. It will give a hair a luster like sheen and enhance its golden colour also. This can be used for all hair types.

Rosemary Hair Rinse

Rosemary tops/leaves	60 gm
Water	1 litre

Procedure : Put the ingredients in a pan and slowly simmer it for 10-15 minutes. Strain the mixture and get the rinse. When it gets cool use it after shampooing. This application used by all hair types gives a lustrous and beautiful look to your hair.

Hair Setting Preparations for All Hair Types

Hair setting preparations are needed to aid styling of your hair. This helps in easy handling of hair, especially, those which tend to be flying and highly unmanageable. Try either of the under mentioned preparations.

Bay-Rum Hair Setting Preparation

Bay leaves	500 gm
Rum	500 ml
Water	500 ml

Procedure : Mix the first two and let the mixture stand for 10-15 dyas. Strain and add the water. Pour it in an airtight bottle and use when required. But this mixture should be kept under refrigeration.

Clove Hari Setting Preparation

Almond oil	1 cup
Palm oil	2 tsp
Benzoated lard	500 gm
Lemon juice	2 tsp
Oil of cloves	1 tsp

Procedure : Heat the benzoated lard and mix it with rest of the ingredients. It will make a pleasantly scented cream to set the hair.

Gum Tragacanth Hair Setting Preparation

Gum tragacanth	15 gm
Alcohol	20 ml
Castor oil	2 tbsp
Glycerine	1 tbsp
Water	250 ml
Perfume	as required

Procedure : Dissolve the gum in alcohol. Stir it over a very of low folame and add castor oil and glycerine to it. Keep stirring and add water. Cool and bottle it. If desired, a few drops of perfume can be added.

Anti-Dandruff Preparation

Sesame oil	1 tbsp
Bilavan	3 tbsp

Procedure : Blend the two together and apply it on the head. Leave it on for 2-3 hours and wash it off with a shampoo in lukewarm water.

Anti-Dandruff Rosemary Preparation

Rosemary leaves	1 handful
Water	1 litre
Vinegar	2 tsp

Procedure : Boil the water and soak rosemary leaves in it. Let it stand for one night. Strain and add vinegar to it. After shampooing wash your hair with this prepartion. It treats the hiar very fast.

Anti-Dandruff Lemon Preparation

Lemon juice	8 tbsp
Water	1.5 cup

Procedure : Mix both the ingredients together and apply it on the head. Leave it on for 2-3 hours then wash off. This treats the dandruff miraculously.

Anti-Dandruff Lemon Preparation

Lemon Peels	1 handful
Saptala	1 handful
Water	500 ml

Procedure : Soak lemon peels and saptala in boiling water. Let it stand for 5-6hours then strain it. Use this prepration for rinsing your hair after shampooing.

Anti-Dandruff Egg Preparation

Egg white	1 egg
Lemon juice	1 tbsp

Procedure : beat the egg white and mix lemon juice in it. Apply it and have to soak for about an hour before washing the hair with a shampoo.

Anti Dandruff Vinegar Preparation

Vinegar	2 tbsp
Water	0.5 bucket

Procedure : Mix the vinegar in the water. When you have shampoed your hair wash your hiar with this mixture if troubled with dandruff.

Anti Dandruff Sesame Preparation

Sesame oil	500 ml
Bhangra leaves	100 gm

Procedure : Both Bhangra leaves in sesame oil for 15 minuts. Let it stand for an hour, than starch it. Massage this oil in your head. leave it for an hour then shampoo your hair.

Chapter - 21

PLANT ECONOMICS ON HERBAL COSMETICS

Rated Plant Capacity = 305.00 Kgs/Day

LAND & BUILDING (Land 2000 sq.mt.) = Rs. 26,50,000.00

PLANT & MACHINERY

1. Stainless Steel Tank with agitator
2. Stainless Steel Tank (closed top)
3. Tray Dryer
4. Pulveriser
5. Crusher
6. Filter Press
7. Homogeniser
8. Percolator
9. Grinding machine
10. Sterilization unit
11. Storage Tank (SS)
12. Bottle filling & sealing machine
13. Automatic filling & sealing machine
14. Laboratory and testing equipments
15. Miscellaneous viz weighing balance, screen etc.

FIXED CAPITAL

1.	Land & Building	Rs.	26,50,000.0
2.	Plant & Machinery	Rs.	12,35,000.0
3.	Other Fixed Assets	Rs.	3,20,000.0
	TOTAL	Rs.	42,05,000.0

RAW MATERIALS

1. Til Oil
2. Motha, Kankol
3. Thus, Charrila
4. (Sailag) Nagar
5. Chandar
6. Long, Dalchine
7. Ratanjot
8. Kapur Kachure
9. Sat bar
10. Tejpal
11. How bar
12. Bahara
13. Amla Oil
14. Harral
15. Clampa
16. Keora (Keya)
18. Alachi,
19. Pudeena
20. Perfume
21. Menthol
22. Ouotl water
23. Ouillaya bark powder
24. Ammonium Carbonate
25. Borax
26. Bay leaf oil
27. Heena powder
28. Sodium Carbonate
29. Potassium Carbonate
30. Soap powder
31. Perfume
32. Calcium Carbonate
33. Sodium Carboxy Methyl Cellulose
34. Glycerin
35. Preservative
36. Soda Lauryl Sulphate
37. Herbal Extract (Flower)
38. Annar ke phul (Pomegranate flamer)
39. Annar ke chilke (Pomegranate skin)
40. Bhuna Huwa suhaya (Roasted Borax)
42. Bhuna Huwa Fitkari (Roasted alum)

Plant Economics on Herbal Cosmetics

43. Akarkara
44. Majuphal (Gall Nut),
45. Rume Martage
46. Samendra Thag
47. Supari Bhuni Huwi (Roasted tal Nut)
48. Lanolin
49. Emulsifying wax
50. Beer wax
51. Almond
52. Herblotion
53. Powdered Mehandi leaves
54. Powdered Caanill flamer
55. Walnut bark
56. Kohl Powder
57. Indigo Leaves

TOTAL WORKING CAPITAL/MONTH

1.	Raw Material	Rs.	4,60,644.45
2.	Salary & Wages	Rs.	63,000.00
3.	Utilities & Overheads	Rs.	41,500.00
	TOTAL	Rs.	5,65,144.45

TOTAL CAPITAL INVESTMENT

Total Fixed Capital	Rs.	42,05,000.00
Total Working Capital for 3 Months	Rs.	16,95,433.35
TOTAL	Rs.	59,00,433.35

TURN OVER/ANNUM

Herbal Hair Oil 15,000 litres
Herbal Hair Shampoo 30000 litre
Herbal Tooth Paste 15000 kgs
Herbal Tooth Powder 1500 kgs
Herbal cleansing cream 1500 kgs
Herbal Henna 15000 kg

TOTAL	Rs.	1,08,75,000.00

PROFIT SALES RATIO = 23.47 %
RATE OF RETURN = 43.25 %
BREAK EVEN POINT (B.E.P) = 44.46 %

Chapter - 22

PLANT ECONOMICS ON HERBAL SHAMPOO AND CREAMS

Rated Plant Capacity = 750.00 Bottles/Day
1.250 Bottles SHAMPOO/Day
(100 ML. PACK)
500 Bottles SKIN TONING
CREAM/Day (50 gms PACK

LAND & BUILDING (Land required 500 Sq.mt.) = Rs. 16,40,000.00

PLANT & MACHINERY

1. Storage tank
2. Reaction vessel
3. S.S. Homogeniser
4. Bottle washing, cleaning & drying.
5. Filtering unit
6. Pumps & accessories.
7. Heating & other miscellaneous electrical appliance.
8. Lab testing equipment.
9. Mixing tank
10. Filling Machine
11. General Equipments piping & instrumentation.
12. Lab testing equipment.
13. Weighing machine equipment.
14. Other miscellaneous tools etc.
15. Pumps, fans, blowers, etc.

FIXED CAPITAL

1.	Land & Building	Rs.	16,40,000.00
2.	Plant & Machinery	Rs.	4,50,000.00
3.	Other Fixed Assets	Rs.	1,10,000.00
	TOTAL	Rs.	22,00,000.00

RAW MATERIALS

1. Sodium lauryl sulphate
2. Coconut diethanolamide
3. Glycol stearate
4. Methyl p-hydroxy benzoate
5. Formaldehyde
6. Sodium benzoate.
7. Phosphoric acid.
8. Sodium chloride
9. Yellow dye
10. Perfume
11. Egg powder
12. Gainda flower
13. Motir flower petals
14. Anarpeel
15. Pudina
16. Potato meal
17. Kheera
18. Orange peel
19. Tulsi
20. Nimboo peels
21. Chandan powder
22. Neem leaves
23. Chironji
24. Shakti chur
25. Multani mitti
26. Glycerine
27. Methyl-p-hydroxy benzoate

TOTAL WORKING CAPITAL/MONTH

1.	Raw Material	Rs.	69,600.00
2.	Salary & Wages	Rs.	69,520.00
3.	Utilities & Overheads	Rs.	59,000.00
	TOTAL	Rs.	1,98,120.00

TOTAL CAPITAL INVESTMENT

Total Fixed Capital	Rs.	22,00,000.01
Total Working Capital for 3 Months	Rs.	5,94,360.00
TOTAL	Rs.	27,94,360.01

TURN OVER/ANNUM

Sale of 75000 Nos. of shampoo bottles (100 ml pack)
Sale of skin toning cream 15000 bottles

TOTAL	Rs.	44,25,000.00

PROFIT SALES RATIO = 34.75 %
RATE OF RETURN = 55.03 %
BREAK EVEN POINT (B.E.P) = 42.29 %

Chapter - 23

PLANT ECONOMICS OF TOILET SOAP AND HERBAL SOAP

Rated Plant Capacity = 500.00 Kgs/Day

LAND & BUILDING = Rs. 42,50,000.00
(Land required 1000 sq.mt.)

PLANT & MACHINERY

1. Boiling Kettle
2. Mixing & Kneading Machine
3. Chilling rolls
4. Dryer
5. Plodder Machine
6. Cutting machine
7. Semi-automatic stamping press
8. Miscellaneous like pipe fitting, conveying system etc.
9. Complete Plant for Manufacturing of Herbal Toilet Soap with Cosmetics Products

FIXED CAPITAL

1.	Land & Building	Rs.	42,50,000.00
2.	Plant & Machinery	Rs.	7,52,500.00
3.	Other Fixed Assets	Rs.	27,500.00
	TOTAL	Rs.	50,30,000.00

RAW MATERIALS

1. Neem Oil, Castor Oil, Soap Noodles, Common Salt etc. for Herbal Soap
2. Coconut oil

3. Castor oil
4. Caustic Soda lye
5. Carbolic acid
6. Colour
7. Palm Rosa oil and other perfume

TOTAL WORKING CAPITAL/MONTH

1.	Raw Material	Rs.	5,71,225.00
2.	Salary & Wages	Rs.	51,750.00
3.	Utilities & Overheads	Rs.	73,850.00
	TOTAL	Rs.	6,96,825.00

TOTAL CAPITAL INVESTMENT

Total Fixed Capital	Rs.	50,30,000.00
Total Working Capital for 3 Months	Rs.	20,90,475.00
TOTAL	Rs.	71,20,475.00

TURN OVER/ANNUM

By sale of 1,50,000 Kg. of Toilet
Soap and Herbal Soap   Rs.   1,09,50,000.00

PROFIT SALES RATIO = 13.34 %
RATE OF RETURN = 20.51 %
BREAK EVEN POINT (B.E.P) = 54.24 %

Chapter - 24

PLANT ECONOMICS OF HERBAL HAIR OIL (AYURVEDIC)

Rated Plant Capacity = 14700.00 Bottles/Day

LAND & BUILDING = Rs. 12,75,000.00
(Land required 3000 Sq.Mtrs.)

PLANT & MACHINERY

1. Stainless steel kettle
2. Pulverizing
3. S.S. Vessel fitted with agitator
4. M.S. Tanks
5. Mixer
6. Filter
7. Packing machine
8. Til oil storage tank
9. Lab equipments.

FIXED CAPITAL

1.	Land & Building	Rs.	12,75,000.00
2.	Plant & Machinery	Rs.	9,30,000.00
3.	Other Fixed Assets	Rs.	2,23,000.00
	TOTAL	Rs.	24,28,000.00

RAW MATERIALS

1. Hartago (harar) fruit
2. Bahera fruit
3. Til oil
4. Manjisht twigs

5. Turmeric (haldi)
6. Kapur (camphor)
7. Amla oil
8. Lawanga (clove oil ext.)
9. Chandan (sandal wood oil)
10. Kewara ext.
11. Jatamansi oil ext.
12. Pudina salts
13. Almond oil
14. Packaging material

TOTAL WORKING CAPITAL/MONTH

1.	Raw Material	Rs.	53,43,609.90
2.	Salary & Wages	Rs.	77,750.00
3.	Utilities & Overheads	Rs.	67,000.00
	TOTAL	Rs.	54,88,359.90

TOTAL CAPITAL INVESTMENT

Total Fixed Capital	Rs.	24,28,000.00
Total Working Capital for 3 Months	Rs.	1,64,65,079.70
TOTAL	Rs.	1,88,93,079.70

TURN OVER/ANNUM

By sale of 44,10,000 bottles (100 ml each) of herbal oils (ayurvedic) like banphool oil   Rs. 7,93,80,000.00

PROFIT SALES RATIO = 12.35 %
RATE OF RETURN = 51.90 %
BREAK EVEN POINT (B.E.P) = 31.01 %

Chapter - 25

PLANT ECONOMICS OF ANTISEPTIC CREAM

Rated Plant Capacity = 200.00 Kgs/Day

LAND & BUILDING = Rs. 15,25,000.00
(Land 750 sq. mts.)

PLANT & MACHINERY

1. Stainless Steel Jacketted Vessel
2. Stainless steel tank
3. S.S. filling tank
4. Automatic weighing filling, tube sealing machine
5. Conveyor
6. Cardboard Pack, filling sealing machine
7. Electronic weighing balance
8. Electronic balance small
9. Carton sealing machine
10. Laboratory Equipments

FIXED CAPITAL

1.	Land & Building	Rs.	15,25,000.00
2.	Plant & Machinery	Rs.	35,95,000.00
3.	Other Fixed Assets	Rs.	8,20,000.00
	TOTAL	Rs.	59,40,000.00

RAW MATERIALS

1. Extract of Calendula
2. Extract of Chandan
3. Extract of Ushir

4. Extract of Ghritkumar
5. Extract of Tulsi
6. Extract of Jatamansi
7. Extract of Saussurea Lappa
8. Extract of Aguru
9. Extract of Daruharidra
10. Zinc Oxide
11. Absolute Alcohol
12. White petroleum jelly
13. Lanoline
14. Mineral Oil
15. Packaging Tubes, Printed cardboard packs, cartons etc.

TOTAL WORKING CAPITAL/MONTH

1.	Raw Material	Rs.	6,61,725.00
2.	Salary & Wages	Rs.	1,09,500.00
3.	Utilities & Overheads	Rs.	1,65,500.00
	TOTAL	Rs.	9,36,725.00

TOTAL CAPITAL INVESTMENT

Total Fixed Capital	Rs.	59,40,000.00
Total Working Capital for 3 Months	Rs.	28,10,175.00
TOTAL	Rs.	87,50,175.00

TURN OVER/ANNUM

By sale of 30,00,000 Packs of Antiseptic cream in 20 gms size packs (60000 kgs. total cream)   Rs.   1,80,00,000.00

PROFIT SALES RATIO = 22.85 %
RATE OF RETURN = 47.01 %
BREAK EVEN POINT (B.E.P) = 49.09 %

Chapter - 26

PLANT ECONOMICS OF KESH KALA TEL

Rated Plant Capacity = 5000.00 Bottles/Day
100 gm each bottle

LAND & BUILDING (Land area 500 Sq.Mts.) = Rs. 12,50,000.00

PLANT & MACHINERY

1. Mixing vessel (S.S.) with stirrer
2. Reaction vessel
3. Baby boiler
4. Automatic bottle filling, sealing & weighing machines.
5. Lab equipments.

FIXED CAPITAL

1.	Land & Building	Rs.	12,50,000.00
2.	Plant & Machinery	Rs.	18,95,000.00
3.	Other Fixed Assets	Rs.	6,70,000.00
	TOTAL	Rs.	38,15,000.00

RAW MATERIALS

1. Paraffin oil
2. Triethanolamine
3. Glyceryl monolaurate
4. Gum tragacanth
5. Stearic acid
6. PPD dye

7. Methyl parahydroxy benzoate
8. Water (distilled)
9. Perfumes
10. Packaging material
11. Card board boxes
12. Miscellaneous packaging materials viz. cartons etc.

TOTAL WORKING CAPITAL/MONTH

1.	Raw Material	Rs.	8,93,775.00
2.	Salary & Wages	Rs.	64,625.00
3.	Utilities & Overheads	Rs.	76,000.00
	TOTAL	Rs.	10,34,400.00

TOTAL CAPITAL INVESTMENT

Total Fixed Capital	Rs.	38,15,000.00
Total Working Capital for 3 Months	Rs.	31,03,200.00
TOTAL	Rs.	69,18,200.00

TURN OVER/ANNUM

Sale of 15,00,000 bottles of Kesh Kala Tel (100 gm. each bottle)	Rs.	1,87,50,000.00

PROFIT SALES RATIO = 24.26 %
RATE OF RETURN = 65.76 %
BREAK EVEN POINT (B.E.P) = 35.12 %

Chapter - 27

PLANT ECONOMICS OF KALI MEHANDI

Rated Plant Capacity = 20.00 Kgs./Day

LAND & BUILDING = Rs. 1,79,500.00
(Land required 150 sq.mts)

PLANT & MACHINERY

1. Pulverizer-cum-mixer
2. Storage vessel
3. Mixing vessel
4. Homogeniser
5. Drier
6. Grinding machine
7. Bottle filling machine
8. Powder packaging machine
9. Lab-Equipments
10. Baby boiler
11. Screening Machine
12. Weighing Machine
13. Generator
14. Erection and others

FIXED CAPITAL

1.	Land & Building	Rs.	1,79,500.00
2.	Plant & Machinery	Rs.	2,29,000.00
3.	Other Fixed Assets	Rs.	80,000.00
	TOTAL	Rs.	4,88,500.00

RAW MATERIALS

1. Mehandi Powder
2. Lecithin
3. E.D.T.A.(Ethylene diamine tetracetic acid tetrasodium salt)
4. Water
5. Sodium sulfite
6. Ammonium hydroxide
7. Isopropanol
8. Para-phenylenediamine
9. Para amino phenol
10. 2-Hydroxy 1:4 naphthaquinoze
11. Pyrogallol
12. Hydroquinone
13. Perfume

TOTAL WORKING CAPITAL/MONTH

1.	Raw Material	Rs.	1,46,425.00
2.	Salary & Wages	Rs.	11,125.00
3.	Utilities & Overheads	Rs.	9,950.00
	TOTAL	Rs.	1,67,500.00

TOTAL CAPITAL INVESTMENT

Total Fixed Capital	Rs.	4,88,500.00
Total Working Capital for 3 Months	Rs.	5,02,500.00
TOTAL	Rs.	9,91,000.00

TURN OVER/ANNUM

Receipt By sale 6000 kg in packed Kali Mehandi powder	Rs.	29,10,000.00

PROFIT SALES RATIO = 20.77 %
RATE OF RETURN = 61.00 %
BREAK EVEN POINT (B.E.P) = 39.62 %

Chapter - 28

PLANT ECONOMICS ON HAIR OIL AND FORMULATION

Rated Plant Capacity = 60.00 Kgs./Day

LAND & BUILDING (Land Required 200 sq.mt.) = Rs. 3,00,000.00

PLANT & MACHINERY

1. Stainless steel tank with stirrer
2. Filling machine manually operated
3. Sealing machine
4. Bottle washing machine pump, motors etc.,
5. Bottle dryer
6. Filter press
7. Laboratory equipments

FIXED CAPITAL

1.	Land & Building	Rs.	3,00,000.00
2.	Plant & Machinery	Rs.	1,62,000.00
3.	Other Fixed Assets	Rs.	62,000.00
	TOTAL	Rs.	5,24,000.00

RAW MATERIALS

1. Castor oil (Deodorised)
2. Colour
3. Tincture cantheridine
4. Oil rosemary
5. English lavender
6. Heiko Tuberose

7. Coconut oil
8. Amla oil
9. Benzoic Acid
10. Oil colour
11. Lemon oil
12. Bergamout oil
13. Rosemary oil
14. Nerole oil
15. Lavender oil
16. Bela (Jasmine) oil
17. Refined coconut oil
18. Alkanet root
19. Oil lavender
20. Oil geranium rose
21. Clores oil
22. Oil cinnamon
23. Oil bergmol

TOTAL WORKING CAPITAL/MONTH

1.	Raw Material	Rs.	1,05,706.55
2.	Salary & Wages	Rs.	12,878.75
3.	Utilities & Overheads	Rs.	11,460.00
	TOTAL	Rs.	1,30,045.30

TOTAL CAPITAL INVESTMENT

Total Fixed Capital	Rs.	5,24,000.00
Total Working Capital for 3 Months	Rs.	3,90,135.90
TOTAL	Rs.	9,14,135.90

TURN OVER/ANNUM

Sale of Amla oil 6000 kgs.
Sale of Jasmine oil 6000 kgs
Sale of catheridine oil 6000 kgs.

TOTAL   Rs.   24,30,000.00

PROFIT SALES RATIO = 27.21 %
RATE OF RETURN = 72.32 %
BREAK EVEN POINT (B.E.P) = 32.97 %

Chapter - 29

PLANT ECONOMICS OF BABY OIL

Rated Plant Capacity = 500.00 Kgs./Day
2500 Bottles/Day OF 100 ML
1250 Bottles/Day OF 200 ML

LAND & BUILDING = Rs. 14,00,000.00
(Land Area 500 sq.mt)

PLANT & MACHINERY

1. Mixer (M.S)
2. Filter
3. Storage Tanks
4. Boiler
5. Bottle filling & scaling machine
6. Laboratory Testing Equipment
7. Misc. pipe & pipe fitting, tools etc.

FIXED CAPITAL

1.	Land & Building	Rs.	14,00,000.00
2.	Plant & Machinery	Rs.	5,00,000.00
3.	Other Fixed Assets	Rs.	1,00,000.00
	TOTAL	Rs.	20,00,000.00

RAW MATERIALS

1. Mineral oil light
2. Olive Oil
3. Hexachlorophene

4. Antioxidant(tocopherol)
5. Perfume
6. Packaging Materials (Glass/Plastic/PET Bottle) Labels & other Misc. Consumables (L.S)

TOTAL WORKING CAPITAL/MONTH

1.	Raw Material	Rs.	10,94,995.00
2.	Salary & Wages	Rs.	1,00,415.00
3.	Utilities & Overheads	Rs.	53,550.00
	TOTAL	Rs.	12,48,960.00

TOTAL CAPITAL INVESTMENT

Total Fixed Capital	Rs.	20,00,000.00
Total Working Capital for 3 Months	Rs.	37,46,880.00
TOTAL	Rs.	57,46,880.00

TURN OVER/ANNUM

Sale of Baby Oil	Rs.	2,06,25,000.00

PROFIT SALES RATIO = 21.79 %
RATE OF RETURN = 78.19 %
BREAK EVEN POINT (B.E.P) = 29.53 %

Chapter - 30

ESTABLISHMENT OF A HERBAL BEAUTY PARLOUR

Herbal beauty parlour can be established in a very small investment by ladies in their own residences. The awareness of looking beautiful is growing not only in big cities but also in small towns and the ladies are taking the services of professional beauticians in beauty parlours. Before establishing a beauty parlour following considerations are important :

1. Present status and viability of beauty parlours.

2. Training for beauticians, consultancy and franchisee assistance for beauty parlours.

3. Requirement of funds and the sources of financial assistance.

1. Present status and viability of beauty parlours

The conventional beauty parlours normally use chemical based cosmetics in the form of skin bleaching creams and hair dyes which are harmful in long run, which the herbal beauty products used in herbal beauty parlours do not have any side effects and therefore the herbal beauty parlours are not only beauty parlours but beauty clinics where the beauty problems are diagnosed and given natural treatment, so that such problems have a permanent cure instead of a temporary one. Due to this fact the future of such herbal beauty parlours is very bright. The services of beaty parlours include hair cutting & setting, facial bridal make-up etc. which requires the services of well trained beauticians.

2. Training for beauticians, consultancy and franchise assistance for beauty parlours.

Professional training of beauticians for various services like hair cutting, hair treatment, hair dressing/styling, beauty culture, make-up beauty therapy, thermolyses, Electrolysis, Manicure, Padicure, Peeling etc. are available from reputed institutes like Shahnaz Herbal and training institute and others. In the training institute various diploma and crash courses are available.

It is advisable to associate with some reputed beauty parlour like Shahnaz Hussain and act as their franchisee. This not only enhances the credibility of beauty parlour but also ets the various beauty products from the parent unit and also follows their procedures and rules. The parent unit also helps the ranchisee in the publicity of its franchisee.

3. Requirement of Funds and the sources of Financial Assistance.

A small level beauty pariour can be setup within an investment of Rs. One lakh and the funds are available from various Government agencies, banks and government shchemes viz. Pime Minister Rozgar Yojna. A brief profile giving the funds required and profitability of such beauty parlour is as under:

Project Economics

A. Fixed Costs :

Land and building

Semi furnished room of area about 30 sq. mtr. at a monthly rent of Rs. 2,000/-

Equipments

Hydro Dryer	1 No.	
Ozone Machine	1 No.	
Vibrating Messagers	2 Nos.	
Hair Dryers	2 No.	
Wax heater	1 No.	Rs.50,000
Steamer	1 No.	
Peeling Machine	1 No.	
Termolysis Machine	1 No.	
Steamozore	1 No.	

Furnitures & Fixtures

Partition Wall	1 Set
Show Cases	2 Nos.
Dressing Tables	2 Nos.
Hydraulic Chairs	1 Nos.
Revolving Chairs	2 Nos.
Ordinary Chairs	4 Nos.
Mirrors	4 Nos.

B. Running Costs (Monthly)

Raw Materials

Cosmetics, Hairdyes, Talcum Powder & Face Powder Creams, Oils, waxes ec.	Rs. 8000

Salaries of staff:

Beautician (Enterpreneur)	Rs. 4,000
Assistant Beautician	Rs. 3,000
Assistant (General)	Rs. 2,000

Misc. Expenses:

(insurance, Advertisement, Stationery, & Maintenance	Rs. 2,000

Electric Power — Rs. 1,000

Working Capital (per month):

Rent of premises	R. 2,000
Raw Materials	Rs. 8,000
Salaries	Rs. 9,000
Electric Powder	Rs. 1,000
Misc. Expenses	Rs. 2,000
Total	Rs. 22,000

(C) Total cost of project

Fixed Cost	Rs. 90,000
Working capital per month	Rs. 22,000
Total	Rs, 1,12,000

(D) Means of finance

Loan from bank (75%)	Rs. 84,000
Equity (25%)	Rs. 28,000
Total	Rs. 1,12,000

(E) Annual cost of production

Working capital per year (Rs. 22000x12)	Rs. 2,64000
Depreciation on fixed assets(@20%)	Rs. 18,000
Interest on loan(@15%)	Rs. 12,600
Total cost of production per annum	Rs. 2,94,600

(F) Monthly Revernue :

	Beauty Services	Nos./Month
1.	Eyebrow	75
2.	Maicure	25
3.	Padicure	25
4.	Head message	25
5.	Hair bleaching	25
6.	Arm bleaching	25
7.	Face bleaching	25
8.	Stomach bleaching	15
9.	Waxing	25
10.	Facial	25
11.	Hair setting	50
12.	Hair Cutting	50
13.	Hair dye	15
14.	Bridal make-up	02
15.	Purming	05
16.	Ozone treatment(for hair)	05

17.	Ozone treatment (for face)	05
18.	Thermoherb treatment	05
19.	Vegetable peeling	05
20.	Eye treatment	10
(for removing blmishes)		10

Lumpsum monthly Revenue	Rs.35,000/-
Annual Revenue	**Rs. 4,20,000**

(G) Profitablity:

Profit per year -- Rs. 420000-Rs,294600=Rs,1,25,400/-

Profit per monh: Rs.10,450

(This profit is in addition to the monthly salary of the Beautician Entrepreneur --Rs.4,000/-)

OTHER USEFUL PUBLICATIONS

★HANDBOOK OF SYNTHETIC & HERBAL COSMETICS
★COSMETICS PROCESSES & FORMULATIONS HANDBOOK
★HAND BOOK OF PERFUEMS WITH FORMULATIONS
★ESSENTIAL OILS PROCESSES & FORMULATIONS HAND BOOK
★HAND BOOK OF ESSENTIAL OILS MFG. & AROMATIC PLANTS
★HANDBOOK OF PERFUMES & FLAVOURS
★HAND BOOK OF HERBS, MEDICINAL & AROMATIC PLANTS CULTIVATION

AVAILABLE AT :

ENGINEERS INDIA RESEARCH INSTITUTE

Regd. Off. : 4449, Nai Sarak (S1), Main Road, Delhi-6 (India)
Ph. : 3918117, 3916431, 3960797, 3920361 Fax : 91-11-3916431
E-mail : eirisidi@bol.net.in Website : startindustry.com

Chapter - 31

HERBAL BEAUTY PRODUCTS MANUFACTURE

With the growing awareness of consumer towards natural products and increased health consciousness, the inclination towards herbal beauty products is on the rose.

The natural & herbal beauty products being free form any harmful side effects and soft to the body ae gaining importance in current times. These herbal beauty products are bases upon herbs, minerals, fruits, vegetables, honey, milk, lemon, vinegar, heena, eggs etc.

Product Mix

It is proposed to set up a unit to manufacture following herbal beauty products:-

1. Skin (cleansing, cold & vanishing) creams & face lotions
2. Pomades
3. Beauty masks
4. Face powders & talcum powders
5. Hair washes & shampoos
6. Hair oils & hair lotions
7. Cosmetics for make-up

Formulations & Process of Manufacture

The Formulations as given in chapter 4 'Different herbal cosmetis preparations' are selected for diferent herbal beauty products.

The process of manufature of various herbal beauty products involves, taking of different ingredients in the predetemined quantities as per the formulations, theri heating grinding, sieving mixing (dry or wet), emulsification or homogenization, filtering and packing. The packaging is done as per the products characteristics and requirements.

Quality control tests are conducted from raw material stage to processing and finished products.

Project Economics

A. Fixed Costs :   Rs. lakhs

    Land : 400 sq mtrs @ Rs. 600/sq mtrs.   2.40

    Site development expenses   0.60

    Building :

    (a) workshed & store 200 sq. mtrs.

    @ Rs. 4000/sq.   8.00

    (b) office & lab 60 sq. mtr. @ Rs. 5000/sq.   3.00

    Plant & Machinery

    1. Micro Pulversiers/Grinders

    2. Sifter

    3. Paddle/Drum mixers

    4. Homogenizer/Emulsification equipment

    5. Strainer or filter   Rs. 25.00 lakhs

    6. Jacketed/non jacketed kettles

    7. Filling & sealing machines

    8. Labelling machines

    Misc. Fixed Assets

    Electricals, furniture, weighing, scales,
testing and material handling accessories Rs. 5.00 lakhs.

    Running Costs (Monthly)

(A) Raw Materials

    Herbal & Natural Products

    (i)   Herbal extracts

    (ii) Essential oils

    (iii) Vegetable oils

(iv) Aromatic waters   Rs. 3.00 lakhs
(v) Natural waxes
(vi) Lanoline
(vii) Case in

Non herbal products
(i) Stearic acid
(ii) Glycerine
(iii) Emulsifiers
(iv) Boric acid
(v) Perfumes
(vi) Titanium oxide
(vii) Petroleum jelly

Packing material

(B) **Salaries of staff : (monthly)**

	No.	Amount in Rs. per month
Production Incharge	1	5000
Sales/purchase assistant	1	4000
Skilled operators	2	6000
Helpers	4	10,000
Total	8	25,000

Monthly Salary   Rs. 0.25 lakhs

Misc. Expenses.
(Insurance, Advertisement,
Stationery & Maintenance)   Rs. 0.15 lakhs

Electric Power   Rs. 0.35 lakhs

Working Capital (per month):   Rs. lakhs

Raw Materials	3.00
Packaging	0.25
Salaries	0.25
Electric Power	0.35
Misc. Expenses	0.15
Total	4.00 lakhs

(C) Total cost of project

Fixed Cost	Rs. 44 lakhs
Working capital per month	Rs. 4 lakhs
Total	Rs. 48 lakhs

(D) Means of finance

Loan from bank (75%)	Rs. 36 lakhs
Equity (25%)	Rs. 12 lakhs
Total	Rs. 48 lakhs

(E) Annual cost of production

Working capital per year (Rs. 4 lakhs×12)	Rs. 48 lakhs
Depriciation of fixed assets (@20%)	Rs. 6 lakhs
Interest on loan (@15%)	Rs. 5.4 lakhs
Total cost of production per annum	Rs. 59.4 lakhs
	(say Rs. 60 lakhs)

(F) Monthly Sales Revenue :

Following finished products in different quantities will be sold.

1. Skin creams & lotions
2. Pomades
3. Beauty masks
4. Face powders & Talcum powders
5. Hair washes & shampoos

6. hair oils & hair lotions

7. Cosmetics for make-up.

Total quantity : 3750 kg/month

Lumpsum monthly revenue Rs. 3750kg/monthly @ Rs. 200 per kg (average price)   Rs. 7.5 lakh/month

Annual Sales Revenue	Rs. 90 lakhs

(G) Profitability :

Profit per year - Rs. 90 laksh - Rs. 60 lakh = Rs. 30 lakhs

Profit per month : Rs. 2.5 lakh

OTHER USEFUL PUBLICATIONS

★ HANDBOOK OF SYNTHETIC & HERBAL COSMETICS
★ COSMETICS PROCESSES & FORMULATIONS HANDBOOK
★ HAND BOOK OF PERFUEMS WITH FORMULATIONS
★ ESSENTIAL OILS PROCESSES & FORMULATIONS HAND BOOK
★ HAND BOOK OF ESSENTIAL OILS MFG. & AROMATIC PLANTS
★ HANDBOOK OF PERFUMES & FLAVOURS
★ HAND BOOK OF HERBS, MEDICINAL & AROMATIC PLANTS CULTIVATION

AVAILABLE AT :

ENGINEERS INDIA RESEARCH INSTITUTE

Regd. Off. : 4449, Nai Sarak (S1), Main Road, Delhi-6 (India)
Ph. : 3918117, 3916431, 3960797, 3920361 Fax : 91-11-3916431
E-mail : eirisidi@bol.net.in Website : startindustry.com

Chapter - 32

LIST OF HERBS SUPPLIERS

A.S.R. Company
Punalur-691305
Kerala

A.V.V. Satyanarayna
A.P. Residential School
Pedabayalu-531040
Visakhapatnam
Andhra Pradesh

Abhuday Industries
27 Market Yard
Sidhpur-384151
Gujarat

Abirami Botanical Corporation
55,P.S.S. Nadar Street
Tuticorin-628001
Tamilnadu
Senna & Crude Merchant

Academy of Development Sciences
Karjat Taluka
District Raigad Kashela
P.O. - 410201
Maharashtra

Adcco Ltd.
District Hoogli Adcconagar
P.O.-712121
West Bengal
Adco Corporation
67-69 Mohammedan Road
2nd Floor, Dada Manzil,
Mumbai-400003
Maharashtra

Ahmedali Jafferjee Gandhi
24, Pollock Street
Kolkata-700001
West Bengal

All India Drug Supply Company
11, Dariyasthan Street,
Masjid Bunder Road,
Mumbai-400003
Maharashtra

Aman Impex Pvt. Ltd.
14, Roop Chand Roy Street
Kolkata-700007
West Bengal

Amar Ji
330 Katra Hussain Baksh
Khari Baoil
Delhi-110006

A.M.K. Mohammed Ibrahim Rowther
Davapuram Road,
Tuticorin-628003
Tamil Nadu

Amrutha Kesari
364, Avenue Road
Bangalore-56002
Karnataka

Amsar Pvt. Ltd.
2, Hormuz Mansion

72-B, Desai Road
Mumbai-400026
Maharashtra

Andaman & Nicobar Fores Development Corporation Ltd.
P.O. Haddo Port Blair-744103
Andaman & Nicobar
Island (Government)

Arun & Company
Arun Chamber, P-38
Indian Exchange Place
Kolkata-700001
West Bengal

Aruna Brothers
J-27A, Jangpura Extension
P.B. 352, Delhi-110001
Delhi
Arunachal Pradesh Forest
Development Corporation Ltd.
District Tirpa Deomali-786629
Arunachal Pradesh
(Government)

Arya Vastu Bhandar
46, Dispensary Road
Dehradun - 284001
Ph.:0135-654994
E-mail :
aryavastubhandar@hotmail.com

Arya Vastu Bhandar
2308/203 Sapna Kaushik,
Market Gali Hinga Beg
Tilak Bazar
Delhi-110006
Ph.:011-3916958, 2926850
Delhi

Ashish Overseas Corporation
34, Sarvodaya Industrial Estate
Mahakali Road
Andheri East Mumbai-400093
Maharashtra

Ashok Industries
Higway, Bhandu,
District Mehsana Bhandu
Gujarat

Asian Drug Company
1244, Chah Rahat
Delhi-110006
Delhi

Asian Trading Corporation
38/40, Veer Vithal Das
Chandan Street
Mumbai-400003
Maharashtra

Assam Physiochemical Industries
R.K. Bose Road
Dhubri-793301
Assam

Aurora Export Trading Agency
6-A, 3rdFloor, Saklat Place,
Kolkata-700072
West Bengal

Babu Ram Harish Chand
2114, Khari Baoli,
Delhi-110006
Delhi

Babulal & Brother
Premnagar Dehra-Dun
Uttar Pradesh

Balisana Isabgol
GIDC Industrial Estate,
Dist. Mehsana Balisana-384110
Gujarat

Bamboo Basket
Delhi

BAN MARC
Kamdar Mansion,
Dhedar Road
Rajkot-360001
Gujarat

List of Herbs Suppliers

Banoushadi Jari-Buti Bhandar
S-19, Budh Vihar,
Delhi-110041
Delhi

Banwari Lal Shree Ram
545, Katra Ishwar Bhawan,
Khari Baoli, Delhi-110006
Delhi

Baskar Company
34, New Thandavaraya Frammi St.
Washrmenpet
Madras-600021
Tamil Nadu

Beharilal Hemraj
176 Jamuna Lal Bajaj Street
Kolkata-700007
West Bengal
Beshaj Bhawan
6668, Khari Baoli,
Delhi-110006

Bharat Crude Drug Supply Company
Ravji Mansion,
Kazi Syed Street
Mumbai-400009
Maharashtra

Bharat Drug & Extracts
13, Jail Road,
Dewas City-455001
Madhya Pradesh

Bharat Vasthu Bhandar
Dhamawala Dehradun
Uttar Pradesh

Bharati Salai
Triplicane Madras
Tamil Nadu
West Bengal

Bhartia Sons Ltd.
12, Government Place
East Calcutta-700069
West Bengal

Bhogilal C. Shah & Company
8/1, South Tukoganj,
Nabhodip, Indore-452001
Madhya Pradesh

Biddle Sawyer & Co. (India) Pvt. Ltd.
25, Dalal Street,
Fort Mumbai-400001
Maharashtra

Bisco Company
P.B.5002, 12/14,
Kazi Sayeed Street
Mumbai-400009
Maharashtra

Biyanis
25, Ganesh Chandra Avenue
Kolkata
West Bengal

Brij & Company
567-A, Katra Ishwar Bhawan
Khari Baoli, Delhi-110006
Delhi

Brij Bhushan Lal Gupta
Sarafa Bazar
Saharanpur
Uttar Pradesh

C.M. Jain
1, Carter Road,
9-A, Dhavalgauga
Bandra West Mumbai
Maharashtra

Catholic Hospital Association of India Community Health Department
P.B.2126, 157/6, Staff Road
Gunrock Enclave
Secunderabad-500003
Andhra Pradesh

Central Council for Research in Unani Medicine

Central Herb Garden & Museum National Botanical Research Institute
Campus, Lucknow-226001
Uttar Pradesh

Central Research Institute for Unani Medicine
11/4/625, Dilkhusha
A.C. Guards, Hyderabad-500004
Andhra Pradesh

Chandigarh Herbal Drug Seller's Association
Chandigarh

D. Jamnadas & Company
207, Samuel Street,
Vadgadi, Mumbai-400003
Maharashtra

Dashrathlal Ramjibhai Patel
Hari Cotton Mills Compound
Sidhpur-384151
Gujarat

Deepak Bawa & Company
Majith Mandi
Amritsar-143001
Punjab

Deepan Trading Corporation
A-47, Maskati Market, Ist Floor,
Ahmedabad-380002
Gujarat

Devi Prasad Ashish Kumar
2772, Gali Arya Samaj
Bazar Sita Ram
Delhi-110006

Devi Sahai Banwari Lal & Sons
2089-90, Katra Tambacoo,
Khari Baoli,
Delhi-110006.

Devi Sahai Mohan Lal
2210-1, Aggarwal Market,
Katra Tambacoo,
Khari Baoli,
Delhi-110006

Dinesh Gurbase Bawa Sons
Majith Mandi Amritsar
Punjab

Directorate of Cinchona & other Medicinal Plants, Government of West Bengal
10/1A, Indian Mirror Street
Kolkata-700013
West Bengal

Directorate of Forests, Government of West Bengal Minor Forests Produce Division
Siliguri
West Bengal

Directorate of Indian Medicine, Dhanvanthari Vana
GCIM, Near Bangalore University
Bangalore-560009
Karnataka

Dogra Drugs Pharma
29, Industrial Estate
Bilaspur-174001
Himachal Pradesh

Doon Trading Company
Panetitari, Premnagar P.O.
Dehra Dun-24807
Uttaranchal

Dr. Jain's Special Herbs
A-10, Raj Complex,
2nd Floor, Military Road
Marol Andheri,
East Mumbai-400059
Maharashtra

Drug & Alkaloid Company
4127, Naya Bazar,
P.B. 1297
Delhi-110006

List of Herbs Suppliers

Duncans Agro Industries Ltd.
31 Netaji Subhash Road
Kolkata
West Bengal

Durga Prasad & Company
2080/81, Katra Tambacoo
Khari Baoli,
Delhi-110006

Eastman & Company
3, Southern Avenue,
Kolkata-700026
West Bengal

Essential Oil Industries
District Sibsagar Sepon
P.O. 785673
Assam

Exel Drug House
18-B, Sukeas Lane
Kolkata-700001
West Bengal

Expo International Exporters & Supplies
20, Old Court House Street
Kolkata-700001
West Bengal

Export Enterprises
4, Bhagwan Bhawan
196/198, Samuel Street
Mumbai-400009
Maharashtra

Fairdeal Corporation Pvt. Ltd.
66, Lakshmi Building,
Sir P.M. Road,
Fort Mumbai-400001
Maharashtra

Fakirchand Jagdish Chand Mistry
Village Kahari-Kalam,
District Ambala Bhambhol
Haryana

Faqir Chand & Sons
6704, Khari Baoli,
Near Fatehpuri
Delhi-110006

Foundation For Revitalization of Local Health Traditions
50 MHS Layout 3rd Main
2nd Stage, Anandnagar,
Bangalore-560024, Karnataka

G.Dass & Company Pvt. Ltd.
27 W. Great Cotton Road,
Tuticorin-628002
Tamilnadu

Gadodia Kirana Company
2084, Katra Tambacoo
Khari Baoli,
Delhi-110006

Gaindamal Babulal & Company
Block B Pocket, W Flat,
74, Shalimar Bagh,
Delhi-110052

Gajraj Mehandi Udyog
Manufacturers : Henna Powder
& Herbal Henna Hair Colours
28, Pali Road, "Gajraj House"
Sojat City-306104
Ph.:0091-2960-22152
Fax : 0091-2960-22545
Rajasthan

Gauri Shankar & Company
532, Katra Ishwar Bhawan
Khari Baoli
Delhi-110006

Gautam Export Corporation
506, Surat Sadam, 5th Floor
Surat Street
Mumbai-400009
Maharashtra

Genex Corporation
29, New Colony,

Tuticorin-628001
Tamilnadu

Girdharilal Vithaldas Patel
S.T. Road, Sidhpur-384151
Gujarat

Girijan Co-op. Corporation Ltd.
East Point Colony
Visakhapatnam-530017
Andhra Pradesh

Giriraj Enterprises
Highway Unjha
Gujarat

Giya Exports
60, Sir Hari Ram Goenka Street
Kolkata-700007
West Bengal

Gopal Brothers
578, Katra Ishwar Bhawan
Khari Baoli,
Delhi-110006

Govind Prasad Raut
8th Mile District Dibrugarh
Mandi Sadiya
Assam

Gulab Chand Laduram
Attar Naya Bazar,
Ajmer
Rajasthan

Gutti Ram Sukhanand
290/2, Katra Pedan,
Khari Baoli,
Delhi-110006

Hari Ram & Company
2045, Aggarwal Market,
Katra Tambacoo,
Khari Baoli, Delhi-110006

Hari Ram & Sons
412, Katra Medgran
Khari Baoli, Delhi-110006

Hemant & Company
509, Gordia House,
100-102, Kazi Syed Street
Mumbai -400003
Maharashtra

Herb & Drug India
29, Nattukottai Chetty Street,
Tutticorin-628001
Tamilnadu

Herbal Drug Vendors
Interstate Bus Terminus,
Sector-17, Chandigarh
Punjab

Herbal Stores
P.B.5047, 23, Khadak Street
Mumbai-400009
Maharashtra

Herbas Indica
351, Industrial Area,2
Chandigarh
Punjab

Herbs Exporters
D-49, Defence Colony,
New Delhi-110024

Herbs India Inc.
15A/16, Damodar Park,
Dilshad Park,
Shahdara, Delhi-110095

Hillgreen Company
17, 13th Croos Vasanthanagar
Extension, Bangalore-560052
Karnataka

Himalya Drug Company
Saharanpur Road
Clement Town, Dehradun,
Uttaranchal

Himalya Herb Stores
Madho Nagar,
P.B.130,

List of Herbs Suppliers

Saharanpur-247001
Uttar Pradesh

Himalyan Drugs
Herbs & Alkaloids Syndicate
C-4/33-A, Lawrence Road,
Delhi-110035

Himalyan Traders
Katra Dulo, Amritsar-143001
Punjab
Hindustan Trading Corporation
Sidhpur-384151
Gujarat

Hiralal Gajdharlal
24, Maktaram Babu Street,
Kolkata-700007
West Bengal

Indian Drugs (Crude) Distributors
12-B, Clive Row, P.B.2836
Kolkata-700001
West Bengal

Indian Drugs House
6669, Khari Baoli, Delhi-110006
Delhi

Indian Herbs Research & Supply Company
Saharanpur
Uttar Pradesh

Indian Institute of Ayurveda for Drug Research
Near Ranikhet
Tarikhet-263645
Uttar Pradesh

Indian Marine Service Pvt. Ltd.
6/1, Lurdsay Street,
Kolkata-700016
West Bengal

Indo Exports
Bindu Sarover Road,
Sidhpur-384151
Gujarat

Indo World Trading Company Ltd.
10, Armanian Street,
Kolkata-700001
West Bengal

Indo World Trading Corporation
303, Prakash Chambers
6, Netaji Subhash Marg
Daryaganj, New Delhi-110002

Innovations Pharma International
62/12, Old Rajinder Nagar,
Delhi-110050

Institute of Alternative Medicine & Research (in progress)
Ambala-Shimla Highway
Panchkula.
Haryana

International Traders
Ramesh Chambers, 2nd Floor
14 Garibdat Street,
Vadgadi, Mumbai-400003
Maharashtra

International Traders
Gopinath Building,
Gali Batashan, Khari Baoli,
Delhi-110006,

J.P. Mills
Sidhpur-384151
Gujarat

Jadavali Lallubhai & Company
247, Kalbadevi Road,
P.O. Box 2034, Mumbai
Maharashtra

Jai Hind Trading Corporation
28, New Rohtak Road,
Delhi-110005

Jai Industries
Highway Khali

Sidhpur-384151
Gujarat

Jai Trading Corporation
11 Barboume Road Kolkata-70001
West Bengal

Jain Brothers
Neemuch-458441
Madhya Pradesh

Jammu & Kashmir Forest Development Corporation Ltd.
Chief Conservator of Forests
Jammu & Kashmir

Jawahar Industries
46 North Cotton Road Tuticorin
Tamilnadu

Jawahar Lal Nehru Ayurvedic Medicinal Plants Garden & Herbarium
Kothrud Pune-411029
Maharashtra

Jay Kay & Company
8 Gopinath Building Khari Baoli Delhi-110006
Delhi

Jenson Enterprises
34 New Thandavaraya Street,
P.B. 905 Madras-600021
Tamilnadu

Jiwanram Sheoduttrai
Block D, Chowringhee Mansion
30 Jawaharlal Nehru Road
Kolkata-700016
West bengal

John Trading Corporation
P.B. 5503 Bombay-400014
Maharashtra

Juna Gandhi
515-517 Maulana Azad Road,
Nuli Bazar Bombay-40004
Maharashtra

K. Uttam Lal (Exports) Ltd.
Bhagwan Bhawan Ist Fl.
196-198 Samuel Street
Mumbai-400009
Maharashtra

K.D. Shah Enterprises
49/15 Sir C.v. Raman Road P.B. 1457,
Alwarpet Madras-600013
Tamilnadu

K.M. Abdul Kadhar
145/2 Ettayapuram Road
Tuticorin-628002
Tamilnadu

K.P. Edthapanose & Sons
Exporters & Importers
Box 9 Alwaye-683101
Kerela

K.V. Patel & Company
S.T. Road Sidhpur-384151
Gujrat

Kadmi International
Kashi House, 7-A Connaught Place Delhi-110001
Kalidas Gandhi
Centre Street Camp pune-411001
Maharashtra

Kamalkant Chotalal & Company
106 Bhandari Street, Narainarao
Koli Marg Mumbai-400003
Maharashtra

Kanilal Ram Kumar
178 Harrison Road Kolkata-70007
West Bengal

Kantilal Joitaram Patel
Kakosi Road Sidhpur
Gujarat

Kamataka Foresh Development

List of Herbs Suppliers

Corporation Ltd.
"Vanavikas" 18th cross
Malleswaram Bangalore-560003
Karnataka

Kashmir Ayurvedic Works
Azad Nagar,
Putlighar Amritsar-143001
Punjab

Kerela Agricaltural University & Medicinal Plants Research Station
P.O. Asamanoor, District
Emakulam, Odakkali-683549
Kerela

Keshavlal Vithaldas Patel
Gulab Park, S.T. Road
Suidhpur-384151 Gujrat

Kolaba Business Centre
C 25/5 Middle Circle Cannaught
Place Delhi-110001
Delhi

Kothari Phytochemicals (International)
766 Annanagar Madurai-625020
Tamilnadu

Kothari Plantations
Madurai Tamilnadu

Krishna Kapoor & Company
Woodlands, The Mall Amritsar
Punjab

Krishna Traders
20 Harichandra Mullick Street
Kolkata-70005
West Bengal

L. Nanalal Bros.
New Anand Bhawan, rm. 303, 3rd fl
257 Narshi natha Street P.B. 5022
Mumbai-400009
Maharashtra

Laxmidas Haridas Tanna & Company
Gulabi House 3rd Fl.,
111/115 Kazi Syeed street
Mumbai-400009
Maharashtra

Lehri Mal Anoop Kunar & Company
576 Katra Inshwar Bhawan Khari
Baoli, Delhi-110006
Delhi

M.S. Hoda
Piska Farm Piska Nagri
Ranchi-835303

M.S. Vawda & Company
67, B.R.B.B. Road
Canning Street
Kolkata-700001
West Bengal

Madhura Industries,
107, Rippon Street
Kolkata-700016
West Bengal

Madhya Pradesh State Minor Forest Product (T&D)Cooperative Federation Ltd.
38-B, Vikas Bhawan
4th Floor Bhopal-462011
Madhya Pradesh

Magan Lal & Company
Paltan Bazar, Dehradun
Uttar Pradesh

Majumdar Consultants
21, Shiv Mandir Shopping
Complex
Chittaranjan Park, Delhi-110019

Mangal Commercial Corporation
215/88, Panjrenpole Road
Mumbai-400004
Maharashtra

Manilal & Lallu Bhai & Company
P.B.2008, Kalbadevi Road
Near Narain Mandir,
Mumbai-400002
Maharashtra

Matadin Bhagwan Dass
548, Katra Ishwar Bhawan
Khari Baoli, Delhi-110006

Maxo Laboratories Pvt. Ltd.
35-E, Kamla Nagar
P.O. Box 2156
Delhi-110007

Meghalaya Forest Development Corporation Ltd.
Laohumiera Shillong-703001
Meghalaya

Mehta Pharmaceuticals(P) Ltd.
Chheharata Amritsar-143001
Punjab

Merchants & Traders Pvt. Ltd.
32, Armencences Street
Kolkata-700001
West Bengal

Miller & Co. Pvt. Ltd.
24, Netaji Subhash Road
G.P.O. Box 2567,
Kolkata-700001
West Bengal

Minex Agencies
71, Ganesh Chandra Avenue
Kolkata-700013
West Bengal

Modern Agricultural Services
Opp. Plot 60
Jai Hind Colony
Deopur, Dhule-424002
Maharashtra

Modi Industres
Sidhpur
Gujarat

Mohammad Hussain Ajmal Hussain
6681/82, Khari Baoli,
Delhi-110006

Mohan Kumar & Company
158-187, Samuel Street
Mumbai-400009
Maharasthra

Mohal Lal Laxmikant
Safdarganj, Norther Railway
Barabanki
Uttar Pradesh

Money Corporation
T.C.27/979, Srikandeswaram
East Road,
Thiruvananthapuram-695023
Kerala

Murugan & Bros
78, South Raja Street
Tuticorin-628001
Tamil Nadu

Muthuswami, S.P.
Great Cotton Road,
Tuticorin-628001
Tamil Nadu

Mutual Traders
449, Naya Bans Khari Baoli
Delhi-110006
Delhi

Mysore Sales International Ltd.
MSIL House, 36,
Cunningham Road
Bangalore-560052
Karnataka

Nadar P.P.M. Thangayaiah
972/2, North Third Street
Pudukottai
Tamil Nadu

List of Herbs Suppliers

Nathimal Ruganmal
6689/90, Khari Baoli,
Delhi-110006

Nathubhai Cooverji & Company
Arna Bhawan
87-C, Broach Street
Mumbai-400009
Maharashtra

Navin Bharat Manufacturers
D-373, Defence Colony,
Delhi-110024

Navneeth Lal Savilal
64, Mudi Bazar,
Mandavi, Mumbai-400003
Maharashtra

New Kiryana Store
2565, Tilak Bazar,
Khari Baoli, Delhi-110006

New Udaya Pharmacy & Ayurvedic Laboratories
Kadavanthara
Cochin-682020
Kerala

Niyogi & Company
352-354, Samuel Street,
Vadgadi, Mumbai-400003
Maharashtra

North Gujarat State Isabgol Industries
Highway Unjha
Gujarat

Organon India Ltd.
Himalya House,
38 Chowringhee Road
Kolkata-700016
West Bengal

Orient Traders
615/VI, Bagh Jhanda Singh
Amritsar-143001
Punjab

Oriental Herbs
E-26, Saket, New Delhi-110017
Delhi

Orissa Forest Development Corporation Ltd.
Bhubaneswar-750002
Orissa

P.A.V. Sundaram
166, New Colony,
Tuticorin-628001
Tamil Nadu

P.L. Associates
Botwala Building, Top Floor,
8, Horniman Circle Fort
Mumbai-400001
Maharashtra

P.P.M. Thangayaiah Nadar
South Cotton Road,
Tuticorin-628001
Tamil Nadu

P.S. Jammal & Sons
Street 16, 430 Patel Nagar,
Talab Tillo, Jammu & Kashmir
Jammu & Kashmir

P.S. Nathan & Company
48, Auna Nagar,
Tuticorin-628008
Tamil Nadu

P.S. Sankaralinga Nadar
50, P.S.S. Nadar Street,
Tuticorin-628001
Tamil Nadu

P.S.S. Ganeshan
P.S.S. Nadar Street,
North Cotton Road,
Tuticorin-628001
Tamil Nadu

Palanichamy V.M.P.K.
T.R. Naidu Street
Tuticorin
Tamil Nadu

Pandian, J.R.
North Cotton Road,
Tuticorin-628001
Tamil Nadu

Pandit & Company
D-49, Street 11, MIDC
Nasik-422007
Maharashtra

Parvatia Sahkari Bhesaja Vikas Evum Karya Vikraya Sangh
Pithoragarh
Uttar Pradesh

Patel Corporation
Highway, Khali
Sidhpur-384151
Gujarat

Pearl & Company
Dr. Babasaheb Ambedkar Road,
Byculla, Mumbai-400027
Maharashtra

Pharma Impex
10, Middleton Road,
Kolkata-700071
West Bengal

Pharmaceutical Crude Drugs Enterprises
Kosi Road, Opp. State Bank,
Dist. Nainital, Ramnagar-244715
Uttar Pradesh

Pharmachem International
361, Maulana Azad Road
Mumbai-400004
Maharashtra

Phyto-Biotech Internationl
GNB Road, Ambari
Guwahati-781001
Assam

Pillay S.P.M. Pirama Nayagam
South Raja Street,
Tuticorin-628001
Tamil Nadu

Poneselvan Traders
312, South Cotton Road,
Tuticorin-628001
Tamil Nadu

Ponnu Saw Mills
316, South Cotton Road,
P.B.105, Tuticorin-628001
Tamol Nadu

Prasad & Sons
4771, Bharat Ram Road,
23, Daryaganj, Delhi-110002

Premji Haridas & Company
Bhanushali Chambers,
166-170, Sant Tukaram Road,
Mumbai-400001
Maharashtra

PSPK Jayarajapandiyan
Tuticorin-628001
Tamil Nadu

Punj Traders
2087, Aggarwal market,
Katra Tambacoo,
Khari Baoli,
Delhi-110006
Delhi

Quality Seeds Producer & Marketer
Shivaji Chowk,
Parabhani-431401
Maharashtra

R.G. Herbal Pvt. Ltd.
M-53, Palika Bhawan,
Opp. Hotel Hyatt Regency,
R.K. Puram, Delhi-110066.

List of Herbs Suppliers

Radharam Sohal Lal
3 Mallik Street
Kolkata-700007
West Bengal

Radhey Shyam Rajinder Kumar & Co.
532, Katra Ishwar Bhawan
Khari Baoli, Delhi-110006

Radhey Sons
367/3, Katra Hussain Baksh
Khari Baoli, Delhi-110006
Delhi

Raj & Company
Deals in : Henna leaves & powder,
Shikakai, Amla, Neem, Bahera,
Tulsi & All other herbal R/M
Dasshera Maidan,
Neemuch-458441
Ph.:07423-21600
Fax : 07423-25341
E-mail:rajspice@bom4.vsnl.net.in
Madhya Pradesh

Rajendra Brothers
Highway, Khali
Sidhpur-384151
Gujarat

Ram Narayan Raj Narayan
Perfume Manufactueres
Makarand Nagar, Kannauj
Ph.: 05694-34716 (O)
05694-34286 (F)
Fax ; 05694-34286, 34297
Kannauj

Rameshwar Das Chhottey Lal
2091, Aggarwal Market,
Katra Tambacoo,
Khari Baoli, Delhi-110006
Delhi

Regional Research Centre (Ayurveda)
Sankai View Itanagar-791110
Arunachal Pradesh

Regional Research Centre (Ayurveda)
Gwalior Road,
Jhansi-248003
Madhya Pradesh

Regional Research Centre (Ayurveda)
Madhav Vilas Palace
Amer Road
Jaipur-302002
Rajasthan

Regional Research Institute of Unani Medicine
Aligarh Muslim University,
Department of Research in Unani
Medicine Aligarh-202001
Uttar Pradesh

Regional Research Institute of Unani Medicine
District Balasore,
Bhadrak-756100
Orissa

Regional Research Institute of Unani Medicine
1 West Mada Church Street,
Royapuram,
Chennai-600013
Tamilnadu

Regional Research Institute of Unani Medicine
Nawab Manzil,
Guzri
Patna-800008
Bihar

Regional Research Institute of Unani Medicine
University of Kashmir
University Health Centre,
Hazratbal, Srinagar-190006
Jammu & Kashmir

Robinsomar & Company
2 Mission Row Extension
Kolkatta-700001
West Bengal

Roshan Lal Sham Sunder
50-51, Akali Market,
Amritsar
Punjab

S. Bhattacharjee & Company
Circular Road,
Serampur
West Bengal

S.Chandra Enterprises
82/2 (33),
Chandni Chowk,
Delhi-110006

S.Sangyong Corporation
206, Arunachal Building,
19 Barakhamba Road
Delhi-110001

S.Sattara & Company
1399, Tilak Bazar,
Khari Baoli, Delhi-6

S.K. Dutta & Company
215, Old Dalanwala
Dehradun-248001
Uttar Pradesh

S. Lachman Singh & Sons
Katra Hari Singh
Amritsar-143001
Punjab

S.S. Trading Company
15, Nehru Market,
P.O.B.21,
Bijapur-586010
Karnataka

Sahkan Vikas Sangh Ltd.
Chamoli
Uttar Pradesh

Saiba Industries Pvt. Ltd.
129-131 4th Floor,
Kazi Sayed Street,
Mumbai-400003
Maharashtra

Sanjay Kumar Shankar Lal & Company
208, Surat Sadan,
88/89 Surat Street,
Mumbai-400009
Maharashtra

Sanjay Traders
Highway, Khali Sidhpur-384151
Gujarat

Santosh Ayurvedic Drug Supply Company
33, Daryansthan Street
Majit Bhandar
Mumbai-400003
Maharashtra

Satpal Kamal & Sons
Bindu Sarover Road,
Sidhpur-384151
Gujarat

Shankar & Company
519, Katra Ishwar Bhawwan
Khari Baoli
Delhi-110006

Sheikh Nazir Ahmed
15, New Iddgha Building,
Park Road, Baramulla
Jammu & Kashmir

Shekherco
P.B. 256, Muzaffarnagar-251001
Uttar Pradesh

Shell India
P.B.-1, Sheratallay
Thayakal, P.O. Ernakulam-688530
Kerala

List of Herbs Suppliers

Shiba Pada Kundu & Sons
168-B, Cotton Street,
Kolkata-700023
West Bengal

Shree Ganesh Aushadhi Bhandar
229, Kalbadevi Road,
Mumbai-400002
Maharashtra

Shree Ramajayam Corporation
50 P.S.S. Nadar Street,
North Cotton Road
Tuticorin-628001
Tamilnadu

Shree Suvas Industries
Highway, Chaurasta
Palampur-385002
Gujarat

Shree Swastik Industries
Deesa Highway,
Chaurasta Palanpur-385002
Gujarat

Shree Swastik Industries
Manasnun Rajpur-492001
Madhya Pradesh

Shree Swastik Export Corporation
Highway, Chaurasta
Palampur-385002
Gujarat

S.S. Trading Company
M.G. Road, P.B. No.-21,
Bijapur-586101
Karnataka
PH.:08352-51443
Telefax : 08352-50992
E-mail : sureshnihalani@hotmail.com

Shyam Sunder Gupta
2032, Aggarwal Market,

Tambacoo Khari Baoli
Delhi-110006

Sidhpur Isabgol Processing Company
Bindu Sarover Road,
Sidhpur-384151
Gujarat

Sidhpur Sat-Isabgol Factory
Bindu Sarover Road,
Sidhpur-384151
Gujarat

Sigma Trading Company
Nafees Chambers,
3rd Floor Lokmanya Tilak Marg,
Mumbai - 400001
Maharashtra

Simlipahar Foresh Development Corporation Ltd.
Kolkatta-700012
West Bengal

Solai Program
Christianpet,
N.A. District Katpadi-630027
Tamilnadu

Suman Trading Company
10-2/32/1, Pamuvair Street
Ramaraopeta,
Kakinada-533004
Andhra Pradesh

Superb Fascinations Importers Exporters Indentors
Sanjauli Shimla
Himachal Pradesh

Survey of Medicinal Plants & Collections Unit (Homoeopathy)
112, Government Arts College Campus
Udhagamandalam-643002
Tamilnadu

Swami Corporation
4, Hari Niwas,
C. Road Church Gate
Mumbai-400020
Maharashtra

Swaroop & Company
330, Katra Hussain Baksh,
Khari Baoli, Delhi-110006

Swastic Traders
394, Kuth Bazar
Mamaya Chambers
Mumbai-400009
Maharashtra

**Swastic Medical Store
(Atul R. shah)**
177-178, Laxmi Road,
Pune-411002
Maharashtra

Taj Trading & Company
6681, Khari Baoli,
Delhi-110006

**Tamilnadu Government
Cinchona Department**
Nilgiris
P.B.6,
Udhagamandalam-643001
Tamilnadu

Thenammal & Company
54.P.S.S. Nadar Street
Tuticorin-628001
Tamilnadu

**Tibetan Medical & Astro
Institute
(Men-Tsee-Khang)**
Khara Danda Road,
District Kangra
Dharamsala-176215
Himachal Pradesh

Timex Agencies
9/48, Punjabi bagh,
Delhi-110026

Tirkha Ram Om Prakash
585, Katr Ishwar Bhawan
Khari Baoli
Delhi-110006

Tola Ram India Ltd.
68, Nalini Sett Road
Kolkata-700070
West Bengal

**Tribal Cooperative Marketing
Development Federation of
India Ltd.**
Savitri Sadan 2
Preet Vihar Community Centre
Vikas Marg
Delhi-110092

Trimurti Enterprises
3 Satya Niketan,
Moti Bagh 11
Delhi-110021

**Tripura Forest Development &
Plantation Corporation**
Kunjabad Agartala-799001
Tripura

Tropical Trading Company
Tuticorin-628001
Tamilnadu

Universal Carbon Company
46, Ezra Street
Kolkata-70001
West Bengal

**V. Nathan Herbal & Cosmetics
Pvt. Ltd.**
Manfacturers : Herbal Bath Soaps,
Agarbathis, Laundry Soaps
Shed No.72, SIDCO Industrial
Estate, Kappalur, Madurai-625008
Ph.:0452-882675, 884901, 534601
Fax : 04627367
e-mail : vnathansoap@vsnl.com

V.S. Arulangadam & Sons
35, Ginfactory Road

P.O.B. 47
Tuticorin-628002
Tamilnadu

V.V. General Traders
1, Sutharashahi Kundanpura
Muzaffarnagar-251002
Uttar Pradesh

Vadilal Vithaldas Patel
S.T. Road,
Sidhpur-384151
Gujarat

Vishal Traders
Sahadat Ganj
Lucknow-226003
Uttar Pradesh

Visharam
306 Shaikh Menon Street
Mumbai-400002
Maharashtra

World Trading Corporation
Opposite Parda Bagh,
Daryaganj, New Delhi-110002

OTHER USEFUL PUBLICATIONS

★ HANDBOOK OF SYNTHETIC & HERBAL COSMETICS
★ COSMETICS PROCESSES & FORMULATIONS HANDBOOK
★ HAND BOOK OF PERFUEMS WITH FORMULATIONS
★ ESSENTIAL OILS PROCESSES & FORMULATIONS HAND BOOK
★ HAND BOOK OF ESSENTIAL OILS MFG. & AROMATIC PLANTS
★ HANDBOOK OF PERFUMES & FLAVOURS
★ HAND BOOK OF HERBS, MEDICINAL & AROMATIC PLANTS CULTIVATION

AVAILABLE AT :

ENGINEERS INDIA RESEARCH INSTITUTE

Regd. Off. : 4449, Nai Sarak (S1), Main Road, Delhi-6 (India)
Ph. : 3918117, 3916431, 3960797, 3920361 Fax : 91-11-3916431
E-mail : eirisidi@bol.net.in Website : startindustry.com

Chapter - 33

SUPPLIERS OF PLANT, MACHINERY AND EQUIPMENTS

CONSULTANTS

JEJU CHEMICALS
2248, Gali Hinga Beg,
Tilak Bazar,
Delhi - 110 006
Ph : 3921790, 3919246, 3918689
Resi : 7014316, 7010388
Fax : 91-11-3283643
E-Mail : jeju@bol.net.in
Contact : Mr. Narender Gupta
Specialists and Consultants for Perfumes, Cosmetics, Agarbatties, Soaps and Gutka Pan Masala.

COMPLETE PLANT SUPPLIERS FOR COSMETIC UNIT

Adam Fabriwerk Pvt. Ltd.
203, Rajguru Apts, New Nagar Das Road,
Andheri (E),
Mumbai - 400069
Phone : (022)-8380548, 8384173
Fax : (022)-8390195
E-Mail : adamfab@vsnl.com
Website:
www.adamfabriwerk.com

Chemac Equipments Pvt. Ltd.
M.J.D'souza Compound,
Safedpool,Sakinaka,
Mumbai - 400072
Phone : 8510777,8592352

Fax : 8516986
E-Mail :
chemac@bom4.vsnl.net.in
Website :
www.chemacequipments.com

Asoka Enterprises
49, Jhawtala Road, 4th Floor,
Kolkata- 700019
Phone : 2409048
Fax : 91-33-247-9750/280-4268
E-Mail :
asoka_cal@hotmail.com
Website:
www.calcuttayellowpages.com/adver/100832.html

Harrisons Pharma Machinery Pvt. Ltd.
4648/21, Shedumal Building,
Darya Ganj,
New Delhi - 110002
Phone : 3275631, 2216431
Website: www.acpl.com/pharma

Gem Pharma Machineries
Plot No. A/82, Road No. 16,
Towards Kishan Nagar,
Wagle Ind. Estate,
Thane - 400064
Tel : 022-5820257/022-5814158
E-Mail :
gemmumbai@hotmail.com.

L & M Automatics
T-47, Sector XII,
Noida- 201301,
Phone : 011-8-4553476

Pharmech Engineering Corporation
117, Vasan Udyog Bhavan,
Senapati Bapat Marg,
Lower Parel.
Mumbai - 400013
Phone : 4935968,4975102
Fax : 91-22-4975102

Indo German Pharma Pvt. Ltd.
Kothari House, Plot A-13,
Street No.5,
Off Cross Rd. B, M.I.D.C.
Andheri (E),
Mumbai - 93 (India)
Phone : 8323615,8342338. 8372500
Fax : 91-22-8374426
E-Mail :
indogmbh@bom3.vsnl.net.in
Website :
www.indogermanpharma.com

AGITATOR

Adam Fabriwerk Pvt. Ltd.
203, Rajguru Apts.
New Nagardas Road,
Andheri (E),
Mumbai - 400069.
Phones : 83 80548, 8384173,
Telefax: 022-8390105,
E-Mail:adamfab@vsnl.com

Burman Plant & Machinery Co (P) Ltd.
36, Sarkar Lane,
Kolkata-700007.
Phones : 2411340.
Fax : (91)(33) 296077.

Instruments & Equipments
35, Chittaranaj Avenue,
Kolkata-700012.

Modern Scientific Industries
199-A, Saket, Meerut-250001 (U.P).
Phone-(0121) 644086,
Gram:INDUSTRIES.

Multitech Services
221-226, Gala Complex,
2nd Floor,
D. Upadhyaya Marg,
Mulund (W),
Mumbai - 400080.
Phones :
5613136,5611291,5650593,
Fax- (91) 022-5646325.

Pharma Machinery (The)
1092, M.B.Road,
Mahajati Nagar,
Kolkata-700051.
Phones : 5513779.

WEIGHING BALANCES

Anamed Instrument Pvt. Ltd.
7 Sita Estate, First Floor,
133/136, Mahul Road,
Chembur,
Mumbai - 400074
Phones : 5516908,5555137,
Fax:022-5563356.

Bombay Burmah Trading Corpn. Ltd.
334, A-Z, Industrial Estate,
G. Kadam Marg,
Lower Parel,
Mumbai - 400013.
Phones : 4938218/19.
Fax :4951384.

Instrument & Equipment
35, Chittaranjan Avenue,
Kolkata - 700012.

Labman Industries
24/1 B, Manmath Nath
Ganguly Road,
Kolkata - 700002.

Modern Scientific Instruments Co.
48/A, 48/B, Sadashiv Cross Lane,
Shri Girdhari Bhavan,
Kandewadi,
Mumbai - 400004.

Zenith Surgical Co.
Central Building No.1
1st Floor,
Bomaji Master Road,
(New Silk Bazar),
Opp. Kalbadevi Post Office.
Mumbai - 400002.
Phones : 259526/310157

BLISTER PACKING MACHINE

Ajit Foils & Allieds
No. 50, Mookatkal Street,
Opp. Roxy Theatre,
Puraswalkam,
Chennai - 600007
Phones : 6422246,6424391,
567700, 562400

C.C.Engineering Co.
B-4/401, Veena Nagar,
Opp. Gabriel (India) Ltd.,
L.B.S. Marg,
Mulund (W),
Mumbai - 400080.
Phones : 91-22-5680731,
Fax : 91-22-5677883.

Elmach Packages (India) Pvt. Ltd.
410, Hill View Co-op.
Industrial Estate.
Off. L.B.S. Marg,
Ghatkopar (W),
Mumbai - 400086
Phones : (022) 5008007,
5008071, 5007217, 5951703
Gram. 'BLISTERPACK',
Fax : (022) 5008684,
5951702
E-Mail : elmach@vsnl.com,
http.//www.elmach.com

Jemco Chuck Mfg. Works,
Nirmal House, 128-B,
Govt. Industrial Estate
Ghatkopar, Kandivli (W),
Mumbai - 400 067
Phones : 8682621.

Karnavati Engineering Ltd.
Dist. Mehsana (Gujarat)
Phones : 02764-62463,
Fax : 0764-42608
E-Mail : kel-irm@
wilnetonline.net,
Website :
www.karnavatiengineering.com.

Larson & Toubro Ltd.
L.& T. House,
Narotham Morarji Marg,
Ballard Estate,
Mumbai - 400001,
Phones : 022-268121 (9 Lines).

Pam-Pac Machines Ltd.
127, Kandivli Industrial
Estate, Kandivli (west),
Mumbai - 400067
Phones : 8682650/8930/
8931, 8689109/7110/
7112/3111.
Fax : 91-22-8683091,
E-Mail:
pam.ppamc.@gems.vsnl.net.in

Santosh Industries
76, Adarsh Co-Op. Industrial
Estate. Chakudia Mahadev
Road, Rakhial,
Ahmedabad-380023 (Gujarat)
Phones : 2740284,279376.

Serwell Instruments Inc.
"Sukruthi", 149, First 'R'
Block, Chord Road,
Rajajinagar,
Bangalore-560010.
Phones : 3320309,3325697
Gram. TEKSALES,
Telex. 080-8921 RSE-IN,
Fax : 3325697

BOTTLE FILLING MACHINE

Acmevac Sales Pvt. Ltd.
109, Unique Industrial
Estate. Chakala Road,
Andheri (E),
Mumbai - 400093
Phones : 8329647, 8375837,
Telefax. 022-8390195,
E-Mail : adamfab@vsnl.com.

Suppliers of Plant, Machinery and Equipments

Armstrong Smith Ltd.
Brady House, 12/14,
Veer Nariman Road,
Mumbai - 400023

Beekay Pharma Mach Industries
Plot No.11, Bidg. No-A-41,
Sector No. 3, Shantinagar,
Mira Road-401107 (W.Rly)
Dist. Thane (Maharashtra).
Phone (Offi) 022-8105686,
8116416.
(Fact) 022-022-8521608,
Fax : (0788) 357307

Bright Pharma Machinery
37-A, New Empire Industrial
Estate Kondivita Road,
Pipe Line
J.B. Nagar Andheri (E),
Mumbai - 400059
Phones : 8214341, 8398359,
8327150
Fax : 91-22-8210190,
E-Mail : panchal@brightxee
bom.xeemail.com.

Chitra Engineers
23, Narmada Estate Near
Khodiyarnagar Police Station.
South Chali, N. H. No.8,
Odhav (Viratnagar),
Ahmedabad- 382415
Phones : (Off) (079) 2891666,
2876516, 2890136, 2873052
Fax : (079) 2891666,
2874194
E-Mail : chitrmt@vsnl.com

EEE CEE & Co.
1. Anant Estate Opp Comet
Estate. Rakhial.
Ahmedabad-380023
(Gujarat)
Phones : 079-2743075,
Fax : 079.2743075

L & M Automatics
60/7, Old Dal Mandi,
Kanpur-208001 (U.P)
Phones : 352367,352570,
Fax : 91-512-316788.

Mixo Fill (India)
1351, Street No.45, Jafrabad.
New Seelampur, Shahdara,

Delhi - 110053.
Phones : (Fact) 2263446,
2263362,
(Off) 3274460, 3270735,
Fax : 011-3265278

Pharam Fab Industries
B-11, Hariyali Industrial
Estate, L.B.S. Marg,
Vikhroli (W)
Mumbai - 400083
Phones : 5792116, 5791504
Fax : 022-5791504,
E-Mail :
pharmacab@pharmabiz.com.

Scientific Apparatus Co. (The)
1/H/10, Kalimaddin Sarkar
Lane.
Kolkata-700010.
Phone -357036

BOTTLE WASHING & DRYING MACHINES

Adrian Engineering Works
11-A, Nirmala Colony,
St. John Baptist Road.
Bandra,
Mumbai - 400050.
Phone-6824783

Armstrong Smith Ltd.
Brady House, 12/14,
Veer Narman Road,
Mumbai - 400023

Central Industries
Ashok Villa,
Vallabhbhai Road,
Vile Parle, (west)
Mumbai - 400056
Phones : 6127074

Ganesh Engineering Works
1507, Ganesh Pura,
Main Market, Tri Nagar.
Delhi - 110035
Phones : 7117972

Indo German Pharma Pvt. Ltd.
Kothari House, Plot No. A-13
Off. Cross Road B,
Street No. 5,
MIDC, Andheri (E)
Mumbai - 400093

Phones : 8342338,
8323615, 8373500
8387411, 8219251,
Fax : 91-22-8374426
E-Mail :
indogmbh@bom3.vsnl.net.in

Jayvir Industries
D-15, Ambica Estate,
Nr. C.T.M. Mills,
Behind Ambica Hotel,
Highway, Amraiwadi,
Ahmedabad-380026
(Gujarat)
Phones : 91-79-2775322

K. Mahadev & Company Pvt. Ltd.
Datta Mandir Road, Bhandup,
Mumbai - 400078
Phone : 5610920

Master Mechanical Works Pvt. Ltd.
Pushpanjali, S.V. Road,
Santacruz (W)
Mumbai - 400054
Phones : 6493459,
6491680,6490619
Gram. ROLLSEALER.
Telex. 78283MMW IN.
Fax: 91-22-6494781

Navjivan Engineering Works
Panchal Nivas,
Pupapari Naka,
Opp. Futy Masjid, Daripur,
Ahmedabad-380001.
Phones : 337012, Gram.
CROWNWHELL.

Paneser Engg. Works
230, Chowk Katra Karam
Singh,
Amritsar - 143001 (Punjab)

CAP SCREWING MACHINE
(P.P Cap Sealing Machine)

Adrian Engineering Works
11-A, Nirmala Colony,
St. Baptist Road.
Bandra,
Mumbai - 400050.
Phones : 6824783.

Allied Sales Corporation
37 Ground Floor,
Swastik Industrial Estate,
178, Vidyanagari Marg,
Kalina, Mumbai - 400098
Phones : 6105906,6162745,
Fax : 91-22-6105906

Amar Engineering Works
B-6, Gupta Pala ,
A-2/42, Opp. M.C.D. Office.
Rajouri Garden,
New Delhi - 110027.
Phones : 5431105,5938670
Fax : 5469291

Central Scientific Supplies Co. Ltd.
2, Agaram Road, Tambaram.
Chennai.
Phones : 89223,
Gram. SYPHON.

Excel-Techno Engineering Pvt. Ltd.
21, Stadium House,
Navrangpura,
Ahmedabad-380009
Phones : (079)(Off)
6427866,4412351,
(Fact) 2744174,
Telex. 0121-6853 SARA IN.
Fax : 079-6427866/469101.

Master Mechanical Works Pvt. Ltd.
Pushpanjali, S.V. Road,
Santacruz (W),
Mumbai - 400054
Phones :6493459,6491680,
6490619,
Gram. ROLLSEALER,
Telex. 78283 MMW IN.
Fax : 91-22-6494781

Neomachine Mfg. Co. Pvt. Ltd.
39/2A, Purna Das Road,
Kolkata-700029
Phones :
4644568,4640457,4647253
Gram. TECHPHARMA.
Fax : 91-33-4643473
4647254.

Quality Engineering Works
554-55, Navjeeven.
Schoolwali,

Chauhan Bangar,
Seelampur, Delhi - 110053.

United Engineering Co. (The)
Sweekar, V.B. Road,
Vile-Parle (W),
Mumbai - 400056
Phones : 6105701,
Fax : 91-22-6712246

COLLAPSIBLE TUBE SEALING AND CRIMPING MACHINES

Allied Sales Corporation
37, Ground Floor,
Swastik Industrial Estate,
178, Vidyanagari Marg,
Kalina,
Mumbai - 400098,
Phones : 6105906,6162745,
Fax : 91-22-6105906

Ashok Machine Tools
Mavdi Plot,
Rajkot-360001 (Gujarat)

Beekay Pharma Mach Industries
Plot No.11, Bldg. No. A-41,
Sector No.3, Shantinagar,
Mira Road-401107 (W.Rly)
Dist. Thane (Maharashtra)
Phones : (Off) 022-8105686,
8116416
(Fact) 022-8521608
Fax : (91-22) 8113673.

Caelsons Industries
4610, C-Type, GIDC,
Phase IV,
Vatwa, Ahmedabad
(Gujarat)
Phones : 5835372

Ganesh Engineering Works
1507, Ganesh Pura,
Main Market, Tri Nagar,
Delhi - 110035
Phone . 7117972.

Magnose Engineering Company
19, Ashoka Industrial Estate,
L.B. Shastri Marg, Mulund
(West) Mumbai - 400080

Phones :
5617373,5612165
Gram. STEVSYL
Fax : 91-22-
5914218,5644511,
E-Mail
:leoscor@bom3.vsnl.net.in

Peojee Bottling Co.
63,Bangur Avenue,
Block D,
Kolkata-700055

Shivalaya Machinery Mfg. Co.
1, Shivaji Nagar, Mittal
Compound,
Indore-452003 (M.P)
Phones : (0731)
530699,545541
Fax : 533274

CRUSHING & GRINDING MACHINES (Disintegrators)

Adair Dutt & Co. (I) Pvt. Ltd.
5,B.B.D. Bagh East.
Kolkata-700001

Frederick Herbert
10, Second Pasta Lane,
Colaba,
Mumbai - 400005

Ganesh Engineering Works
1507, Ganesh Pura,
Main Market, Tri Nagar,
Delhi - 110035
Phones : 7117972

Industrial Scientific Corporation
BA-148B, Janakpuri
New Delhi - 110058.

Metrex Scientific Instruments Pvt. Ltd.
WH-20, Mayapuri Industrial
Area,
Phase-I,
New Delhi - 110064
Phones : 5130702,5138271

Monarch Engineering Works
13, Kharwa Gali,
6th Kumbharwada,
Mumbai - 400004

Suppliers of Plant, Machinery and Equipments

Raman & Well Pvt. Ltd.
Chateau Marine,
3rd Floor,
133, Netaji Sabhash Road,
Mumbai - 400020
Phones :
2049164,2049527,2856397
Gram. RAMANWELL.
Fax : 2023042

Talson Industries (India)
Shed No. 128, Block B,
Sector II, Noida,
Ghaziabad-201207 (U.P)

Toshniwal Brothers Pvt. Ltd.
Industrial Estate, Makhupura,
Ajmer-305002 (Rajasthan)

DRYERS & DRYING OVENS

Adair Dutt & Co. (I) Pvt. Ltd.
5, B.B.D. Bagh East,
Kolkata-700001

Alpha Scientific & Surgical Co.
18, St. John's Church Road,
Bangalore-560005
(Karnataka)
Phones : 5565945

Andhra Scientific Co. Ltd.
3rd Floor, Janambhoomi
Chambers.
Fort Street, Ballard Estate,
Mumbai - 400001

Associated Instrument Manufacturers (India) Pvt.Ltd.
India House, Fort Street,
P.O.Box 119,
Mumbai - 400001

Altanto Enterprises
Gala No. 15, 3rd Floor,
Jogani Estate, J.Ramji
Boricha Marg.
Opp. Kasturba Hospital.
Mahalaxmi,
Mumbai - 400001
Phones : 3096098
Fax : 91-22-3073537

Bhuvaneswari & Co.
4-3-314, (3464) 1st Floor,
Dundoho Vihar,
Rashtrapathi Road.
Secunderabad - 500003 (A.P)
Phones : 7713632,
Gram. TRADEBOOM.
Telex. 0425-6333 PCO IN-TMB 237,
Fax : 7713632

B.P. Industries
B-103, G.T.Karnal Road.
Industrial Area.
Delhi - 110033
Phones : 7125184, 7115196,
7123501

Create Industries
C/7, Anup Estate,
N.H.8, Near Bharat
Party Plot, Amraiwadi,
Ahmedabad-380026
Phones : 2874085
Fax : (790) 6302607

D.K. Scientific Industries
4,5, Ashoka Chember.
Rasala Marg.
Near Lions Hall, Ellisbridge.
Ahmedabad - 380006
(Gujarat)
Phones : 079-6469471 to 74
Fax : 6469471
E-Mail :dksipttd@icenet.net

Eastern Scientific Machinery Corp.
12-A, Peermohamed Manzil,
Colaba,
Mumbai - 400005

EXPERIMENTAL COSMETIC TESTING EQUIPMENTS

Armstrong Smith Ltd.
Brady House, 12/14,
Veer Nariman Road,
Mumbai - 400023

Instruments & Chemical Pvt. Ltd.
Modal Town.
Ambala City - 134
(Haryana)
Phones : 56079,56690,
Gram INCO

Jayron Electronics
7, Mihir Park Society,
Near Dollars Avenue,
Old Padra Road,
Baroda - 390020 (Gujarat)
Phones : 342487,
Fax : 340850

LABELLING AND GUMMING MACHINE

Adrian Engineering Works
11-A, Nirmala Colony,
St. John Baptist Road.
Bandra, Mumbai - 400050
Phones : 6824783

Beekay Pharma Mach Industries
Plot No. 11, Bldg. No. A-41,
Sector No.3 Shantinagar,
Mira Road - 401107
(W.Rly) Dist. Thane
(Maharastra).
Phones : (Off) 022-8105686,8116416
(Fact) 022-8521608
Fax : (91-22) 8113673

Chemtronick Enterprises
16-11-20/4/1/2, Saleem
Nagar Colony,
St. Domnic's School Lane,
New Malakpet,
Hyderabad-500036
Phones : 548461.

Hemson Private Limited
60, Mistry Ind, Complex,
M.I.D.C. Cross Road, A
Andheri (E), P.B.No. 9409,
Mumbai - 400093
Phones :
8321820,8325841,8326148
Gram. HEMSEAL

Indo-German Pharma Pvt. Ltd.
Kothari House,
Plot No. A-13,
Off. Cross Road B,
Street No.5
MIDC, Andheri (E),
Mumbai - 400093
Phones : 8342338, 8323615.

8372500, 8387411, 8219251
Fax : 91-22-8374426
E-Mail
:indogmbh@bom3.vsnl.net.in.

Kailash Machine Tools
12, Harshad Estate,
(Margha Farm), Mamtanagar,
Near Viratnagar Char Rasta,
Rakhial (Bapunagar),
Ahmedabad-380024.
Phones : 2744697,
Fax : (079) 2744394

KNK Engineering Works
A/135, Ghatakopar Industrial
Estate,
L.B.Shastri Marg,
Ghatkopar,
Mumbai - 400086

Mahdav Machinery
B-22, Rajbaug Society,
Canal Road, Ghodasar,
Ahmedabad-380008
(Gujarat)
Phone: 079-2772431

LABORATORY EQUIPMENTS

Astronix Enterprises
199-A, Sake,
Meerut,
(U.P)

D.R. Surgicals
A-56, Gandhi Nagar,
Moradabad
(U.P)

Electronic Instrumentation
12, Mahesh Nagar,
Ambala Cantt. 133001
(Haryana)
Phone : 171-
643087.641797,643057
Telex: 392-214 MIT IN. Fax.
91-171-6425595

Gordhandas Desai Pvt. Ltd.
Court Chambers,
35 Sir V. Thackersey Marg,
Mumbai - 400020
Phone: (022)-
2004208,2001418.
Telex: 011-83065,
Fax. (91-22) 2000581

Indequip Scientific Enterprises
10/12, Jamboolwadi,
Kalbadevi Road,
Mumbai - 400002

Instruments & Chemical Pvt. Ltd.
Model Town,
Ambala City-134003
(Haryana)
Phone : 56079,56690
Gram. INCO

Lawrence & Mayo
Instruments Division,
274 D.N.Road,
Mumbai - 400001

Santosh Medical & Surgical Centre
Opp. B.L.D.E. Hospital,
Bijapur-586101
(Karnataka)

BALL MILL

Kumar Sales Corporation
10, Santok House, Dady
Santok Lane,
2nd Floor, Dhobi Talao,
Mumbai - 400002
Phone : 2062776,2084749
Fax : 022-8873345

L & M Automatics
60/7, Old Dal Mandi,
Kanpur-400098
Phone : 6122928,6127440
Gram. LANAFLOR.

Rank & Co
A-95/3, Wazirpur Industrial
Estate,
Dehli-110052
Phone : 7456101-2-3-4,7441958,
Garm. MIXKING
Fax : 7234126,7471905

Saran Brothers
87/362, Jarib Ki Chowki,
G.T.Road, Kanpur-208003
(U.P)
Phone : 246790,220180

S.S. Engineering
Plot. No.C-2/8,
Mayapuri Industrial Area,
Phase II ,
New Delhi - 110064.

MIXERS/BLENDERS
(Cone, Double Cone, Drum,
Mass, Paste,
Planetary, Powder, Ribbon,
Roto-cube,
Sigma-blade)

Accumax Engineering
C-5A/184, Janakpuri,
New Delhi - 110058,
Telefax. 5501092

Alliance Engineering Co
Trisandhya Building,
97, D. Phalke Road,
Dadar CR, Mumbai - 400014,
Phones : 4112461,4156510
Gram. QUICKMIX.
Fax: (022) 4138307,4137648

Amit Trading Co
21, Chewool Wadi,
Dr. M.B.Velkar Street
(Kolbhat Lane),
Kalbadevi Road,
Post Box No. 2691,
Mumbai - 400002
Phone : 2056895

Bectochem Engineers
B-202, Rising Sun
Apartment,
Juhu Tara Road,
Opp.Palmgrove
Hotal, Santa Cruz.
Mumbai - 400009
Phones :
8500300,8500057,8502400
Gram. BECENG
Fax: 022-8506785

Burman Plant & Machinery Co.(P) Ltd.
36, Sarkar Lane,
Kolkata-700007
Phone : 2411340
Fax : (91) (33) 296077

Dalal Engineering Pvt. Ltd.

Suppliers of Plant, Machinery and Equipments

Post Box. No. 63,
Thane-400601 (Maharashtra)
Phones : 022-
5343577,5343528
Fax. 022-5345570,
E-Mail: dalalfac@vsnl.com.

Flora Engineering Corporation
28-A, Phool Bag, Rampura
(Near Railway Crossing)
Delhi - 110035

Gem Pharma Machineries
Plot No. A/82, Road No.16,
Towards Kisan Nagar,
Wagle Estate,
Thane-400604 (Maharashtra)
Phones : 022-5820257,
5814158
Telex : 91-022-5826387
E-Mail :
Gemmumbai@hotmail.com.

**OVER-PRINTING MACHINE
(Batch Numbering & Date
Printing on Cartons &
Labels)**

Amar Engineering Works
B-6, Gupta Palace,
A-2/42, Opp. M.C.D. Office,
Rajouri Garden,
New Delhi - 110027
Phone : 5431105,5938670
Fax: 55469291.

Gowtham Pharma Distributors
1st Floor, 111, Nyniappa
Naicken Street,
Chennai-600003,
Phone : 5357700,5352400
Gram. GOWTHAM CAPS,
Telex : 41-5189 SPSI IN,
Fax : 91-44-5352401
Pagar No. 9610-107700.

L & M Aotomatics
60/7, Old Dal Mandi,m
Kanpur-208001 (U.P),
Phone : 352367,352570
Fax : 91-512-316788.

Mixo Fill (India)
1351, Street No. 45,

Jafrabad, New Seelampur,
Shahdara, Delhi - 110053
Phones : (Fact)
2263446,2263362,
(Off) 327460,3270735
Fax : 011-3265278

Patel Engineering Works
Bhajiwala Chawl, Ram Nagar
Chincholi Bunder Road,
Malad (West)
Mumbai - 400058
Phone : 8815065

Push Pack Industries
J-149, GIDC,
Killa-Pardi-396125,
Valsad (Gujarat)
Phone : 026352-680,
Gram. PUSHPACK

Techno-Blist
65/5, F Road, GIDC
Phase-I Vatva
Ahmedabad-382445 (Gujarat)
Phone : 5834253
Fax : 91-079-5834253.

PASTE FILLING MACHINES

Armstrong Smith Ltd.
Brady House, 12/14,
Veer Nariman Road,
Mumbai - 400023

Frederick Herbert
10, Second Pasta Lane,
Colaba,
Mumbai - 400005

Gowthem Pharma Distributors
1st Floor, 111, Nyniappa
Naicken Street,
Chennai-600003.
Phones : 5357700,5352400,
Gram. GOWTHAM CAPS
Telex. 41-5189 SPSI IN
Fax : 91-44-5352401
Pagar No. 9610-107700

Square Pharma Machineries
Gala No. 30/31
Arihant Industrial Estate,
Off. Saki Vihar Road,

Saki Naka,
Mumbai - 400072
Phone: 8528306,8500201,
Fax : 022-8378552

Sreeniwas Engineering Works
2-1-460/1, Nallakunta,
Hyderabad-500044,
Phone : Off. 7662606
Fact . 7619475
Gram. SREENEX

Supar Pharma Indl.Severice
20, Mahalaxmi Industrial
Estate,
Near Bombay Conductor,
GIDC, Vatva,
Ahmedabad-382445 (Gujarat)
Phone : 079-5833849,390407

United Engineering Co. (The)
35-A, Hazra Road,
Kolkata-700029
Phones : 4759744
Gram. UNIENGCO
Fax : 91-033-4757727

POWDER FILLING MACHINE

Amba Engineers
6, Laxmi Industrial Estate,
Navnit Prakashan
Compound,
Ajod Dairy Road, Rakhial,
Ahmedabad-380023
Phone : (079) 2743948,
Gram. AMBAFILL
Fax : (079) 2743948

EEE CEE & Co.
1, Anant Estate,
Opp. Comet Estate,
Rakhial,
Ahmedabad-380023
(Gujarat)
Phone : 079-2743075
Fax : 079-2743075

Machino Medicinia Pvt. Ltd.
WZ-12, Phool Bagh,
Rampur More,
Delhi - 110035

354 Herbal Cosmetics & Beauty Products with Formulations

Phone: 91-11-5447399,5430672
Gram. ASIAN SALE
Fax: 91-11-5156151

N.K.Engineering Co
Plot No. 1808
Phase-III, GIDC,
Vatva,
Ahmedabad-382445
Telefax. 91-79-5891746

Supar Seals Company
WZ-12, Phool Bagh,
Rampura More,
Delhi - 110035
Phones : 91-11-5447399,5430672,
Gram. ASIAN SALE
Fax: 91-11-5156151

Virajka Machinery Mfg Co
5, Shrine Industrial Estate,
Rakhial,
Ahmedabad-380023

REACTION VESSELS/ STORAGE TANKS

Burman Plant Machinery Co. (P) Ltd.
36, Sarkar Lane,
Kolkata-700007
Phone : 2411340,
Fax : (91)(33) 296077

Dalal Engineering Pvt. Ltd.
Post Box No. 63,
Thane-400061 (Maharashtra)
Phone : 022-5343577,5343528,
Fax: 022-5345570
E-Mail: dalalfac@vsnl.com.

Machino Medicinia Pvt. Ltd.
WZ-12, Phool Bagh,
Rampur More,
Delhi - 110035
Phone : 91-11-5447399,5430672
Gram. ASIAN SALES
Fax : 91-11-5156151

Neomachine Mfg.Co. Pvt. Ltd.

39/2A, Purna Das Road,
Kolkata-700029
Phones :
4644568,4640457,4647253
Gram. TECHPHARMA
Fax : 91-33-4643473,4647254

Rank & Co
A-95/3, Wazipur Industrial Estate,
Delhi - 110052
Phone : 7456101-2-3-4,7441958
Gram. MIXKING
Fax :7234126,7471905

Sainath Boilers & Pneumatics
18-A, Minerva Industrial Estate,
Mulund (West)
Mumbai - 400080
Phones : 5613239

Sehgal Industrial Works
T-1698, Malka Ganj Road,
Subzi Mandi, Delhi - 110007
Phone : 3953823,3970381,
Fax : 011-3970381

Textiles Art Machinery
Unit No. 145, Adarsh
Industrial. Estate,
Sahar Road, Chakala,
Andheri (E),
Mumbai - 400093
Phone : 8322721,8325957
Gram. TAMHYDRO
Telex. 011-71933 TAM IN.

STERILISING PLANTS

Dalal Engineering Pvt. Ltd.
Post Box No. 63,
Thane-400601
(Maharashtra)
Phones : 022-5343577,5343528,
Fax : 022-5345570
E-Mail : dalalfac@vsnl.com

Grovers Pvt. Ltd.
4-F4, Shankardham
Sundervan Complex.

Off Lokhandwala
Complex Road,
Andheri (W),
Mumbai - 400058
Phones : 6293092,6294079,
Fax : 91-22-6293014,
E-Mail :
groversgple@aems.vsnl.net.in

Jainsons (I) Regd
P.O.Box 37,
Jain Temple Bldg. Dal Mandi,
Ambala Cantt-133001
(Haryana)
Phone : 171- 644198/633157
Fax : 643485.

Lab. Instruments
78-C, J.S.Seth Road,
Ratnadeep. Near Roxy.
Opera House,
Mumbai - 400004
Phones : 3690973, 3681316
Fax : 3690973

Modern Scientific Industrial
199-A, Saket, Meerut-250001
(U.P)
Phone: (0121) 644086
Gram. INDUSTRIES

N.V.Industrial Pvt Ltd.
Shudha Park,
Raja S.C.Malik,
Garia, 24-Parganas
(West Bengal)

Rank & Co
A-95/3, Wazipur Industrial Estate,
Delhi - 110052
Phone : 7456101-2-3-4,7441958
Gram. MIXKING
Fax : 7234126,7471905

Reva Pharma Machinery
Plot No. 942/4, GIDC,
Makarpura, Baroda-390010
(Gujarat)
Phone : 0265-640082

STRIP PACKING MACHINE

Bhuvaneswari & Co

Suppliers of Plant, Machinery and Equipments

13, Old Trunk Road,
Pallavaram,
Chennai-600043.

Hindco Brothers
Plot No. 6120, C/1 Type,
GIDC, Vapi-396195
Dist. Valasd (Gujarat)

Hindco India
11, A.B.Aradhana
Industrial Estate,
Navghar Road,
Post Box No. 32
Bhyandar (East) 401105
Dist. Thane (Maharashtra)
Phone : 6982423

**Kulbindra Engineering
Works (Regd)**
AA/7B-1, Gali No. 4G,
Anand Parbat,
Industrial Area,
New Rohtak Road,
New Delhi - 110005
Phones : 5765749,5743222

**Magnose Engineering
Company**
19, Ashoka Industrial Estate,
L.B.Shastri Marg. Mulund
(West) Mumbai - 400080
Phones : 5617372,5612165,
Gram. STEVSYL
Fax : 91-22-
5914218,5644511,
E-Mail:
leoscor@bom3.vsnl.net.in

Mahajan & Company
17, M.K. Brothers Industrial
Estate,
Kurla-Andheri Road,
Mumbai - 400072

Metal Fabs
2-1-460/1, Nallakuntha,
Hyderabad-500044
Phones : 7662606,
Fax : 91-040-7619475
Gram. SREENEX.

Rupa Industries
3840, Kanhiya Nagar,
Tri Nagar
Delhi - 110035
Phones : 7222471

**TANKS
(Storage, etc)**

Adam Fabriwerk (P) Ltd.
203, Rajguru Apts.
New Nagardas Road,
Andheri (E),
Mumbai - 400069
Phones : 8380548,8384173,
Telefax : 022-8390195,
E-Mail: adamfab@vsnl.com

Alankar Industries
Post Box : 27371,
Andheri (west)
Mumbai - 400058

Anup Engineering Limited.
Behind 66 Kv Electric Sub
Station, Odhav Road,
Ahmedabad-382415
(Gujarat)
Phones: 2870622,2872823,
Gram. ANUPAM.
Telex : 121-6327
ANUP IN.
Fax : 079-2870642

Atomplant Industries
52, Angol Road,
Tilakwadi, Belgaum-590006
(Karnataka)
Phone : 22024, 22910
Gram. ATOMPLANT

Bhuvaneswari & Co
13,Old Trunk Road,
Pallavaram,
Chennai-600043

**Burman Plant & Machinery
Co (P) Ltd.**
36, Sarkar Lane.
Kolkata-700007
Phone : 2411340,
Fax : (91)(33) 296077

**Chemitex Engineering
Enterprises**
Plot 277-278, GIDC
Odhav-382415 (Gujarat)
Phone : 2871180,2871280

Cosywo Engg. Co
15, Laxmi Co-op,Industrial
Estate Ltd.

Amraiwadi Road, Near
Nagarvel Hanuman Mandir,
Ahmedabad-380026
Telefax : 2748168,2748001,
E-Mail: cosywo@usa.net,
Website: www.indianic.com/
cosywo

Eureka Engineering
E-13,14, Industrial Area,
Site No. 1, Bulandshahar
Road,
Ghaziabad -201001 (U.P)
Phone :
722712,711916,713905
Gram. EUREKA
Fax : 0575-712136

Fillopack Industries
Unit No.2, Vijay Industrial
Estate
I.B.Patel Road.
Goregaon (E)
Mumbai - 400063
Phones : 6122399

Gopinath Engg.Co
9/C, Archana Industrial
Estate,
No.2 Beside Anil Synthetic,
Behind Rakhial P.O. Rakhial,
Ahmedabad-380023
Phones : 362711,367080,
Gram. EMBEETRUCK
Telex : 121-7002
EMBE IN .

Hospital Supply Company
111, Chittranjan Avenue,
Kolkata - 700012

**Iadlab Equipment
Corporation**
403, 4th Floor,
Binu Aptt, Section 25,
Behind Venus,
Ulhasnagar-421004.
Phones : 0251-534246
Fax : 0251-530254

**Pay Rs. 1200/-
for Classified
Advertisement**

Chapter - 34

PACKAGING MATERIALS

BOTTLES

TOURO TRADES
809, Katra Neel,
Chandni Chowk,
Delhi - 110006
Phones: Off: 3975346
Resi. 2814781
Fax : 011-3924988
Deals in : Aluminium
Bottles 5 ml. to 25 kg,
Aluminium Fancy Caps
(Golden) Aerosole &
Refilable Spray mist
devices, Glass
Bottles for perfume &
cosmetics
Contact Person :
Varun Seth

Apanjan Glass Industries
3-A, Chowranghee Place,
Room No. 17, (1st Floor)
Kolkata - 700013

Bajaj Commercial Corporation
B-5/11, Mahesh Nagar,
S.V.Road,
Goregaon (W),
Mumbai - 400062
Phone : 6723867

Barkha Bottle Bhandar
Sukhadiya Gram,
Behind Sector-D,
Indore-452003 (M.P)
Phone : 442141

Borosil Glass Works Ltd.
44, Khanna Construction
House,
Dr. R.G. Thadani Marg,
Worli, Mumbai - 400050
Phone : 4930362/0360/0370
Gram. BOROSIL
Telex. 011-75351 BOROSIL
Fax : 4948161

East India Glass Industries
Jessore Road, P.O.
Ganganagar,
24-Parganas-743 250
(West Bengal)
Phone : 5522383

Flamingo Blow-Pack
57, Laxmanbhai Estate,
Near Revabhai Estate,
Near Shreeji Hotel,
Amraiwadi,
Ahmedabad-380026 (Gujarat)

Gier Trading Company (Agency)
Gier House 4,
Chatawala Lane,
Kolkata - 700012
Phone : 269810/267303/
267968

Haldyn Glass Ltd.
Off Western Express
Highway,
Goregaon (East)
Mumbai - 400063
Phone : 8730311-
14,8742480-2,
Gram. PILFERPROOF
Telex : 011-70047
HGWL IN
Fax : 91-22-8735231,

E-Mail:
vintar@giashm0.1.vsnl.net.in.
Website: chttp://
ww.infoindia.com/haldyn.

Indian Scientific Glass Industries
4A, Luis Annexe,
Pandurang Budhkar Marg,
Mumbai - 400013
Phones : 4309556,4222870,
Gram. KHEMKAPLUS.
Telex : 011-73684 ISGI IN
Fax : 91-22-
4304379,4309556

Japan Bottle House
312, Tilak Bazar,
Delhi - 110006
Phone : 3963057, 3942812

CAPS
(Aluminium, etc)

Touro Trades,
809, Katra Neel,
Chandni Chowk,
Delhi - 110006
Phones: Off: 3975346 Resi.
2814781
Fax : 011-3924988
Deals in : Aluminium
Bottles 5 ml. to 25 kg,
Aluminium Fancy Caps
(Golden) Aerosole &
Refilable Spray mist
devices, Glass
Bottles for perfume &
cosmetics
Contact Person : Varun
Seth

Packaging Materials

Aar Es Pharma
5, Lakhpat Rai Lane,
Bahadur Gunj,
Allahabad-211003 (U.P)

Bengal Metal Industries
10, Chaulpatty Road,
Beleghata,
Kolkata-700010
Phone : 359448

Bombay Glass Blowing Industries
7, J.K.Industrial Estate,
Off. Mahakali Caves Road,
Andheri (East)
Mumbai - 400093
Phone : 8329530
Fax : 8363208,
E-Mail :
bomglass@bom5.vsnl.net.in.

Bottle Closures
16, Keytuo Industrial Estate,
Kondivita Road,
Andheri (E)
Mumbai - 400059
Phone : 8387366

Central Tin Works
Chinchpokli Corner Lane,
Mumbai - 400027
Gram. TINOBOXES

Container & Commodities Trading Co
108, D. New Chinch Bunder,
Mumbai - 400009

Datta Tin Works Pvt. Ltd.
Srikandath Road,
Ernakulam,
Cochin-682016 (Kerala)
Phone : 35199.

Everest Glass Emporium
No.D-39, 2nd Floor,
P-36, India Exchange Place,
Kolkata-700001
Phone : 2429417
Gram. PRINTOGLASS.

Friend's & Co
'Kailash', 320,
Sir Bhalchandra Road,
Matunga (C.Rly)
Mumbai - 400019

Ghanshyam Das Somani & Co
Somani Bhawan, 2060,
Ramlalaji Ka Rasta,
Jaipur-302003
Phones : 568060,568061
Gram. GHANSHAM CO.
Fax : 91-141-565505

CLOSURES & SEALS
(Pilfer Proof)

Alpine Packers & Closurs
C-3/98, Ashok Vihar,
Phase II,
Delhi - 110052
Phone : 7226151

Bharati Engineers
3727-28/29,Dariba Pan.
Opp. Shtiela Cinema,
New Delhi - 110055
Phone : 7524749

Chempion Packaging Industries
29 RE/4, Street No. 4 ,
Anand Parbat Industrial Estate,
New Rohtak Road,
New Delhi - 110005.

Goleria Rubber Products
3, Manisha Bldg.
Mathuradas Cross Road,
Irani Wadi,
Behind Asian Bakery,
Kandivli (W)
Mumbai - 400067
Phone : 022-
8616004,8016720,807315
Fax : 022-8073151,8616004

Harison & Co
23/25, Paradise Lane,
L.J.Road,
Mahim
Mumbai - 400016

Indian Glass Agency
39/1, Site No. IV.
Industrial Area,
Sahibabad (Ghaziabad)
(U.P)
Phone : 201385

Indopack
9/110, Anand Parbat

Industrial Area,
(Opp. Anand Parbat Police Station),
New Delhi - 110005,
Phones : 5729308,5742695
Fax : 5752330

Jeffrey & Basack Pvt. Ltd.
29, Madan Mitter Lane.
Kolkata-700006

Kiv Group Industries
Sunmill Compound,
Lower Parel,
Mumbai - 400003

Larsons & Toubro Ltd.
L & T House, Narotham
Morarji Marg,
Ballard Estate,
Mumbai - 400001
Phones : 022-268121
(9 Lines)

Lion Engg. Polymer Products
D/3, Surjit Sangam,
Mathuradas Road,
Kandivili (W)
Mumbai - 400067
Phone : 8078876

CONTAINERS (Cardboard, Glass, Plastic etc.)

Agra Bottle Stores
17/37, Prayag Market,
Old Banaras Bank,
Phulatti Bazar,
Agar-282003 (U.P)
Phone : 367158,368116

Alpha Containers
1, Jash Market, Ring Road,
Surat-395002 (Gujarat)
Phone : 0261-638100 (5 Lines)
Fax : 0261-
623545,623546,633217
E-Mail : alpha@alphage.com.
Website : http://
www.alphage.com.

Anand Timber Traders
170, Reay Road,
Mumbai - 400010
Phones : 8725768, 8121224,
8514650, 8512098

Arora Metal Industry
Ist Floor, 66,Ezra Street,
(G.P.O Box No. 2289),
Kolkata-700001
Phone : (033)
2254367,2254170
Gram. Metal Seal.

Bajaj Glass Enterprises
B-5/10, Mahesh Nagar,
Goregaon (w),
Mumbai - 400062
Phones : 6723867

Bhagwandas Devshi Pvt. Ltd.
87, Shamaldas Gandhi Marg.
Mumbai - 400002
Phones : 311084
Gram. EMBOT

Bharat Associated Industries
P-5, B.R.B. Basu Road,
2nd Floor,
Kolkata-700001
Phones : 317470

CORKS

Delhi Bottle Stores
142, Tilak Bazar,
Delhi - 110006

Injecto Pack (India)
G-49, City Centre, 570,
M.G. Road,
Indore-452001 (M.P)
Phones : 531343,472802

J.H. Mehta & Brothers
Dev Ashish,
1st Floor,
Near Klassic Gold Hotel,
Ellisbridge,
Ahmedabad-380006
Phones : 6564949,404824
Fax : 91-6446646
E-Mail : jhmehta@ghahd
.gbblobalnet.ems.vsnl.net.in

Mukherjee Bottle & Co
105, Akhil Mistry Lane,
Kolkata-700009
Phones : 033-3508906

New Bottle & Pasti Stores
Chhotelal's Chawl,
Outside Delhi Gate
Ahmedabad-380004

Nitco (Glassware) Pvt.Ltd.
36, Brabourne Road,
Kolkata-700001

Peojee Bottling Co
63, Bangur Avenue,
Block D.
Kolkata-700055

FILM BLISTER

Flexible Packaging Co
128/129, New Sadguru Nashik
Industrial Eate,
Western Express Highway,
Goregaon (East)
Mumbai - 400063
Phone : 8733602,
Telexfax : 8734856
E-Mail :
vilam@bom4.vsnl.net.in

Sudharma Polymers Pvt.Ltd.
11, Sufalam Flats
Jaihind Press,
Ashram Road,
Ahmedabad-380009 (Gujarat)
Phone : 079-6587786
Fax : 079-5831994

Vij Packaging
Opp. Kalupur Chakla,
P.O. Tankshal Road,
Kalupur,
Ahmedabad-380001
(Gujarat)
Phone : 079-380109,338932,
Fax : 079-2121614

FILM PLASTIC
(Flat,Tubular)

Aryan Chemicals
Maharshi Dayanand Marg,
Near Railway Line,
Saijpur Bogha,
Ahmedabad-382345
Phone : 2816331-32-2822933,
Fax: 91-79-2821541

Bhandari Industries Ltd.
Gate No. 1028,
Village Shirol,
Tal Rajgurunagar
Distt Pune-410505
(Maharashtra)

Phones : 91-2135-24065,24066
Fax : 02135-24068
E-Mail : bilcare@ip.eth.net.in

Unipharma Rotographics & Scientifics Pvt.Ltd.
A-18, Naraina Industrial Area,
Phase-I, New Delhi - 110028
Phones :
5793386,5795163,5795164
Gram. HOTMELT IN
Fax : 5795164

FOILS

Ajit Foils & Allieds
No. 50, Mookatkal Street,
Opp. Roxy Theatre,
Puraswalkam.
Chennai-600007
Phones : 6422246, 6424391, 567700, 562400

Aryodaya Plastic Industries
Arya Printing
Press Compound,
Saijpur Bogha,
Ahmedabad-382345

Central Drug Syndicate
2068/5, Chuna Mandi,
Paharganj,
New Delhi - 110055
Phones : 7510806,6418285
Fax : 91-11-7523433

Chaso Associated
CB-33/2, Ring Road, Naraina,
New Delhi - 110028.

Flexible Packaging Co
128/129, New Sadguru
Nashik Industrial Estate,
Western Express Highway,
Goregaon (East)
Mumbai - 400063
Phone : 8733602,
Telefax : 8734856
E-Mail :
vilam@bom4.vsnl.net.in

LABLES

Agra Bottle Stores
17/37, Prayag Market,
Old Banaras Bank
Phulatti Bazar,
Agra-282003 , (U.P)
Phone : 367158,368116

Packaging Materials

Delhi Bottle Stores
142, Tilak Bazar,
Delhi - 110006

Divya
25, Band Street,
Fort, Mumbai - 400023
Phone : 2664396

Kiv Group Industries
Sunmill Compound, Lower Parel,
Mumbai - 400003

Open Foils Enterprises
Plot No. 403/1,
Opposite Gurukul,
Sector 22, Gandhinagar-382022
(Gujarat)
Phone : 91-0-2712-24422

Reliable Printers
170, Mahatma Gandhi Road,
Kolkata-700007

PAPER WAXED

Aryan Chemicals
Maharshi Dayanand Marg,
Near Railway Line,
Saijpur Bogha,
Ahmedabad-382345
Phone : 2816331-32-2822933
Fax : 91-79-2821441

Arya Printing Press
Maharshi Dayanand Marg,
Near Rly. Line,
saijpur Bogha,
Ahmedabad-382345
Phone :2816331-32-2822333,
Gram. ARYAPRESS,
Fax : 91-79-2821441
E-Mail :
aryanChemicals@hotmail.com.

Manish Printing & Packaging
Maharshi Dayanand Marg.
Saijpur Bogha,
Ahmedabad-382345
(Gujarat)
Phones : 816331-32-33-34,
Fax : 91-79-8515441,

STRIP PACKING MATERIAL

Flexible Packaging Co
128/129, New Sadgur Nashik

Industrial Estate,
Western Express Highway,
Goregaon (East)
Mumbai - 400063
Phones : 8733602,
Telefax : 8734856
E-Mail
:vilam@bom4.vsnl.net.in

Indopack
9/110, Anand Parbat
Industrial Area,
(Opp. Anand Parbat Police Station)
New Delhi - 110005
Phones :5729308,5742695
Fax : 5752330

Metalpack
S-238, Greater Kailash,
Part-II,
New Delhi - 110048
Phone : 6431427

Reliable Printers
170, Mahatma Gandhi Road,
Kolkata-700007

TUBES COLLAPSIBLE

Chandra Extrusion Products
Navneet Bhavan,
Teli Bagh,
Lucknow.

Grinar Extrusion (P) Ltd
1/4, Madhapura Market,
Shahibag Road,
Ahmedabad-380004
Phones : 386120-23-24

Kiv Group Industries.
Sunmill Compound,
Lower Parel,
Mumbai - 400003

Pharma Bottle Distributors,
Chotalal's Chakla,
O/S. Delhi Gate,
Ahmedabad-380004
(Gujarat)
Phone : 079-5624865,
Fax : 079-5625841

Shalimar Textile Mfg. Pvt Ltd.
(Tube Divn),117-AB, Govt.

Industrial Estate,
Kandivli (W)
Mumbai - 400067
Phones :693504,692251/52
Gram. SARATUBE

Zenith Tin Works Pvt. Ltd.
Opp. Race Course,
Cherk Road,
Mahalaxmi.
Mumbai - 400034

VIALS

Adit Containers
34/133, Laxmi Industrial Estate,
Faizabad Road,
Lucknow-226016
Phone :(0522) 386876, 386704
Fax : 0522-380147

Amrut Industries
VIII, Vikas Estate,
Vishweshwarnagar.
Off Aarey Road,
Goregaon (East)
Mumbai - 400063

Anupam Glass Works
2, Hazi Banku Lane,
Konnagar-712235,
Hooghly (West Bengal)
Phones : 6622576,6621181,
Gram. AMPOULE

Bombay Glass Blowing Industries
7, J.K. Industrial Estate,
Off. Mahakali Caves Road,
Andheri (East)
Mumbai - 400093
Phone : 8329530
Fax : 8363208,
E-Mail :
bomglass@bom5.vsnl.net.in

Cap Seals India
184, Subhash Colony,
Near Khandelwal College,
Shastri Nagar, Jaipur-302016
Phones : 301440,301394,
Fax : 302658,
Gram. C.S.I. CAPS

Container & Commodities Trading Co.
108, D.New Chinch Bunder,
Mumbai - 400009

Durga Agencies
184, Subhash Colony,
Near Khandelwal College,
Shastrinagar,
Jaipur-302016
Phone :
301440,301394,302658

Esschem (Pvt) Ltd.
19th Floor, Centre-1,
World Trade Centre, Cuffe
Parade,
Mumbai - 400005
Phones : 2182485,2182339,
Telex : 11-86975
ESCM. 11-81161 ESCM.
Fax : 91-22-2183045/
2184351

Garg Glass Works Pvt. Ltd.
86/1, Dr. Sundari Mohan
Avenue,
P.O.Entally,
Kolkata-700014,
Phones : 2448665,2447465,
Gram. GARGAMPULE
Fax : 033-2448665

General Trading Corporation
Walkhiwala Bldg.
24, First Dhobi Talao Lane.
P.O. Box No.2743
Mumbai - 400002

Govind Prased & Sons
66, Ezra Street,
Kolkata-700001

Hindusthan Thermostatics,
5, Industrial Estate,
Ambala Cantt-133001
(Haryana)
Phone : 642816,21216
Fax : 640391

Indo Glass Trading Corporation
3/119-B, Shivaji Service
Industries,
Manmala Tank Road,
Mahim, Mumbai - 400016
Phones :
4305669,4307130,4221632
Fax : 022-4301131

Jaisons (I) Regd.
P.O.Box 37,
Jain Temple Bldg.
Dal Mandi,
Ambala Cantt-133001

(Haryana)
Phones :171-644198/633157
Fax : 643485

Jg.Glass Industries Pvt.Ltd.
Air India Bldg. Nariman Point,
Mumbai - 400001
Phone : 298355,
Gram,. NUTRALGLAS

Kamal Glass Bottle Supplying Co.
K-14, Opp. Manva Ashram,
Tonk Road, Jaipur-302018
Phone : 397034,395455,
Fax : 0141-517967

Kejriwal Industries
45, Rajasthani Udyog Nagar,
G.T.Karnal Road,
Delhi - 110033
Phone : 7210910
Fax : 3263449

**WASHERS
(Rubber, Cork, Cardboard)**

Bengal Metal Industries
10, Chaulpatty Road,
Beleghata,
Kolkata-700010
Phone : 359448

Govind Prasad & Sons
66, Ezra Street,
Kolkata-700001

Meenakshi Metal Caps
V-19A, Budh Vihar,
Delhi - 110041

Mukherjee Bottle Co.
14, New Colony
(Paschim Para)
Rahara-743186,
North 24-Parganas
(W.Bengal)
Phone : 033-5530574

National India Rubber Works Ltd.
Katni-483501 (M.P)
Phone : (07622) 2406,2360,
Gram. RUBBER

R.K.Desai & Co.
Bentinck Street.
Ist Floor,
Kolkata-700069

Shish Hari Enterprises
3rd, Floor, 198,
Kalbadevi Road,
Mumbai - 400002
Phones: 2014341,2086877
Fax : 022-2014341

WRAPPERS

Flexible Packaging Co.
128/129,
New Sadguru Nashik
Industrial Estate,
Western Express Highway,
Goregaon (East)
Mumbai - 400063
Phone : 8733602,
Telefax : 8734856
E-Mail :
vilam@bom4.vsnl.net.in

Paper Products Ltd.
120, Dinshaw Wacha Road,
Mumbai - 400001

Subnil Packing Machines Pvt. Ltd.
Shed NO.37, Road, No.1, IDA
Mallapur, Nacharam,
Hyderabad-500076 (A.P)
Phone : 91-40-7176810,
Fax : 91-40-7176841
E-Mail : works@subnil.com

Super Scientific Glass Industries
E-66, Sardar Estate,
Ajwa Road,
Vadodara-390019
(Gujarat)
Phone : 462088,
Fax : 0265-461032.

PET BOTTLES/ CONTAINERS

Ruptex Mineral Water Pvt. Ltd.
14, Rani Jhansi Road,
New Delhi - 110055
Ph: 3631280, 3552349

Varahi Plastics Pvt. Ltd.
WZ-8/1, Industrial Area,
Kirti Nagar,
New Delhi - 110015
Ph: 5107300, 5107301
Fax : 5451504,
E-Mail: varahi@vsnl.com

Chapter - 35

SUPPLIERS OF RAW MATERIALS

NEW BHARAT CHEMICAL WORKS
4908, Phoota Road,
Sadar Bazar,
Delhi - 110 006
Ph : 3613307, 3538310
Telefax : 3523602
Resi : 5437208
Estd. : 1929
Contact : Mr. P.S. Arora
House for widest range of Chemicals. Specialist in Cosmetic Raw Materials including Herbal Cosmetics Raw Materials.

SHANKAR DYES AND CHEMICALS
1209, Shankar Building,
Gali No. 11, Sadar Bazar,
Delhi - 110 006
Ph : 3673462, 3558239, 3616830
Fax : 91-11- 3558239
Branch :
119, Tilak Bazar,
Delhi - 110 006
Ph : 3970589, 3959574
Resi : 7492678
E-Mail : djeswani@sattiya.net.in
Website : www.shankardyesandchemicals.com
Contact : Dr. Nirmal Kumar and Dilip Kumar
Specialists in All Type of Chemicals and Dyes Products, All Kinds of Chemicals and Dyes Pigments.

K K Trading Company
1-A, Goela Lane,
Under Hill Road,
Civil Lines, Delhi-54
Ph: 3941380, 3956222, 3945829
Fax : 91-11-3945829
E-Mail : Kkt@satyam.net.in
Contact for full range of Cosmetic raw materials and also refer our advertisement in the back page for full details of our products

HERBS AND HERBS EXTRACT

Natural Herbs
The Ayurvedic People
Correspondence at:
147, New Rajdhani Enclave,
Preet Vihar, Delhi-110092
Phone : 2448184
Phones:
3975938,3935938,3936938
E-mail :
naturalherbs@rediffmail.com
Regd. Office
73/40, Ishwar Market,
Gandhi Gali, Fateh Puri,
Delhi-110006
Deals In.
Herbs, Roots, Gums,
Leaves, Bark & Heena etc.
Contact Person. R.S.Sahu

S.V.Marketing
2210/19, Aggarwal Market,
Khari Baoli, Delhi- 110006
Ph. 3933003,3915500

Pansom Herbals Pvt. Ltd.
Export Extracts Herbs
Aroma/ayur@vsnl.com
H-38, South Ext. Part-I,
New Delhi-110049
Phone : 4648034

Sunjay Pharma
Best Quality Herbs & Ayurvedic Raw Materials
6093, F.Flr, Gali Batashan,
Khari Baoli,
New Delhi-110006
Phone : 3921335

Nathi Mal Rugan Mal
6689, Khari Baoli,
Delhi- 110006
Ph. 3924664,3944527,
C.E.Mr. Devender

Sood Brothers
Khari Baoli,
Delhi - 110006
Ph. 3961551,
Mr. Sudhir Sood

Karan Enterprises
6644, Khari Baoli,
Delhi - 110006
Ph. 3961551

Devi Sahai Mohan Lal
2087, Katra Tobacco,
Khari Baoli,
Delhi - 110006
Ph.
3924455,3962916,3962767
C.E. Mohan Lal

Devi Sahai Banwari Lal,
Katra Tobacco,
Delhi-6
Phone : 3979238

Taj Trading Co.
6682, Khari Baoli,
Delhi- 110006
Ph. 3952184,
C.E. Mr. A.Hasan

Mohd. Husain Ajmal Husain,
6681-82, Khari Baoli,
Delhi-6
Ph.3954516,3955069
C.E.Mr. Tahir

Indian Drug House,
6669, Khari Baoli,
Delhi-110006
Ph. 3942792,3981039
C.E. Mohd Afag.
(Only crude Drugs and Indian Herbs Suppliers)

M.M. Herbo Global,
G-21, Laxman Path,
Off Janpath, Shyam Nagar Ext.
Jaipur-302019,
Ph. 367000,291000,294000

Chemloids
40-15-14 Brindavan Colony
Vijayawada-520010
Phone : 473468,475278
Telex : 0475-270 CHEM IN
Products: Herbal concentrates
in pastes/powder form

Goodwin Pharma Chem Laboratories
13-1-10, Ground Floor
Old Bank Road
Guntur-522001
Phone : 22566
Products: Herbal extracts in the form
of thick paste and dry powder

Indo World Trading Corporation
303, Prakash Chambers
F, Netaji Subhash Marg
NEW DELHI-110002
Phone: 3278059,3283480
Fax : 3274521
Products: Herbal extracts

Jagdish Kumar Hari Om And Company
485/2, Katra Ishwar Bhawan
Khari Baoli
DELHI-110006
Phone : 2910274
Fax : 2514221

May Fair Aromatics
D-15, Nizamuddin East
NEW DELHI-110013
Phone : 4634073
Products: Herbal extracts

Abhyuday Industries
27, Market Yard, PO 006
Sidhpur-384151
Phone :20534,20529
Fax : 21034
Products: Crude drugs,
psllium husk and seeds,
husk powder

Ansar Industries
P.O.Box No-365
4/3367, H.K.Street
Zampa Bazar ASD3
Surat - 395003
Phone : 3352,32645
Gram : Ansar
Products. Herbal extracts
in paste and powder form

MENTHOL

Rajhans Aromatics
201, Inderprostha Tower,
Commercial Complex
Wazirpur Industrial Area,
Delhi-110052
Tel : 91-11-7134004,
7139697,
Fax : 91-11-7254501,
7483638
E-Mail :
rajhans@nda.vsnl.net.in
Website :
www.rajhansaromatics.com

Vishal Chemicals
Subhash Road,
Chandausi - 202412
Distt. Moradabad (U.P)
Phone : (05921) Off : 51246,
51370

Sheetal Exports
Old Central Bank Building.
Gopi Chowk
Budaun - 243601 (U.P.)

India
Ph : 91-5822-
24257,24827,24427
Fax : 91-5832-24068
E-Mail :
sheetalexports@usa.net.

Natural Agro Chem Overseas
B-27, Somdatt Chamber-I,
5, Bhikaji Cama Palace,
New Delhi- 110066
Ph : 6191465, 6191356
Fax : 011-6196922
E-Mail :
naco@mantraonline.com

Arora Aromatics
Near Kalki Temple,
Sambhal - 244302 (India)
Ph . Off. 05923-24624,24914
E-Mail :
menthol@mickyonline.com

BALSUM PERU

Desai Chemical Co. Pvt. Ltd.,
11, Ezra Street,
Kolkata - 700 001
Ph : 033- 2479541
Fax : 2479738
E-Mail :
pratap@satyam.net.in

S. Zhaveri & Co.
109, Shiv Smruti Chambers,
49, Dr. Annie Besant Road,
Worli, Mumbai - 400018
Phone : (022)-4932949,
4932044,
Fax : (022)-4930300
E-mail :
szhaveri@bom3.vsnl.net.in

COCONUT OIL

M.P.Dyechem Industries
59 & 63, Sector A,
Sanwer Road Industrial Area,
Indore - 452003,
Madhya Pradesh,
Phone : (0731)-
420325,420775
Fax : (0731)-420136

Suppliers of Raw Materials

Nataraj Traders
Big Street,
Ambajipeta - 533214
Andhra Pradesh
Phone : (08856)-43216
Fax : (08856)-43016

Prakesh Trading Co.
216, 10th Khetwadi Lane,
Dinath Compound,
Mumbai - 400004
Phone :(022)-
3852748,3885573
Fax : (022)-3801719

Virendra Oil Mills
C/29, Vijay Smruti,
19th Road, Chembur,
Mumbai - 400071.
Phone : (022)-5281875,
5280366,
Fax : (022)-5281732

CINNAMON LEAF OIL

Leela Aromatics
1st Floor, Devkaran Mansion,
24, Mangaldas Road,
Princess Street,
Mumbai - 400002.
Phone : (022)-2050558,
2057314
Fax : (022)-8351601

TMV Aromatics P. Ltd.
3rd Floor, Srinivas Colony,
M.G. Road, Cochin,
Ernakulam - 682035,
Kerala.
Phone : (0484)-381330,
350528
Fax : (0484)-373121

HERBAL EXTRACTS

Sears Phytochem Ltd.
55/1/2C, New Palasia,
Indore-452001.
Madhya Pradesh
Phone : (0731)-
540215,431035,533920
Fax : (0731)-431168,538226
E-Mail : sears@vsnl.com
Website : http://
www.searsphytochem.com

Indo World Trading Corp
303, Prakash Chambers,
6, Netaji Subhash Marg,
Darya Ganj,
New Delhi- 110002
Phone : (011)-3278059,
3283480
Fax : (011)- 3274521,
3250434

Shree Shantinath Pharma Chem P.Ltd.
48 & 50, Amrut Niwas,
165, Lohar Chawl,
Mumbai - 400002
Phone : (022)-2005469,
2077092,
Fax : (022)-20964401,
2013276
E-Mail :
synchrotech@vsnl.com
Web : http://
www.sugandhgroup.com

Hindustan Mint & Agro Products Pvt.Ltd
Barehseni Street,
Chandausi - 202412
Phone : 91-5921-50540,
51900
Fax : 50074
E-Mail :
hindustan@nde.vsnl.net.in
Website :
www.hindustanmint.com

Shree Chem Industries
2/4, Kubal Niwas
Gokhale Road (N),
Dadar (West),
Mumbai - 400028
Phone : (022)-
4456868,4453649
Fax : (022)-4376265
E-Mail :
mrl.ltd@bom5.vsnl.net.in

OLIVE OIL

Arian Enterprises
460, Aggarwal Chamber III,
26, Veer Savarkar Block,
Shakarpur, Vikas Marg
Naw Delhi-110002
Phone (011)-2242156,
2217070,
Fax : (011)-2439188

DETERGENTS

Albright & Wilson Chemicals India Ltd.
Rajmahal, 3rd floor,
84, Veer Nariman Road,
Mumbai - 400020
Phone : 2041272/2048270
Fax : 91-22-2041007

Ashoka Industries
14-15, Industrial Area,
1st Phase,
Sojat City - 306104,
Rajasthan,
Phone : (02960)-
22279,22179

Chemox Industrial Corp
33 A, Vatsa House,
Janmabhoomi Marg,
Mumbai - 400001
Phone : (022)-
2870133,2874119
Fax : (022)-8574487

Reena Chem
C-3/15, G.I.D.C. Estate,
Nadiad - 387001
Gujarat.
Phone : (0268)-
65172,65173
Fax : (0268)-65171
E-Mail :
reechem@bom8.vsnl.net.in

ESSENTIAL OILS

Aventa Chemicals
F-12, Gali No. 32,
Mahendra Park,
Delhi - 110033
Ph : 2437988, 7422167
Fax : 91-11- 2412205

Rajhans Aromatics
201, Inderprostha Tower,
Commercial Complex
Wazirpur Industrial Area,
Delhi-110052
Tel : 91-11-7134004,
7139697,
Fax : 91-11-7254501,
7483638
E-Mail :
rajhans@nda.vsnl.net.in
Website :
www.rajhansaromatics.com

Vishal Chemicals
Subhash Road,
Chandausi - 202412
Distt. Moradabad (U.P)
Phone : (05921) Off :
51246, 51370

Sheetal Exports
Old Central Bank Building.
Gopi Chowk
Budaun - 243601 (U.P)
India
Ph : 91-5822-
24257,24827,24427
Fax : 91-5832-24068
E-Mail :
sheetalexports@usa.net.

Natural Agro Chem Overseas
B-27, Somdatt Chamber-I,
5, Bhikaji Cama Palace,
New Delhi- 110066
Ph : 6191465, 6191356
Fax : 011-6196922
E-Mail :
naco@mantraonline.com

Arora Aromatics
Near Kalki Temple,
Sambhal - 244302 (India)
Ph . Off. 05923-
24624,24914
E-Mail :
menthol@mickyonline.com

PERFUMES, FRAGRANCES AND AROMATIC CHEMICALS

MOHAN PERFUMERY CO.
144-A, Tilak Bazar,
Khari Baoli, Delhi - 110
006
Ph : Off. 3925808,
3915808
Fax : 91-11- 3943881
Contact : Mr. Chander
Mohan and Deepak Arora
Deals in : Perfumery
Compounds, Natural
Essential Oils and Attars
etc.

Priya Fragrances Pvt. Ltd.
A-2, Jalalpur Road,
Murad Nagar,
Ghaziabad (U.P)
Ph. 01232-41758, 40901
Fax : 41806

Hindustan Mint & Agro Products Pvt.Ltd
Barehseni Street,
Chandausi - 202412
Phone : 91-5921-50540,
51900
Fax : 50074
E-Mail :
hindustan@nde.vsnl.net.in
Website :
www.hindustanmint.com

Gupta & Company Ltd.
xiv/294-95, Gali Mandi Pan,
Sadar Bazar
Delhi-110006
Phone : 7774742,3528923,
E-Mail :
aroma@de2.vsnl.net.in

Swastik Aromatics
45, H.S.I.D.C. Industrial Area
Jind-128102 (Haryana)
Phone - (01681) 26098,
5550559, 5513858

PERFUMERY COMPOUND

Priya Fragrances Pvt. Ltd.
A-2, Jalalpur Road,
Murad Nagar, Ghaziabad
(U.P)
Ph. 01232-41758, 40901
Fax : 41806

Gupta & Company Ltd.
xiv/294-95, Gali Mandi Pan,
Sadar Bazar
Delhi-110006
Phone : 7774742,3528923,
E-Mail :
aroma@de2.vsnl.net.in

Swastik Aromatics
45, H.S.I.D.C. Industrial Area
Jind-128102 (Haryana)
Phone - (01681)26098,
5550559,5513858

Sheetal Exports
Old Central Bank Building.
Gopi Chowk
Budaun - 243601 (U.P)
India
Ph : 91-5822-
24257,24827,24427
Fax : 91-5832-24068
E-Mail :
sheetalexports@usa.net.

PERFUMERY CHEMICALS

Aventa Chemicals
F-12, Gali No. 32,
Mahendra Park,
Delhi - 110033
Ph : 2437988, 7422167
Fax : 91-11- 2412205

Fine Organics
(Food Chemicals Division)
15/2, Neelkanth Market,
M.G. Road, Ghatkopar (East),
Mumbai - 400077
Ph:. 5116900,02/5154384/
5154380/5154495
Fax: 91-022-5153215,
5162276
(Finacon-Cac-Beverage
Clouding Agent Concentrate,
Food Emulsifiers, Glyceryl
Mono Stearate, Sodium
Stearoyl-2-Lactylate,
Whipped Topping
Concentrates etc.)

Rajhans Aromatics
201, Inderprostha Tower,
Commercial Complex
Wazirpur Industrial Area,
Delhi-110052
Tel : 91-11-7134004,
7139697,
Fax : 91-11-7254501,
7483638
E-Mail :
rajhans@nda.vsnl.net.in
Website :
www.rajhansaromatics.com

Gupta & Company Ltd.
xiv/294-95, Gali Mandi Pan,
Sadar Bazar
Delhi-110006
Phone : 7774742,3528923,
E-Mail :
aroma@de2.vsnl.net.in

Market Survey Cum Detailed Techno Economic Feasibility Reports

Rs. 3675/-

Each Report Rs. 3675/-

EIRI Consultants & Engineers have recently prepared the following "Market Survey Cum Detailed Techno Economic Feasibility Reports" which are having great future prospect. The **Detailed Project Reports** will also help you

- To get Loan/Finance from Banks/Financial Institutions.
- To set up your own Industry/Unit (For SSI/Medium/Large Scale Unit).
- To have Detailed and Exhaustive Data on any required Items/Projects.

'ENGINEERS INDIA RESEARCH INSTITUTE' (EIRI) The Premier and Trusted Industrial Consultancy Organization from last 24 Years, offer Complete Consultancy, Liaisoning Jobs, Foreign Collaborations, Buy Back Arrangements etc. alongwith "Market Survey Cum Detailed Techno Economic Feasibility Reports" to the entrepreneurs as well as established Industrialists.

WHY EIRI ONLY ? Because 'EIRI' is having (1) Well equipped data bank cum library. (2) Fully expertise team of consultants, technocrats & engineers for prepairing "Market Survey Cum Detailed Techno Economic Feasibility Reports" on any items in Small/ Medium/ Large Scale. (3) Record quantity of over **32,000** "Market Survey Cum Detailed Techno Economic Feasibility Reports" readily available. (4) More than thousands satisfied clients. (5) Vast experience of more than 24 years. (6) 'EIRI' is being undertaken plants on turnkey basis and (7) Latest and detailed authentic informations Covered in each "Market Survey Cum Detailed Techno Economic Feasibility Reports" and many more plus points which stands 'EIRI' on top.

BRIEF CONTENTS

BEGINING : Project Introduction, Brief History of the Product, Properties, BIS (Bureau of Indian Standard) Specifications & Requirements, Uses & Applications.

MARKET SURVEY : Present Market Position, Expected Future Demand, Installed Capacity, Actual Production & Demand, Statistics of Imports & Exports, Export Prospect, Names & Addresses of Existing Units (Present Manufacturers), List of Buyers.

MANUFACTURING PROCESS : Detailed Process of Manufacture, Selection of Process, Flow Sheet Diagram, Production Schedule.

RAW MATERIALS : List of Raw Materials, Properties, Availability of Raw Materials, Required Quantity of Raw Materials, Cost of Raw Materials, Suppliers of Raw Materials.

PLANT & MACHINERY : List of Plant & Machineries, Miscellaneous Items & Accessories, Instruments, Laboratory Equipments & Accessories, Plant Location, Electrification, Electric Load & Water Maintenance, Suppliers/Manufacturers of Plant & Machineries, Specifications of Machineries & Equipments.

PERSONNEL REQUIREMENTS : Requirement of Staff & Labour, Personnel Management, Skilled & Unskilled Labour, Manageriol Staff/Expert, Accountant etc.

LAND & BUILDING : Requirement of Land Area, Rates of the Land, Built up Area, Construction Schedule, Plant Layout, Cost of Boundry Wall etc.

FINANCIAL ASPECTS : Cost of Raw Materials, Cost of Land & Building, Cost of Plant & Machineries, Fixed Capital Investment, Working Capital, Project Cost, Capital Formation, Cost of Production, Profitability Analysis, Break Even Point (BEP), Cash Flow Statement for 5 to 10 Years, Depreciation Chart, Foreign Collaboration (if possible), Conclusion, Projected Balance sheet, Land Man Ratio.

ADDRESSES : Present Manufacturers, List of the Buyers, Plant & Equipment Suppliers/ Manufacturers, Raw Material Suppliers/Manufacturers etc.

LIST OF THE READY AVAILABLE DETAILED PROJECT REPORTS @ Rs. 3675/- EACH

AUTOMOBILES, MECHANICAL & METALLURGICAL

1. AGRICULTRAL EQUIPMENTS
2. AGRICULTRAL EQUIPMENTS INCLUDING THRESHERS
3. AIR BRAKE HELICAL COIL
4. AIR COOLER
5. AIR FILTERS(FOR SCOOTER CAR & EXCAVATORS ETC.)
6. ALUMINIUM & ALUMINIUM ALLOYS FROM ALUMINIUM SCRAP TO MAKE UTENSILS (INDUCTION FURNACE MELTED)
7. ALUMINIUM ALLOY WHEELS
8. ALUMINIUM ALLOYS FROM ALUMINIUM SCRAP TO MAKE UTENSILS (INDUCTION FURNACE)
9. ALUMINIUM HOT & COLD ROLLING MILL
10. ALUMINIUM BOTTLE MANUFACTURING (COLD EXTRUSION OF ALUMINIUM)
11. ALUMINIUM/COPPER CABLE LUGS
12. ALUMINIUM CANS FOR BEER PACKAGING
13. ALUMINIUM CANS FOR CAPACITORS
14. ALUMINIUM CAPS FOR INJECTION VIALS
15. ALUMINIUM EXTRUSION
16. ALUMINIUM FURNITURE & HARDWARE
17. ALUMINIUM SHEET ROLLING MILL
18. ALUMINIUM UTENSILS
19. ALUMINIUM UTENSILS & SCHOOL BOXES
20. ALUMINIUM WIRE DRAWING AND SUPER ENAMELLING FOR WINDING
21. ANODISED ALUMINIUM UTENSILS
22. ANODIZING OF ALUMINIUM
23. ANTIMONY OXIDE FROM LEAD SCRAP
24. ARC WELDING FILTER GLASS
25. ALUMINIUM FOIL CUTTING & ROLL MAKING
26. AUTO FLAPS FOR TRUCKS & BUSES
27. AUTOMOBILE WORKSHOP (GARAGE & SERVICE CENTRE)
28. AUTO GEARS
29. AUTO HORNS
30. AUTO LEAF SPRING
31. AUTO TUBES
32. AUTO PISTON RING
33. AUTO PISTON
34. BAKERY AND BISCUITS EQUIPMENTS FABRICATION
35. BALL POINT PEN REFILLS
36. BALL ROLLER & TAPER BEARING
37. BAND SAW BLADES
38. BARBED WIRE
39. BICYCLE SPOKES
40. BRAKE LINING ASBESTOES/ RESIN BASED & ASBESTOES FREE
41. BRASS ARTWARE/HOLLOW WARE CASTING (WITH THE HELP OF PHENOLIC RESIN)
42. BRASS CASTING
43. BRASS PIPES FROM BRASS SHEET WITH LONGITUDINALLY WELDING
44. BRASS WARE BY CASTING METHOD (BRASS ARTICLES VIZ. BRASS POOJA LAMPS AND OTHER CASTED)
45. BRIGHT BARS
46. BUFFING AND POLISHING INDUSTRY (JOB WORK)
47. BUTT HINGE (BRASS SHEET)
48. CARBON BRUSH HOLDER & SLIP RING
49. CO_2 WELDING WIRE ELECTRODES (COPPER/ COPPER ALLOY COATED M.S.WIRE)
50. CARBON FILM RESISTORS
51. CARBURETTORS
52. CAST STEEL PANES FOR MELTING FURNACE
53. CHEMICAL ETCHING OF STAINLESS STEEL
54. CHEMICAL RESISTANT IRON & STEEL
55. COLD FORM SECTION MILL
56. COLD ROLLED FORMING OF SECTION AND OTHER SECTIONS
57. COLD ROLLING OF MS STRIP
58. COLD TWISTED DE-FORMED RIBBED STEEL
59. COMPRESSOR (HERMETIC) FOR AIR CONDITIONERS
60. COMPRESSED NATURAL GAS (CNG KIT) FOR AUTOVEHICLE
61. CONTINUOUSLY CAST STEEL WIRE RODS (5 mm)
62. CONTINUOUS CASTING COPPER WIRE RODS
63. CONVEYOR BELTINGS
64. CONVEYOR BELT, TRANSM -ISSION BELT & V BELTS
65. COOKING RANGES
66. COPPER/BRASS SHEETS, CIRCLE & UTENSILS
67. COPPER FOIL
68. COPPER INGOTS, RODS MAKING & WIRE DRAWING
69. COPPER PRODUCTS FROM COPPER SCRAP
70. COPPER SMELTING PLANT
71. COPPER WIRE RODS FROM COPPER SCRAP
72. CORRUGATED BOX MAKING MACHINERY AND OTHER THEIR PARTS
73. CYLINDER LINER FOR AUTOMOBILES
74. DOOR LOCKS/PAD LOCKS
75. DRILL BITS & TOOL BITS
76. DRUM CLOSURES
77. ERW STEEL CONDUIT PIPE
78. EARTH MOVING EQPT.
79. ENGINE VALVES FOR AUTOMOBILES
80. FABRICATION OF HEAT EXCHANGER
81. FABRICATION OF STORAGE TANKS AND M.S. DRUM
82. FERROUS ALLOY NI-HARDY I.V CASTING
83. FERROUS Mn ALLOY CASTING BY ALUMINA THERMIC PROCESS
84. FERRO ALLOYS
85. FERRO SILICON & FERRO MANGANESE FROM DOLOMITE (SMS GRADE)
86. FIRE EXTINGUISHERS
87. FLIP-TONE CANS
88. FORGED CONECTING ROD
89. FORGING UNIT
90. FOUNTAIN PEN NIBS
91. FOUNDRY SAND
92. FUEL INJECTION SYSTEM
93. GALVANIZED M.S.STRIPS
94. GALVANIZING PLANT
95. GALVANIZED IRON WIRE
96. GAS WELDING TORCHES AND NOZZLES
97. GASKET SHEET
98. GATE GRILLS & WINDOW FRAMES
99. GENERATING SET (DIESEL)
100. HARD ANODISED ALUMINIUM
101. HOSPITAL WARES
102. HOSPITAL FURNITURES
103. HOT DIP GALVANIZING
104. HOT FORGED FASTENERS
105. HOT MIX PLANT
106. INJECTION MOULDED PLASTIC COMPOUNDS WITH TOOL ROOM
107. INJECTION MOULDED PLASTIC COMPONENTS AND METAL PIPE SPINNING UNIT
108. INVESTMENT CASTING
109. IRON/STEEL WIRE GAUGE
110. IRON TAWA
111. KNIVES (S.S.KNIVES)
112. KITCHEN SINK (S.S.)
113. L.P.G REGULATORS
114. MACHINE SCREWS & SELF TAPPING SCREWS
115. MARUTI WORKSHOP CUM SERVICE STATION
116. MAGNESIUM INGOTS & BULLETS CASTING

Price Rs. 3675/- for each "Detailed Project Report" Payable in advance through Draft/Cash/ M.O. in favour of *"ENGINEERS INDIA RESEARCH INSTITUTE"*. 4449, Nai Sarak (D), Main Road Delhi - 110 006 OR Ask by V.P.P. ● Ph : 3918117, 391 6431, 392 0361, 396 0797 ●Fax : 91-11- 391 6431 ●E-Mail : eirisidi@bol.net.in ● WebSite : www.startindustry.com

#	Item	#	Item	#	Item
117.	MANUFACTURE OF TIN CONTAINERS	161.	PRINTED TIN CONTAINERS	205.	STEEL CASTINGS
118.	MANUFACTURE OF STORAGE TANKS, PRESSURE VESSELS, HEAT EXCHANGERS	162.	PRINTING PRESS (CYLINDER MACHINE)	206.	STEEL CHAIN
119.	MARK II HAND PUMPS	163.	PUMPS FOR CHEMICAL INDUSTRY (SPECIAL)	207.	STEEL FOUNDRY
120.	MARUTI WORKSHOP CUM - SERVICE STATION	164.	RAILWAY SLEEPERS (M.S.)	208.	STEEL FURNITURES AND ELECTRICAL APPLIANCES
121.	MECHANICAL JACKS	165.	RAZOR TWIN BLADE	209.	STEEL PLANT (MINI)
122.	METAL CUTTING DIE DESIGN	166.	R.C.C SPUN PIPES	210.	STEEL RODS AND COILS FROM SCRAPS
123.	METAL CUTTING OF AND GRINDING WHEELS (ABBRASIVE CUTTING WHEELS)	167.	RECONDITIONING OF M.S. DRUMS/BARRELS	211.	STEEL ROLLING MILL
		168.	RE-ROLLING COPPER AND BRASS SHEET AND RODS	212.	STEEL STRIPS (COLD ROLLED) SILICON WITH GRAIN RIENTED FOR ELECTRIC USE
124.	METAL HOOKS & CLIPS	169.	RE-ROLLING MILLS		
125.	METAL SEPARATION (COPPER, TIN, LEAD) FROM SPENT WASH ACID	170.	RESIN COATED SAND	213.	STEEL TRANSMISSION LINE TOWERS & ROLLING MILL TO PRODUCE STEEL SECTION
		171.	RESIN CORED SOFT SOLDER WIRES		
126.	METALLIC RING JOINTS	172.	ROLLING MILL (BY INDUCTION FURNACE) & MANUFACTURE OF BARS, ANGLES, SQUARES, TUBES AND OTHERS	214.	STEEL FURNITURES AND ELECTRICAL APPLIANCES
127.	METALLIC GASKET (SPIRAL WOUND)			215.	STEEL WIRE DRAWING AND GALVANIZING
128.	MICROVEE & ABSOLUTE FILTER			216.	STEEL WOOL
129.	MICROWAVE OVEN	173.	ROLLER BEARING & FORGING	217.	SUBMERGED ARC WELDED PIPES
130.	MILD STEEL INGOTS	174.	ROLLING OF STAINLESS STEEL PATTA		
131.	MINI STEEL PLANT	175.	RUBBER INSULATED PLIERS (HAND TOOLS)	218.	SUBMERSIBLE PUMP MANUFACTURING
132.	MODERN VEHICLE WORKSHOP	176.	RUBBING COMPOUND FOR AUTOMOBILES	219.	SUPER ENAMELLED COPPER WIRE
133.	MOPED	177.	SCIENTIFIC LABORATORY EQUIPMENTS	220.	THREE WHEELERS
134.	M.S.HINGES			221.	TIE-ROD ENDS
135.	M.S.INGOT AND HR. STEEL STRUCTURALS	178.	SCOOTER ASSEMBLING	222.	TIN CONTAINERS
		179.	SECONDARY LEAD EXTRACTION BY SCRAP BATTERY PLATES,PIPES & SHEET	223.	TOOLROOM AND SHEET METAL PRODUCTS
136.	M.S.INGOT BY INDUCTION FURNACES			224.	TRACTOR TRAILERS
137.	M.S.PIPES	180.	SEAMLESS M.S. TUBES & PIPES	225.	TRANSMISSION POWER FITTING
138.	M.S. WELDING ELECTRODE				
139.	MUFFLERS & SILENCERS FOR THREE WHEELERS	181.	SELF TAPPING STEEL SCREW	226.	TUBULAR POLES
		182.	SEWING NEEDLES	227.	SUPER ENAMELLED COPPER WIRES
140.	NAIL CUTTER WITH FILER & MANICURE	183.	S.G. IRON & ALLOY STEEL		
		184.	SHEET METAL PRODUCTS, (FERROUS/NON-FERROUS)	228.	TUBULAR POLES FOR ELECTRICAL TRANSMISSION (BY FABRICATION PROCESS)
141.	NICHROME WIRE				
142.	NICKEL LINED SCREENS	185.	SHIP/MARINE CONTAINER		
143.	NON-FERROUS ALLOY ROLLING	186.	SHOCK ABSORBERS	229.	TUBULAR POLES OF M.S. & HIGH TENSILE STEEL
		187.	SHOE EYELETS		
144.	NON-FERROUS FORGING	188.	SHOT AND GRITS BY AUTOMIZATION PROCESS	230.	VACUUM CLEANERS
145.	NON-FERROUS FOUNDRY			231.	VACUUM FLASK (STAINLESS STEEL)
146.	NON PRESSURE	189.	SHOVELS		
147.	INCANDESCENT LAMP	190.	SILICO MANGANESE ALLOYS	232.	VALVES FOR REFRIGERATION AND AIR-CONDITION
148.	NUMBER COMBINATION LOCKS FOR LUGGAGES	191.	SILENCERS (MUFFLERS) EXHAUST & TAIL PIPE FOR ALL TYPES OF VEHICLES		
				233.	VEHICLE WELDING & PAINTING
149.	NUTS & BOLTS				
150.	PAPER COATED ALUMINIUM AND COPPER WIRE	192.	SINTERED BEARING	234.	VENETION BLIND
		193.	SINTERED BUSHES	235.	WASHING MACHINES (AUTOMATIC & COMPUTERISED)
151.	PETROMAX CONTAINER	194.	SINTERED METAL PRODUCTS		
152.	PHOTO ETCHING OF STAINLESS STEEL PLATES	195.	SOFT AND HARD FERRITES		
		196.	SPANNERS	236.	WATER CONTROLLER (AUTOMATIC)
153.	PIPE GALVANIZING PLANT	197.	SPARK PLUGS		
154.	PISTON RING-AUTOMOBILE	198.	STEEL PLANT (ELECTRIC ARC FURNACE BASED- EAF)	237.	WATCH STRAPS/CHAINS/ BRACELETS/BELT BRASS & STAINLESS STEEL
155.	PLANT PROTECTION EQUIPMENTS				
		199.	SPHERIODAL GRAPHITE CAST IRON	238.	WATER COOLERS
156.	PLATINUM LABORATORY APPARATUS			239.	WELDED WIRE MESH
		200.	SPRAY DRYER	240.	WELDING ELECTRODES
157.	PRESSURE COOKER & ALUMINIUM UTENSILS	201.	STAINLESS STEEL HINGES	241.	WICK STOVES
		202.	STAINLESS STEEL SHEET ROLLING TO PRODUCE STAINLESS STEEL UTENSILS	242.	WIND MILL WINDOW FRAME (FERROUS & NON-FERROUS)
158.	PRESSURE COOKER (ALUMINIUM)				
159.	PRESSURE DIE CASTING			243.	WRIST WATCH
160.	PRINTED ALUMINIUM COLLAPSIBLE TUBES	203.	STAINLESS STEEL UTENSILS		
		204.	STAPLE PINS,PAPER PIN, GEM CLIPS ETC.		

Price Rs. 3675/- for each "Detailed Project Report" Payable in advance through Draft/Cash/ M.O. in favour of *"ENGINEERS INDIA RESEARCH INSTITUTE"*. 4449, Nai Sarak (D), Main Road Delhi - 110 006 OR Ask by V.P.P. ● Ph : 3918117, 391 6431, 392 0361, 396 0797
●Fax : 91-11- 391 6431 ●E-Mail : eirisidi@bol.net.in ● WebSite : www.startindustry.com

LIST OF FEW READILY AVAILABLE 'DETAILED PROJECT REPORTS' OUT OF 30,000 REPORTS

CHEMICALS
(ORGANIC & INORGANIC)

244. ACETIC ANHYDRIDE
245. ACETIC ACID FROM ETHANOL
246. ACETYLENE BLACK
247. ACETYLENE GAS
248. ACETYLENE GAS & OXYGEN (INTEGERATED UNIT)
249. ACID SLURRY BY MANUAL PROCESS
250. ACTIVATED ALUMINA
251. ACTIVATED BLEACHING EARTH (ACTIVATED FULLERS EARTH)
252. ACTIVATED CARBON FROM CASHEWNUT SHELL
253. ACTIVATED CARBON FROM RICE HUSK
254. ACTIVATED CARBON FROM RICE HUSK, COCONUT SHELL & COCONUT POWDER
255. ACTIVATED CARBON FROM WOOD
256. ACTIVATED CARBON POWDER & GRANULES FROM COCONUT SHELL
257. ACTIVATED CARBON & SODIUM SILICATE FROM PADDY & RICE HUSK
258. ALUM FOR WATER TREATMENT
259. AEROSOL INSECTICIDES SPRAY (BAYGON, HIT, MORTEIN TYPE)
260. AGARBATTI SYNTHETIC PERFUMERY COMPOUNDS
261. ALCOHOL FROM POTATO
262. ALCOHOL FROM RICE GRAINS
263. ALCOHOL FROM RICE HUSK
264. ALCOHOL FROM MOLASSES
265. ALCOHOL, BEER, STARCH, LIQUID GLUCOSE, DEXTROSE, SORBITOL, VITAMIN-C, GERM OIL, CATTLE FEED ETC. FROM MAIZE
266. ALKYD RESIN
267. ALKYLATED PHENOL LIKE NONYL PHENOL, DODECYL PHENOL
268. ALUM (NON FERRIC)
269. ALUM (FERRIC)
260. ALUMINIUM INGOT BY BAUXITE
261. ALUMINIUM PHOSPHIDE
262. ALUMINIUM PHOSPHATE
263. AMINES & ALLIED PRODUCTS
264. AMMONIA GAS
265. AMMONIA GAS BOTTLING
266. AMMONIA LIQUOR
267. AMMONIUM CHLORIDE (PURE & TECHNICAL)
268. ANILINE
269. ARGON GAS
270. ARIEL TYPE DETERGENT POWDER
271. ANTHRAQUINONE
272. ANTIMONY TRIOXIDE
273. AZODICARBONAMIDE
274. BAKING SODA FROM ASH
275. BARIUM CARBONATE
276. BARIUM COMPOUNDS
277. BARIUM PEROXIDE
278. BARIUM-THIO-SULPHATE BANZENE
279. BARYTE POWDER
280. BEER PLANT
281. BELT PASTE (WITH BFS OIL)
282. BENZYL ACETATE, BENZYL BENZOATE, BENZYL ALCOHOL
283. BETA NAPHTHOL
284. BENTONITE POWDER
285. BENZIDINE
286. BIO GAS PLANT
287. BIO GAS FILLING IN CYLINDER
288. BI-CHROMATE OF SODIUM, POTASSIUM & AMMONIUM
289. BI-FUNCTIONAL BLACK MFGR. REACTIVE DYE (DYE FROM COTTON YARN DYEING)
290. BITUMINOUS ROAD EMULSION
291. BLACK PHENYL
292. BLACK SULPHUR
293. BLEACHING POWDER (STABLE)
294. BONE CRUSHING PLANT
295. BONE MEAL (CALCINED) ENRICHMENT WITH CALCIUM & PHOSPHORUS
296. BORIC ACID
297. B.O.N. ACID
298. BRANDY
299. BUTANOL
300. 1,4, BUTANEDIOL
301. BUTYL ACETATE
302. CAFFEIN FROM TEA WASTE
303. CALCINED LIME (DEAD BURNT DOLOMITE)
304. CALCINING OF MAGNESITE & DEAD BURNT MAGNESITE
305. CALCIUM ALUMINATE
306. CALCIUM CARBIDE
307. CALCIUM CARBONATE
308. CALCIUM CARBONATE (PRECIPITATED) FROM BY PRODUCT (LIME SLURRY & CARBON DIOXIDE)
309. CALCIUM CARBONATE (ACTIVATED & PRECIPITATED)
310. CALCIUM CHLORIDE
311. CALCIUM GLUCONATE
312. CALCIUM NITRATE
313. CALCIUM SILICATE BRICKS
314. CAMPHOR POWDER (SYNTHETIC)
315. CARBON DIOXIDE
316. CARBON BLACK FROM FERTILIZER WASTE
317. CARBOXY METHYL CELLULOSE (CMC)
318. CASEIN AND BY PRODUCTS
319. CASEIN FROM MILK
320. CATIONIC SOFTNER (STEARIC ACID BASED)
321. CAUSTIC SODA
322. CAUSTIC SODA FROM TRONA
323. CAUSTIC SODA, CHLORINE AND HYDROGEN GAS BY ELECTRO-LYSIS OF BRINE SOLUTION
324. CELLULOSE ACETATE MOULDING POWDER
325. CELLULOSE POWDER & MICRO CRYSTALLINE CELLULOSE POWDER
326. CEMENT COLOUR
327. CEMENT FROM FLY ASH & LIME
328. CEMENT TILES (GLAZED)
329. DOUBLE FIRING (HEATING)
330. CHELATED ZINC (ZN EDTA)
331. CHEMICALS FROM PRAWN HEAD
332. CHITIN & CHITOSAN FROM PRAWN SHELL WASTE
333. CHLORAL HYDRATE
334. CHLORAMPHENICOL
335. CHROMIC ACID (WITH POLLUTION CONTROL)
336. CHROMIC ACID (OXIDE) & BLUE OXIDE
337. CHLORINATED PARAFFIN WAX (CPW)
338. CHROMIC ACID
339. CEMENT PAINT & DISTEMPER
340. CITRIC ACID FROM LEMON
341. CITRIC ACID FROM MOLASSES
342. CLEANING OF COOLING SYSTEM AND BOILER
343. COAL TAR DISTILLATION
344. COBALT OCTOATE
345. COMPOST FOR MUSHROOM
346. COPPER OXYCHLORIDE
347. COPPER PHTHALOCYANINE BLUE & GREEN
348. CORRECTION FLUID
349. CYANURIC CHLORIDE
350. DEFOAMING AGENT FOR PAPER INDUSTRY
351. DE-NICKELING (ELECTROLYTIC PROCESS)
352. DETERGENT CAKE & POWDER
353. DETERGENT POWDER
354. DETERGENT CONCENTRATE (IDET 10)
355. DEXTROSE MONOHYDRATE & DEXTROSE ANHYDROUS POWDER FROM TAPIOCA STARCH
356. DI-BASIC LEAD STEARATE
357. DI CALCIUM PHOSPHATE
358. DICLOFENAL SODIUM SLOW RELEASE (SR) TABLES 100MG.

Price Rs. 3675/- for each "Detailed Project Report" Payable in advance through Draft/Cash/M.O. in favour of "ENGINEERS INDIA RESEARCH INSTITUTE". 4449, Nai Sarak (D), Main Road Delhi - 110 006 OR Ask by V.P.P. ● Ph : 3918117, 391 6431, 392 0361, 396 0797
●Fax : 91-11- 391 6431 ●E-Mail : eirisidi@bol.net.in ● WebSite : www.startindustry.com

#	Item	#	Item	#	Item
359.	DI ETHYL OXALATE		BRICK	445.	METHANE GAS BY SODIUM ACETATE & SODA LIME
360.	DI METHYL ORTHOPHTHALATE	409.	HYDRATED LIME FROM SEA SHELL	446.	METHYL ACETYL RICINOLATE
361.	DI-METHYL PHTHALATE			447.	METOL
362.	DICLOFENAC GEL	410.	HYDROCHLORIC ACID	448.	METOL FROM HYDROQUINONE & METHYLAMINE
363.	DIOCTYL PHTHALATE (DOP)	411.	HYDRO FLUORIC ACID		
364.	DI PHENYL GLYCERINE	412.	HYDROGEN PEROXIDE (BY AUTO-OXIDATION PROCESS)	449.	MICANITE
365.	DI PHENYL OXIDE			450.	MICRO NUTRIENT MIXTURE
366.	DINITRO-CHLORO BENZENE	413.	ICE PACKS (SOLUTIONS TYPE, WHITE GEL TYPE, VIOLET SEMI SOLID POLYMER TYPE)	451.	MINERAL WATER
367.	DISTILLED WATER			452.	MINERAL WATER AND PET BOTTILNG PLANT
368.	DODECYL BENZENE SULPHONATE				
369.	DUSTLESS CHALK	414.	IMPROVING DROP POINT PARAFFIN WAX FROM 45-50ºC TO 75-80ºC	453.	MINERAL WATER IN BOTTLES, GLASS AND POUCHES
370.	EDTA & ITS SALTS				
371.	ELECTROLESS NICKEL PLATING ON PLASTICS	415.	INDUSTRIAL ALCOHOL	454.	MINI CEMENT PLANT (BY ROTARY KILN PROCESS)
		416.	INTEGRATED COMPLEX OF EASTER & ALLIED PRODUCTS (D.O.P, D.B.P, ETHYL ACETATE WIRE ENAMEL & CABLE JELLY)	455.	MIXED FERTILIZER
372.	ENDOSULFAN				
373.	EPOXY RESIN BASED COMPOUND			456.	MOSQUITO & FLIES REPELLENT AGARBATTI (INCENSE STICKS)
374.	ETHYL ACETATE	417.	IMFL (WHISKY) & COUNTRY LIQUOR		
375.	EHTYL ETHER			457.	MONO CHLORO ACETIC ACID
376.	ETHYL ALCOHOL (POTABLE LIQUOR)	418.	IRON OXIDE FOR MAKING FERITTE	458.	MONOCROTOPHOS (TECHNICAL)
377.	ETHYL HEXANOL	419.	IRON SULPHIDE	459.	MOSQUITO COIL
378.	EXTRACTION OF ESSENTIAL OILS BY SUGAR CRITICAL FLUID (CARBON DIOXIDE) METHOD FROM FLOWERS, HERBAL & SPICES	420.	JUTE BATCHING OIL	460.	MOSQUITO COIL & MAT
		421.	KESH KALA TEL (HAIR DYE LOTION) (VASMOL 33, BLACK NITE TYPE)	461.	MOSQUITO MAT
				462.	MOTHER TINCTURE & BIO CHEMIC MEDICINES
		422.	L-LYSINE MONOHYDROCHLORIDE	463.	NAPHTHALENE & PHENYL (INTEGRATED UNIT)
379.	FERRIC ALUM				
380.	FERRO CHROME LIGNO SULPHONATE	423.	LACTIC ACID FROM WHITE SUGAR BY FERMENTATION PROCESS	464.	NATURAL MINERAL WATER BY REVERSE OSMOSIS PROCESS
381.	FERRO MANGANESE			465.	NICKEL PLATING BRIGHTNER (PRIMARY OR CARRIER BRIGHTNER & SECONDARY BRIGHTNER)
382.	FERRO SILICONE	424.	LDPE GRANULES FROM VIRGIN (LDPE RESIN)		
383.	FERRO VANADIUM FROM VANADIUM SLUDGE				
		425.	LEAD EXTRACTION FROM BATTERY SCRAP		
384.	FERROUS SILICATE			466.	NICKEL SULPHATE
385.	FERROUS SULPHATE	426.	LEAD OXIDE (A) LEAD MONOXIDE (B) LEAD TETRA OXIDE (C) GREYLEAD OXIDE	467.	NICOTINE FROM TOBACCO WASTE
386.	FERTILIZER FROM ANIMAL BLOOD & LEATHER WASTE			468.	NICOTINE SULPHATE FROM TOBACCO WASTE
387.	FLUORESCENT TUBE LIGHT POWDER			469.	NITRO BENZENE
		427.	LIQUID GLUCOSE & ITS BY PRODUCTS	470.	NITRO CELLULOSE SANDING SEALER/LACQUER
388.	FOAMED PVC COMPOUNDING & ITS PRODUCTS				
		428.	LIQUID OXYGEN BOTTLING PLANT	471.	NITRO MUSK
389.	FORMALDEHYDE			472.	NITROGEN & OXYGEN GAS PLANT
390.	FRACTIONAL DISTILLATION OF D.M.O (DEMENTHOLIZED OIL)	429.	LIQUID SHOE POLISH		
		430.	LIQUID FLOOR POLISH	473.	NON-IONIC SURFACTANT (WETTING AGENT)
391.	FRACTIONAL DISTILLATION OF ESSENTIAL OIL & MEDICINAL PLANT EXTRACT	431.	LUBE OIL VISCOSITY IMPROVED FOR P.P.G/P.E.G.		
				474.	NO-CARB PASTE
		432.	LUBRICANTS ASHLESS 100% COMBUSTION	475.	OCTANOL
392.	FRICTION DUST (LIQUID & POWDER) FROM CNSL			476.	ORTHO NITRO PHENOL
		433.	MAGNESIUM CARBONATE AND MAGNESIUM BICARMONATE	477.	OXALIC ACID FROM MOLASSES
393.	FRUIT FLAVOURS				
394.	FURFURAL FROM RICE HUSK			478.	OXALIC ACID FROMRICE HUSK
395.	GARLIC ACID	434.	MAGNESIUM HYDROXIDE POWDER		
396.	GASKET SHELLAC COMPOUND			479.	OXALIC ACID FROM TREE BARK
397.	GEAR OIL	435.	MAGNESIUM SILICATE		
398.	GIBBERELLIC ACID	436.	MAGNESIUM SULPHATE	470.	OXALIC ACID FROM WASTE VEGETABLES
399.	GLASS PUTTY	437.	MALACHITE GREEN		
400.	GLYCERINE	438.	MALEIC ANHYDRIDE		
401.	GOSSYPOL (POLY PHENOL) FROM COTTON SEED OIL	439.	MANGANESE SULPHATE	471.	OXYGEN GAS PLANT
		440.	MANUFACTURING OF CARBON MONO-OXIDE WATER GAS	472.	OXYGEN GAS PLANT (AIR SEPERATION METHOD)
402.	GUAR GUM POWDER				
403.	HAIR FIXER (HAIR GEL TYPE)	441.	MENTHOL BOLD CRYSTALS FROM FLAKES	473.	PARA-AMINO BENZOIC ACID
404.	H - ACID			474.	PARA-AMINO PHENOL
405.	HENNA PASTE MAKING	442.	MENTHOL CRYSTAL & MENTHA OIL	475.	PARA TOLUENE SULPHONIC ACID
406.	HEPTAL DEHYDE				
407.	HIGH CARBON FERRO CHROME	443.	MERCURIC OXIDE	476.	PECTIN FROM RAW PAPAYA
		444.	METAL PRE-TREATMENT CHEMICALS	477.	PERFUME (LEMON & OTHERS)
408.	HYDRATED CALCIUM SILICATE				

Price Rs. 3675/- for each "Detailed Project Report" Payable in advance through Draft/Cash/M.O. in favour of "ENGINEERS INDIA RESEARCH INSTITUTE". 4449, Nai Sarak (D), Main Road Delhi - 110 006 OR Ask by V.P.P. ● Ph : 3918117, 391 6431, 392 0361, 396 0797
●Fax : 91-11- 391 6431 ●E-Mail : eirisidi@bol.net.in ● WebSite : www.startindustry.com

Pay Rs. 8,000/- Only for Tailor made Report We (EIRI) are fully capable to prepare any report as per your requirements

478. PESTICIDE PREPARATION USING NEEM FRUIT & SEEDS (MARGOSA)
479. PET BOTTLES FROM PRE-FORM
480. PET PREFORM FROM RESIN FOR PET BOTTLES
481. PETROLEUM JELLY
482. PHENOL
483. PHENYL
484. PHENYL (BLACK) IN LIQUID FORM
485. PHTHALIC ANHYDRIDE
486. PHOSPHORIC ACID FROM ROCK PHOSPHATE
487. PHOSPHORUS BY CHEMICAL PROCESS
488. PHOTO EMULSION FOR ROTARY SCREEN PRINTING
489. PHTHALOCYANINE BLUE
480. PIGMENT EMULSION FOR TEXTILE
481. PIGMENT GUM
482. PLANT GROWTH REAGEN BASED CHLOROTHYL TRIMETHYL AMMONIUM CHLORIDE
483. PLANT HARMONES BASED ON 2,4-DICHLORPHENOXY ACENTIC ACID & NAPHTHALENE
484. PLASTICINE (MODELLING CLAY)
485. PLASTIC WASTE REPROCESSING
486. PLASTER OF PARIS BANDAGES
487. POLYESTER RESIN (G.P. GRADE LAMINATE GRADE, ELECTRICAL GRADE)
488. POLY VINYL ACETATE
489. POLYVINYL ACETATE EMULSION
490. POLYURETHENE FOAM
491. POTASSIUM DICHROMATE/ BICHROMATE
492. POTASSIUM IODATE
493. POTASSIUM NITRATE
494. POTASSIUM PERMAGNATE
495. POTASSIUM PER SULPHATE
496. POTASSIUM SULPHATE (FERTILIZER GRADE)
497. POTASSIUM PER OXY DI-SULPHIDE
498. POTASSIUM SILICATE
499. POTASSIUM STEARATE
500. POWER ALCOHOL
501. PVC RESIN FROM ETHYL ALCOHOL
502. PYRIDINE & ITS DERIVATIVES
503. RAPID FAST DYES (ONLY PROCESS)
504. REACTOR (CHEMICAL)
505. RECLAMATION OF USED ENGINE OIL (BY CLAY & VACUUM DISTILLATION PROCESS)
506. RECLAMATION OF SPENT BLEACHING EARTH
507. RECLAMATION OF NICKEL SPENT CATALYST FROM VANASPATI INDUSTRY
508. RECTIFIED SPIRIT FROM MOLASSES & MAHUA FLOWERS
509. RECTIFIED SPIRIT FROM RICE STRAW
510. RED OXIDE PAINT/PRIMER (ANTI CORROSIVE) BASED ORGANIC RED PIGMENTS
511. REMOVAL OF ANTIMONY FROM LEAD SCRAP
512. RESORCINOL
513. ROSIN SIZING AGENT
514. RESORCINOL
515. SALINE AND INJECTION WATER
516. SALICYLIC ACID
517. SANTONIN
518. SENNOSIDES FROM SENNO LEAF
519. SHOE POLISH
520. SILICA GEL (BLUE SELF INDICATING PROCESS)
521. SILICONE EMULSION
522. SILICONE FROM RICE HUSK
523. SILICON FROM SILICA (SEMI CONDUCTOR GRADE)
524. SILICONE RESINS
525. SILICONE SPRAYSILVER BRAZING FOIL
526. SILVER EXTRACTION FROM WASTE HYPO SOLUTION
527. SILVER NITRATE
528. SILVER PARTS FOR CERAMIC CAPACITOR SINGLE SUPER PHOSPHATE & MIXED FERTILIZER (NPK)
529. SINGLE SUPER PHOSPHATE (S.S.P.) & SULPHURIC ACID
530. SODA ASH
531. SODA ASH FROM NATRON
532. SODA WATER BOTTLING PLANT (CARBONATED BEVERAGE)
533. SODIUM ALUMINATE
534. SODIUM BI-CARBONATE (BAKING SODA) FROM SODA ASH
535. SODIUM CHLORITE
536. SODIUM CHROMATE SODIUM CYCLAMATE
537. SODIUM DI-CHROMATE
538. SODIUM DI-CHROMATE & SODIUM SULPHATE AS BYE PRODUCTS
539. SODIUM HEXA META PHOSPHATE
540. SODIUM HYDROSULFITE
541. SODIUM HYPO CHLORIDE (BLEACH LIQUOR)
542. SODIUM ISO-PROPYL XANTHATE
543. SODIUM LAURYL SULPHATE
544. SODIUM LAURYL SULPHATE & SODIUM LAURYL ETHER SULPHATE
545. SODIUM NITRATE
546. SODIUM PETROLEUM SULPHONATE (EMULSIFIER)
547. SODIUM SILICATE FROM SILICA & SODA ASH
548. SODIUM SILICATE FROM (1) PADDY SILK HUSK 2) & SILICA
549. SODIUM CARBONATE & SILICA
550. SODIUM SULPHATE
551. SODIUM SULPHIDE BY BARIUM SULPHATE PROCESS
552. SODIUM SULPHIDE FROM AMMONIA & SODIUM CHLORIDE
553. SODIUM SULPHITE
554. SODIUM TRI-POLY PHOSPHATE
555. SOFTENER (CATIONIC ANIONIC & NON-IONIC)
556. SPIRIT FROM PINE APPLE
557. STANNOUS CHLORIDE
558. STEARIC ACID
559. STEARATES MANUFACTURE (CALCIUM, ZINC, ALUMINIUM, MAGNESIUM STEARATES)
560. SULPHUR FROM PYRITES & SLAG
561. SULPHUR CRYSTALS/LUMPS
562. SULPHURIC ACID
563. SULPHURIC ACID FROM DCDA PROCESS
564. SUPER PHOSPHATE (S.S.P)
565. SYNTHETIC IRON OXIDE (YELLOW)
566. SYNTHETIC RED & WELLOW IRON OXIDE FROM IRON FILLING & PICKLE LIQUOR
567. TARTARIC ACID
568. TOILET CLEANER
569. TOLUENE AND SBP FROM

Price Rs. 3675/- for each "Detailed Project Report" Payable in advance through Draft/Cash/M.O. in favour of "ENGINEERS INDIA RESEARCH INSTITUTE". 4449, Nai Sarak (D), Main Road Delhi - 110 006 OR Ask by V.P.P. • Ph : 3918117, 391 6431, 392 0361, 396 0797
• Fax : 91-11- 391 6431 • E-Mail : eirisidi@bol.net.in • WebSite : www.startindustry.com

	CRUDE NAPHTHA	617. AUTO BULB/LAMPS
570.	TRIMETHYL AMMONIUM CHLORIDE	618. AUTOMATIC VOLTAGE STABILIZER
571.	TRIPHENYL PHOSPHITE (T.P.P)	619. BATTERY PLATES
572.	ULTRAMARINE BLUE (LIQUID)	620. BACK OFFICE (Rs. 5000/-)
573.	UREA FORMALDEHYDE & MELAMINE FORMALDEHYDE POWDER	621. B/W TV & COMPUTER MONITOR PICTURE TUBE
		622. BREAD BOARDS
574.	UNDECYLINIC ACID	623. CALL CENTRE
575.	VINYL ACETATE MONOMER	624. CAMERA (35 MM)
576.	VITAMIN C	625. CAPACITORS
577.	VITAMIN E	626. CARBON ELECTRODE USED FOR BATTERY CELL
578.	WASTE WATER TREATMENT PLANT FOR INDUSTRIAL SECTOR IN INDIA (ONLY MARKER SURVEY)	627. CARBON POTETIOMETERS
		628. CEILING FAN
		629. CERAMIC INSULATOR
579.	WIRE DRAWING LUBRICANT	630. CHILDREN INFOTECH TRAINING INSTITUTE (Rs. 5000/-)
580.	WIRE ENAMEL	
581.	XANTHATES	631. CHOKE AND PATTI
582.	YELLOW DEXTRIN	632. CHOKE AND STARTER
583.	ZINC CHLORIDE	633. CHOKE USED FOR FLUORESCENT LAMPS
584.	ZINC OXIDE	
585.	ZINC PHOSPHATING BY COLD PROCESS	634. COLOUR TELEVISION
		635. COLOUR AND BLACK & WHITE TELEVISION
586.	ZINC SILICATE	
587.	ZINC STEARATE	636. COMPACT DISC
588.	ZINC SULPHATE	637. COMPACT DISC PLAYER (AUDIO/VIDEO)
589.	ZINC SULPHATE MONOHYDRATE	
590.	ACID BLACK	638. COMPUTER EDUCATION INSTITUTE
591.	AURAMINE 'O'	
592.	AZO DYES STUFF	639. COMPUTER ASSEMBLY
593.	DYE & DYE INTERMEDIATE	640. COMPUTER HARDWARE
594.	DYE INTERMEDIATES	641. COMPUTER KEYBOARD
595.	MALACHITE GREEN	642. COMPUTER PERIPHERALS
596.	METHYLENE BLUE	643. COMPUTER PRINTERS
597.	PHTHALOCYANINE BLUE	644. COMPUTER RIBBON
598.	PHTHALOCYANINE BLUE & GREEN	645. COMPUTER RIBBON REINKING OR REFILLING
599.	REACTIVE DYES	646. COMPUTER STATIONERY
600.	SULPHUR BLACK DYE	647. COMPUTER STATIONERY &
601.	VAT DYES	
602.	WATER CHILLING PLANT	
603.	WADDING OIL (100%) FOR WADDING OF COTTON HOSIERY CLOTH IN THE DYEING PROCESS	
604.	WHITE OIL	
605.	WAX FLOOR POLISH	

ELECTRICAL, ELECTONICS, COMPUTERS AND INFOTECH/IT PROJECTS

606.	AIR CONDITIONING
607.	ALUMINIUM ALLOY CONDUCTOR
608.	ALUMINIUM CABLE
609.	ALUMINIUM ELECTROYTIC CAPACITORS
610.	AUDIO CASSETTE ASSEMBLING & RECORDING
611.	AUDIO CASSETTES DUPLICATING RECORDING
612.	AUDIO CASSETTES & AUDIO STUDIO
613.	AUDIO CASSETTES PLANE & RECORDED
614.	AUDIO MAGNETIC HEADS
615.	AUDIO MAGNETIC TAPE
616.	AUDIO/VIDEO CASSETTES

GET DATA BACKUP INSTEAD OF PRINTOUTS & PAY THE SAME COST Rs. 3675/-

Add 5% Service Tax

	IMPORTED HARDWARE PARTS
648.	COMPUTER TERMINALS
649.	COMPUTERISED WASHING MACHINE (AUTOMATIC)
650.	COMPUTER SOFTWARE
651.	CONDENSER FOR MOTOR USING MPP FILM

652.	CONTENT DEVELOPMENT CENTRE (EOU) (Rs. 5000/-)
653.	CONTROL PANEL BOARD
654.	COOLING COIL FOR AIR CONDITIONERS
655.	COPPER STRIP COIL FROM SCRAP
656.	CORDLESS TELEPHONES
657.	CYBER CAFE
658.	CYBERKIOSK (Rs. 5000/-)
659.	DATA PROCESSING CENTRE (Rs. 5000/-)
660.	D.C. MICRO MOTORS
661.	D.G.SETS
662.	DISH ANTENNA AND CABLE T.V. NETWORK EQUIPMENT
663.	DISTRIBUTION TRANSFORMERS & REPAIRS
664.	DOMESTIC ELECTRICAL APPLIANCES- ROOM COOLER, WASHING MACHINE, WATER HEATER, ELECTRIC ROOM HEATER
665.	E-SCHOOL
666.	E-COMMERCE/BUSINESS
667.	ELECTRIC ENERGY METER
668.	ELECTRIC FANS
669.	ELECTRIC HORN FOR AUTOMOBILE
670.	ELECTRIC LAMP/GLS (INCANDESCENT LAMP)
671.	ELECTRIC MIXER
672.	ELECTRIC MOTORS UP TO 10 HP. REWINDING OF ALL TYPES OF MOTORS WATER PUMPS
673.	ELECTRIC MOTOR WINDING (FOR FAN, MIXIES, ETC.)
674.	ELECTRIC STEAM IRON
675.	ELECTRICAL APPLIANCES
676.	ELECTRICAL FIXTURES
677.	ELECTRICAL STAMPING
678.	ELECTROLYTIC CAPACITORS
679.	ELECTROMAGNETIC RELAY
680.	ELECTRONIC BALAST/CHOK
681.	ELECTRICAL CHOKE
682.	ELECTRONIC DIGITAL WATCHES
683.	ELECTRONIC DIGITAL WEIGHING MACHINE
684.	ELECTRONIC FIRE ALARM
685.	ELECTRONIC GAS STOVE LIGHTERS
686.	ELECTRONIC PRESSURE INDICATORS, ELECTRICALS, ELECTRONIC LIQUID LEVEL INDICATORS, ELECTRONIC TEMPERATURE INDICATOR, DIGITAL TACHOMETER
687.	ELECTRONIC TELEPHONE INSTRUMENTS
688.	ELECTRONIC TOYS
689.	ELECTRONIC WATCHES & CLOCKS
690.	FAX MACHINES
691.	F.H.P MOTORS
692.	FLOPPY DISKETTES
693.	FLUORESCENT LAMP STARTER
694.	FLUORESCENT TUBULAR

Price Rs. 3675/- for each "Detailed Project Report" Payable in advance through Draft/Cash/M.O. in favour of *"ENGINEERS INDIA RESEARCH INSTITUTE"*. 4449, Nai Sarak (D), Main Road Delhi - 110 006 OR Ask by V.P.P. ● Ph : 3918117, 391 6431, 392 0361, 396 0797
●Fax : 91-11- 391 6431 ●E-Mail : eirisidi@bol.net.in ● WebSite : www.startindustry.com

	LAMPS WITH INTRODUCTION TO MERCURY VAPOUR LAMP	731.	MULTIPLE RELAY FOR LOW VOLTAGE	781.	TRANSMISSION POWER LINE FITTING
695.	FRANCHISEE COMPUTER EDUCATION CENTRE (Rs. 5000)	732.	NEON INDICATOR	782.	TRANSMISSION TOWER FITTING
696.	GAS DETECTOR (L.P.G)	733.	NEON SIGN MANUFACTURE	783.	TV AUDIO EQUIPMENT CABINETS & THEIR ASSEMBLING UNIT
697.	GENERATOR SET & PUMP SETS	734.	OPTICAL FIBRE CABLES		
698.	GENERATOR (BATTERY OPERATED)	735.	ON LINE SHOPPING MALL (Rs. 5000/-)	784.	UN-INTERRUPTED POWER SUPPLY (U.P.S)
699.	GIS SERVICE CENTRE (GEOGRAPHICAL INFORMATION SYSTEMS)	736.	OPTO MECHANICAL & ELECTRICAL EQUIPMENTS	785.	VARIABLE FREQUENCY
		737.	PHOTO COLOUR LAB	786.	VARIABLE VOLTAGE A.C. DRIVE
700.	HARDWARE FITTING FOR TRANSMISSION LINE OVERHEAD LINE MATERIAL	738.	PICTURE TUBE (B/W)	787.	VIDEO CASSETTES (COMPLETE MANUFACTURING & ASSEMBLING)
		739.	PLAIN PAPER COPIER		
		740.	PLASTIC FILM CAPACITORS		
701.	HEADERS FOR TRANSISTOR ICS SEMI CONDUCTOR	741.	POLYESTER CAPACITORS	788.	VIDEO CASSETTES RECORDER (V.C.R)
		742.	PORTABLE GENERATOR SET		
702.	H.T & L.T INSULATORS	743.	PORTAL	789.	VIDEO FILM STUDIO
703.	H.T & M.V INDUSTRIAL CUBICAL SWITCH BOARD	744.	PORTABLE TELEVISION (TV)	790.	VOLTAGE REGULATOR FOR AUTOMOBILES
		745.	POWER CAPACITORS		
704.	INFORMATION MOVING DISPLAY (L.E.D TYPE)	746.	POWER INVERTERS	791.	VOLTAGE STABILIZERS
		747.	POWER PLANT	792.	VOLTAGE STABLIZER & T.V. GAIN BOOSTER
705.	INSURANCE CLAIM PROCESSING CENTRE (EOU) (Rs. 5000/-)	748.	POWER TRANSFORMERS UP TO 600 KVA		
		749.	PRINTED CIRCUIT BOARD	793.	WAX AND CHEMICAL COATED, BRAIDED TINSEL WIRE
706.	INTEGRATED CIRCUITS	750.	PVC WIRES & CABLES		
707.	INTERNET BASED STOCK TRADING (Rs. 5000/-)	751.	RE-CONDITIONING OF PICTURE TUBE	794.	WEBSITE DESIGN & E-MAIL REGISTERING
		752.	RESIN CAST CT & PT (1 KV)		
708.	INTERNET SERVICE PROVIDER (I.S.P.)	753.	SEMI CONDUCTOR DEVICE	795.	WELDING ELECTRODES
		754.	SEMI CONDUCTORS FOR TRANSISTORS & DIODES	796.	WIND ENERGY POWER PROJECT (10 MW) WIRE WOUND POTENTIOMETERS
709.	JELLY FILLED TELEPHONE CABLES				
710.	LAP TOP COMPUTERS	755.	SETTING UP OF A VIDEO STUDIO		
711.	LEAD ACID BATTERIES	756.	SMOKE DETECTORS		**FOOD, AGRO FOOD, PROCESSED FOOD, AGRO PLANTATION, CULTIVATION, FARMING, DAIRY/MILK, TOBACCO/PAN MASALA, BREWERY & DISTILLERY, EDIBLE OILS, EOU FOOD PRODUCTS AND ALLIED PRODUCTS**
712.	LEAD ACID BATTERY PLATES AND ASSEMBLING OF BATTERY	757.	SOLAR CELLS		
		758.	SOLAR MODULES		
		759.	SOLAR PHOTO VOLTAIC SYSTEM		
713.	LEGAL TRANSCRIPTION & SECRETARIAL SERVICES CENTER (EOU)(Rs. 5000/-)	760.	SOLDER FLUXES		
		761.	SOLAR WATER HEATING PANELS		
714.	LIGHT EMITTING DIODES (L.E.D)	762.	STEEL FURNITURE & ELECTRICAL APPLIANCES	797.	ALCOHOLIC BEVERAGES & VENEGAR FROM COCONUT WATER
715.	LINEAR ICS TRAINER KIT				
716.	LOUD SPEAKER	763.	STEREO AMPLIFIERS	798.	ALCOHOL DRINKS FROM ETHYL ALCOHOL BY MIXING OF VARIOUS FLAVOURS
717.	L.T TRANSFORMER REPAIRING	764.	STEREO CASSETTE RECORDERS/PLAYERS		
718.	MEDICAL TRANSCRIPTION CENTRE	765.	STREET LIGHT FITTINGS SURGE SUPPRESSOR	799.	ANTI SCALE COMPOUND FOR ADDING INTO SUGAR JUICE BOILING
719.	METAL FILM RESISTORS	766.	TANTALUM CAPACITORS		
720.	METALLISED POLYPROPYLENE, POLYESTER FILM CAPACITOR	767.	TEFLON COATED ELECTRIC CABLE	800.	APPLE JUICE CONCENTRATED & DEHYDRATED FRUIT & VEGETABLES
721.	MICA BASE ELECTRONIC COMPONENTS	768.	TELEMEDICINE (DISTANCE HEALTH CARE) (Rs. 5000/-)		
722.	MICA PAPER WASTE PAPER FROM MICA WASTE	769.	TELEPHONE CORD/CABLE	801.	ARTIFICIAL FISH MEAL FOR POULTRY FEED
		770.	TELEPHONE (PUSH BUTTON TYPE)	802.	AUTOMATIC BISCUIT PLANT
723.	MICRO PROCESSORS TRAINER KITS BASED ON MICRO PROCESSORS	771.	TELEPHONE (PUSH BUTTON & CORDLESS)	803.	BABY CEREAL FOOD AND MILK POWDER
724.	MINI COMPUTER (PERSONAL COMPUTER)	772.	TELEVISION (CTV & B/W)		
		773.	TELEVISION (3-D)	804.	BACTERIA FOR CANE JUICE
725.	MINIATURE CIRCUIT BREAKER (M.C.B)	774.	TELEVISION DEFLECTION COMPONENTS	805.	BAKER'S YEAST
726.	MINIATURE WATCH BATTERIES (BUTTON CELL)	775.	TELEVISION SIGNAL BOOSTERS	806.	BAKERY INDUSTRY
		776.	TELEVISION TUNERS	807.	BANANA PUREE
727.	MIXER/GRINDER (MIXI)	777.	TRACTION BATTERIES	808.	BEER & WINE
728.	MONO CHROME COMPUTER MONITOR	778.	TRAINING INSTITUTE OF MEDICAL TRANSCRIPTION	809.	BEER PLANT (BREWERY)
				810.	BIDI
729.	MOTOR START ELECTROLYTIC CAPACITOR	779.	TRANSFORMER FOR B/W TV	811.	BIDI & CIGARETTE
		780.	TRANSFORMER FOR VOLTAGE STABILIZER & E.H.T	812.	BISCUIT PLANT
730.	MULTI LAYER P.C.B				

Choose & Start Your Own Industry Out of 30,000 ready Detailed Project Reports

813. BREAD (AUTOMATIC PLANT)
814. BLACK PEPPER (SPICES)
815. BREAD AND BISCUITS
816. BREEDING FARM
817. BROILER CHICKEN
819. BUTTON MUSHROOM CULTIVATION & PROCESSING
820. CANNING OF RASAGULLAS IN METAL CANS
821. CAFFEIN FROM TEA WASTE
822. CANNING OF FRUITS & VEGETABLES
823. CASEIN AND BY-PRODUCTS
824. CASHEW FRUIT JUICE FROM CASHEW FRUIT APPLE
825. CASHEWNUT KERNEL EXTRACTION FROM CASHEWNUT FRUIT
826. CASHEWNUT SHELL LIQUID & KERNEL PROCESSING
827. CASHEW FENI
828. CATECHEU (BY CHEMICAL PROCESS)
829. CATTLE FEED FROM TAPIOCA
830. CHEWING & BUBBLE GUM
831. CHICKEN/SHEEP MEAT PROCESSING
832. CHOCOLATE (MILK)
833. CIGARETTE AND BEEDIES
834. COCOA BUTTER FROM COCOA MASS
835. COCONUT PRODUCTS & BY PRODUCTS PROCESS COMPLEX
836. COLD/SOFT DRINKS
837. COLLECTION OF MILK AND MILK MAKING POWDER
838. COLLECTION OF MILK AND PACKING IN POLYTHENE POUCH (1/2 KG.1 KG. & 2 KG.)
839. CONDENSED MILK (SWEETNED)
840. CONFECTIONERY INDUSTRY (TOFFEE & CANDY, SEMI-AUTOMATIC PLANT)
841. COUNTRY LIQUOR FROM MOLASSES
842. CIGARETTE
843. DAIRY FARM AND DAIRY (MILK) PRODUCTS (PASTEURISED MILK, BUTTER, GHEE, PANEER)
844. DAIRY FARM TO PRODUCE MILK & PACKING IN POUCHES (50%) & CAN(50%)
845. DAIRY FOR MILK PROCESSING
846. DAIRY FARM (BUFALO)
847. DAL (PULSE) MILL UNIT
848. DEHYDRATION OF CARROT & GARLIC
849. DEHYDRATION & CANNING OF FRUITS & VEGETABLES
850. DEHYDRATION OF FIGS
851. DEHYDRATION OF FRUITS AND VEGETABLES
852. DEHYDRATED ONIONS AND ONION POWDER
853. DRY ICE BY BREAKING OF AIR
854. DRYING OF RED CHILLIES, HALDI, DHANIA, AND GREEN PEAS
855. EGG POWDER (40,000 EGGS PROCESSING PER DAY)
856. EXPORT OF PROCESSED FOODS AND MARINE PRODUCTS
857. FISH CANNING & POUCHING
859. FISH FARMING (PRAWN & OTHER MARINE PRODUCTS)
860. FISH MEAL
861. FLOUR MILL AND MUSTARD OIL
862. FOOD COLOUR & ORASTED GROUNDNUT GRAM PEAS, ETC IN POUCHES
863. FROG LEGS PROCESSING
864. FROZEN MEATS PROCESSING
865. FOOD FLAVOURS (WHISKY) VODKA, GRAPE, BUTTER SCOTCH)
866. FOOD PRODUCTS COMPLEX (DEHYDRATED ONIONS, GARLIC POWDER & FLAKES, CATTLE FEED, TOMATO POWDER, TOMATO PRODUCTS, CANNED FRUITS & VEGETABLES, TOMATO PURE, GROUN NUT OIL, REFIND OIL, DEHYDRATED GRAPES, BANANA POWDER & WAFFERS)
867. FRUIT JUICE, JAM, JELLIES & ALLIED PRODUCTS
868. FRUIT JUICE, PICKLES PROCESSING AND CANNING
869. FRUIT JUICE MAKING & PACKING IN PLASTIC CONTAINER/POUCHES
870. FRUIT PROCESSING (JAM & JELLIES)
871. FRUIT PULP & JUICE CONCENTRATES
872. FRUIT & VEGETABLE DRYING (FREEZE DRYING METHOD)
873. GOAT & SHEEP FARMING
874. GRAM DALL/PULSE MILL
875. GRAPE DEHYDRATION
876. HARD BOILED CANDY (TOFFEE & CANDY)
877. HERBAL CIGARETTES
878. HONEY PROCESSING & PACKAGING
879. ICE CREAM OF DIFFERENT FLAVOURS
880. ICE CREAM STABILIZER
881. ICE MAKING PLANT
882. INDIAN MADE FOREIGN LIQUOR (I.M.F.L)
883. INSTANT FOOD (IDLI MIX, DOSA MIX, GULAB JAMUN MIX)
884. INSTANT FOOD (INSTANT FOOD & FAST FOOD PARLOUR)
885. INSTANT NOODLES
886. INSTANT TEA
887. INSTANT TEA FROM BLACK TEA
888. INTEGRATED STARCH BAKING POWDER/YEAST INDUSTRY
889. IODIZED SALT
890. IODIZED SALT (ORDINARY MOISTURE-LESS/FREE FLOWING IN PLASTIC BAGS AND CONTAINERS)
891. JAM, JELLIES, FRUIT JUICE & ALLIED PRODUCTS
892. KATHA AND CUTCH
893. KHANDSARI SUGAR
894. KHANDSARI SUGAR & IMFL
895. LACTIC ACID FROM WHITE SUGAR BY FERMENTATION PROCESS
896. LACTOSE & BY PRODUCTS PROCESSING FROM MILK
897. LIQUID GLUCOSE AND ITS BYE PRODUCTS
898. MACRONI AND VERMICILLI
899. MALT EXTRACTION FROM BARLEY
900. MANGO PROCESSING (MANGO PULP, JUICE & SLICES)
901. MAYUR BRAND TYPE CHEWING TOBACCO
902. MINERAL WATER
903. MILK PRESERVATION & MARKETING TO WHOLE SELLERS (INPOUCH PACKING BY UHT TECHNOLOGY)
904. MILK PROCESSING AND PACKAGING OF MILK PRODUCTS
905. MILK PRODUCTS (CASEIN, LACTOSE, GHEE & WHEY POWDER)
906. MILK TOFFEE
907. MINI FLOUR MILL
908. MINI SUGAR PLANT
909. MISRI (PEARL SUGAR CANDIES)
910. MODERN RICE MILL
911. MURABBA
912. MUSTARD OIL EXTRACTION & REFINING
913. MUTTON TALLOW
914. NAMKEEN INDUSTRY (BHUJIA, CHANA CHUR ETC.)
915. NAMKEEN & SWEETS
916. NON-BASMATI RICE FROM PADDY
917. OLEORESIN, ESSENTIAL OIL, DYES & POWDER OF SPICES
918. OLEORESIN EXTRACTION FROM DIPTERO-CARPUT TURMINATUS AND PINUS KHASYANA
919. OLEORESIN EXTRACTION FROM CHILLI
920. PAN MASALA AND POUCH

Price Rs. 3675/- for each "Detailed Project Report" Payable in advance through Draft/Cash/M.O. in favour of *"ENGINEERS INDIA RESEARCH INSTITUTE"*. 4449, Nai Sarak (D), Main Road Delhi - 110 006 OR Ask by V.P.P. ● Ph : 3918117, 391 6431, 392 0361, 396 0797
●Fax: 91-11- 391 6431 ●E-Mail : eirisidi@bol.net.in ● WebSite : www.startindustry.com

Apart from the above mentioned reports EIRI is also having other most lucrative projects (as many as 30,000). You just name it and we have that report

- 921. PAN MASALA, TOBACCO, ZARDA & KIMAM MAKING
- 922. PANEER FROM MILK
- 923. PAPPAD PLANT
- 924. PAPAIN FROM PAPAYA (PAPAYA LATEX)
- 925. PECTIN FROM MANGO PEEL PECTIN FROM APPLE POMACE
- 926. PHYTO TEA (HERBAL TEA)
- 927. PICKLES AND SAUCES
- 928. PICKLES MURABBA ETC. (VEG. & NON. VEG. PICKLES)
- 929. PIGGERY MEAT PROCESS
- 930. PINE-APPLE JUICE PREPARATION & PACKAGING
- 931. POTATO CHIPS/WAFFERS
- 932. POTATO POWDER
- 933. POUCH FILLING & PACKAGING OF EDIBLE OIL & GHEE
- 934. POULTRY FEED
- 935. PROCESSED FOODS & SPICES (EOU)
- 936. PROCESSED READYMADE FOOD
- 937. PROCESSING OF FRUITS & VEGETABLES
- 938. RABBIT FARMING
- 939. RASGULLAS MAKING & CANNING IN METAL CANS
- 940. READY TO EAT PROCESSED COOKED FOOD
- 941. READY TO EAT SNACK FOOD (CRAX, ROLL & BALL TYPE)
- 942. RICE & CORN FLAKES
- 943. ROASTED/SALTED/ MASALA, CASHEW NUTS, ALMONDS & PEANUTS
- 944. ROLLER FLOUR MILL
- 945. SALT LICKS FOR CATTLE
- 946. SAUSAGES FOOD CASING
- 947. SOFT DRINKS
- 948. SOFT DRINKS ESSENCES
- 949. SOFT DRINKS (NON CARBONATED) MANGO, LICCHI, PINEAPPLE FLAVOURS FROOTI TYPE IN TETRAPACK)
- 950. SOFTY ICE CREAM CONES (FULLY AUTOMATIC)
- 951. SOFT/COLD DRINKS (COLA, ORANGE, LEMON ETC. FLAVOURS)
- 952. SOYABEAN PRODUCTS
- 953. SOYA MILK & PANEER
- 954. STARCH & ALLIED PROPDUCT FROM BROKEN RICE
- 955. STRAWBERRY CULTIVATION & PROCESSING
- 956. SUGARCANE JUICE PRESERVATION
- 957. SUGAR CUBES FROM CANE SUGAR
- 988. SUGAR PLANT
- 989. SWEET AROMA BETEL NUT
- 990. SYNTHETIC TALLOW
- 991. TAMARIND JUICE POWDER
- 992. TEA & COFFEE PROCESSING & PACKAGING
- 993. TOFFEES, GOLIES, CANDY (HARD BOILED)
- 994. TOMATO PRODUCTS
- 994. TRADING BUSINESS OF SPICES & PAN MASALA
- 995. TUITY FRUITY
- 996. VODKA FROM POTATOES
- 997. WINE, BRANDY, WHISKY & CHAMPAGNE
- 997. WINE FROM DATES
- 998. YEAST FROM MOLASSES
- 999. ZARDA, KIMAM NO. 60,90,120,160,240,300 & 400 (TOBACCO)
- 1000. ZARDA-ZAFRANI (BABACHHAP TYPE)

GUMS & ADHESIVE

- 1001. ACRYLIC ADHESIVE
- 1002. ADHESIVE (FEVICOL TYPE)
- 1003. ADHESIVE BASED ON POLYURETHANE
- 1004. ADHESIVE FOR BAND AID (JOHNSON & JOHNSON TYPE)
- 1005. ADHESIVE INDUSTRIES (LAMINATED, STICKER, DDL & OTHER TYPES)
- 1006. ADHESIVE FOR GASKET (LIQUID/PASTE)
- 1007. GUAR GUM
- 1008. GUM BOTTLE (PVC)
- 1009. GUM FOR PASTING LABELS
- 1010. OFFICE PASTE
- 1011. RUBBER ADHESIVE
- 1012. SURGICAL ADHESIVE PLASTER

LEATHER & LEATHER PRODUCTS

- 1013. HANDMADE LEATHER
- 1014. LEATHER AUXILLARIES & CHEMICALS
- 1015. LEATHER DYES
- 1016. LEATHER WASHERS
- 1017. LEATHER BOARD FROM LEATHER WASTE
- 1018. LEATHER FOR UPHOLSTRY (SOFA)
- 1019. LEATHER GARMENTS
- 1020. LEATHER GOODS
- 1021. LEATHER SHOES
- 1022. LEATHER SHOE & CHAPPAL
- 1023. LEATHER SUITCASES, BRIEFCASES & TRAVELLING BAGS
- 1024. LEATHER GOODS AND GARMENTS
- 1025. LEATHER GARMENTS, SHOE & CHAPPAL
- 1026. LEATHER TANNING
- 1027. LEATHER TANNING & GARMENTS (EOU)
- 1028. SHEEP SKIN PICKLING PLANT
- 1029. SHOE UPPER
- 1030. SPORT SHOES (PLASTIC)

MISCELLANEOUS PRODUCTS

- 1031. AGARBATTI (INSENCE STICK)
- 1032. AGARBATTI (Mosquito Repellent)
- 1033. AGARBATI BAMBOO STICK
- 1034. AGARBATTI SYNTHETIC PERFUMERY COMPOUND
- 1035. AIR FRESHNER (ODONIL TYPE)
- 1036. AIR TAXI
- 1037. AMUSEMENT PARK
- 1038. ANODIC ALUMINIUM LABEL
- 1039. AQUACULTURE PRAWN FARMING (100% EOU)
- 1040. AQUA CULTURE SHRIMP FARMING (100% EOU)
- 1041. ARTIFICIAL FLOWERS
- 1042. ARTIFICIAL JEWELLERY
- 1043. ASBESTOS YARN
- 1044. ASH TRAYS FOR MARUTI VEHICLE
- 1045. AIR BUBBLE PACKAGING
- 1046. ASPHALTIC ROOFING SHEET (METAL COMPONENTS)
- 1047. AUTOMATIC BOOK BINDING
- 1048. ALKYD RESIN
- 1049. APPLE JUICE CONCENTRATE
- 1050. BALL POINT PEN FEFILLS (JOTTER TYPE)
- 1051. BANK BRANCH BUILDING
- 1052. BANQUET HALL
- 1053. BIO-COAL BRIQUETTES FROM AGRICULTURAL CELLULOSE WASTE
- 1054. BOOT CREAM/POLISH
- 1055. BUFFING & POLISHING COMPOUND
- 1056. BRASS BADGES BY ETCHING
- 1057. BRIQUETTED FUEL FROM AGRO WASTE
- 1058. BRIQUETTING OF LIGNITE COAL

Price Rs. 3675/- for each "Detailed Project Report" Payable in advance through Draft/Cash/M.O. in favour of *"ENGINEERS INDIA RESEARCH INSTITUTE"*. 4449, Nai Sarak (D), Main Road Delhi - 110 006 OR Ask by V.P.P. ● Ph : 3918117, 391 6431, 392 0361, 396 0797
● Fax : 91-11- 391 6431 ● E-Mail : eirisidi@bol.net.in ● WebSite : www.startindustry.com

1059.	BUFFALO HORN TIP, HOOF
1060.	BANQUET HALL
1061.	BUTTON
1062.	CALCINED PETROLEUM (C.P) COKE
1063.	CANVAS SHOES
1064.	CANVAS SHOES, JUNGLE BOOTS
1065.	CARBON BRUSH, BRUSH HOLDER & SLIP RING
1066.	CEMENT SHEETS WITH COIR FIBRE & OTHER SEGMENTS
1067.	CERAMIC TILES (GLAZED) BY DOUBLE FIRING/HEATING
1068.	CHILDREN RECREATION CENTRE
1069.	COAL BRIQUETTES
1070.	COLD STORAGE & ICE
1071.	COLD STORAGE FOR FRUITS AND VEGETABLES
1072.	COMPRESSOR (HERMETIC) FOR AIR CONDITIONER
1073.	COSTUME JEWELLERY/ IMITATION JEWELLERY
1074.	DECORATIVE LAMINATED SHEET (SUNMICA)
1075.	DIAMOND CUTTING & EXPORTS
1076.	DRINKING STRAW FROM PROPYLENE
1077.	ENGINEERING COLLEGE
1078.	ENTERTAINMENT CLUB
1079.	FASHION TECHNOLOGY INSTITUTE
1080.	FAST FOOD PARLOUR
1081.	FAST FOOD (INSTANT FOOD & FAST FOOD PARLOUR)
1082.	FIRE EXTINGUISHERS (SODA ACID TYPE)
1083.	FISH NET
1084.	FLORICULTURE (CUT FLOWER ROSE) WITH GREEN HOUSE
1085.	FLOOR COVERING SHEET
1086.	FILM STUDIO (VIDEO)
1087.	FLUSH DOOR, CHIP BOARD, WOOD WOOL & OTHER INSULATING BOARDS
1088.	GAS DETECTORS OF L.P.G
1089.	GEMS MANUFACTURING
1090.	GLASS BOTTLE BY SCRAP
1092.	GOAT & SHEEP FARMING
1093.	GOLD ELECTROPLATING
1094.	GOLD JEWELLERY (E.O.U)
1095.	GOLD PLATED SILVER JEWELLERY & CUTLERY
1096.	GRANITE SLAB AND TILES
1097.	GREEN HOUSE
1098.	HARD CHROMIUM PLATING
1099.	HEALTH CLUB AND BEAUTY PARLOUR CUM HAIR SALOON WITH SONA BATH
1100.	HEALTH CLUB CUM BEAUTY PARLOUR TRAINING INSTITUTE
1101.	HORN TIP, HOOVE BUTTON
1102.	HOSPITAL
1103.	HOSPITAL (100 BEDS)
1104.	HOSPITAL (200 BEDS)
1105.	ICE MAKING PLANT
1106.	IMITATION AND COSTUME
1107.	JEWELLERY (NECKLACE, EARRINGS EAR TOP ETC.)
1108.	INITMATE SCENT CHEMICALS FROM ALL TYPES OF FLAVOUR
1109.	INVESTMENT CASTING
1110.	JUTE, COIR, GLASS ROPE/ SUTLI
1111.	JUTE TWINE
1112.	L.P.G BOTTLING PLANT
1113.	L.P.G REGULATOR (DOMESTIC PURPOSE)
1114.	LAMINATED PARTICLE BOARD & HARD BOARD
1115.	LAMINATED SAFETY AND TOUGHENED GLASS
1116.	LEASING & HIRE PURCHASE
1117.	LICHEN (CHARILA)
1118.	MANILA ROPES
1119.	MEDICAL COLLEGE
1120.	MATCH UNIT FROM WAXED PAPER
1121.	MEDIUM DENSITY FIBRE BOARD
1122.	MELAMINE CROCKERY
1123.	MINERAL WATER
1124.	MINI CEMENT PLANT
1125.	MIRROR SILVER, GOLDEN, PINK, BLACK & SMOKES
1126.	MODERN ADVERTISING AGENCY WITH DTP & FILM STUDIO
1127.	MOTEL/SMALL HOTEL
1128.	MULTI COLOUR PRINTING
1129.	MULTI STOREY COMMERCIAL COMPLEX ALONGWITH RESIDENTIAL AND DELUX FLATS FOR FOREIGN TOURISTS & REVOLVING RESTAURENT AT THE TOP
1130.	MULTIPLE LAMINATION INDUSTRY
1131.	MUSHROOM GROWING AND PROCESSING (BY DEEP FREEZING METHOD)
1132.	NEWS PAPER PRINTING
1133.	NICKEL LINED INDUSTRIAL SCREEN
1134.	OFFSET COLOUR PRINTING PRESS (SIX COLOUR)
1135.	OFFSET PRINTING PRESS
1136.	P.C.C ELECTRIC POLES
1137.	PHOTOGRAPHIC DEVELOPER & FIXER
1138.	PVC EXTRUSION PROFILE (DOOR & WINDOWS)
1139.	POP-CORN
1140.	PHOTO ETCHING OF S.S.
1141.	PRE STRESSED CEMENT CONCRETE PIPES
1142.	PILFER PROOF CAPS
1143.	PILFER PROOF CAPS AND CROWN CAP
1144.	POUCH MAKING & GRAVURE PRINTING (ROTO PRINTING)
1145.	POULTRY & FISH FARMING (INTEGERATED UNIT)
1146.	PRINTING OF TIN SHEETS
1147.	READYMADE GARMENTS
1148.	RESTAURANT
1149.	ROSE PLANTATION AND ROSE OIL EXTRACTION
1150.	ROTOGRAVURE PRINTING
1151.	SAFETY BELTS
1152.	SAFETY MATCHES
1153.	SHOE LACES
1154.	SILK COCOON CULTIVATION (GROWING OF SILK COCOON WARM)
1155.	SILK SCREEN PRINTING FORMULATIONS FOR PLASTIC, PAPER & CLOTH
1156.	SPIKENARD (JATAMANSI)
1157.	STENCIL COATING SOLUTION
1158.	SUGAR CANDY (MISRI)
1159.	SUGAR CANE PLANTATION
1160.	SUGAR CANE JUICE PRESERVATION
1161.	SURAT ZARI
1162.	SYNTHETIC SHOES & SOLES
1163.	TEA PACKAGING INDUSTRY
1164.	TENNIS BALLS
1165.	THREE STAR HOTEL
1166.	TRAVELLING AGENCY
1167.	TRAYS, TROLLEYS FOR HOSPITAL WITH SCRATCHLESS COATING
1168.	WAX EXTRACTS (TANNING POWDER)
1169.	WIRE ROPE SLINGS
1170.	WOOD WOOL SLAB
1171.	WOODEN CANE FURNITURE WITH EXPORT POTENTIAL
1172.	WOODEN FURNITURE
1173.	WOODEN PANEL INCLUDING KILN SEASONING
1174.	WOODEN FURNITURE
1175.	WATCH CASE BUFFING
1176.	WATCH DIAL
1177.	WRIST WATCHES
1178.	WATCHES (ELECTRONIC)
1179.	ZEDOARY (KACHUR)

EDIBLE OILS, ESSENTIAL OILS LURICATIING OILS, GREASES, VEGETABLE OILS, WAXES, CAMPHOR, PERFUMES & PERFUMERY COMPOUNDS AND REFINED OILS ETC.

1180.	AROMATIC PERFUMERY COMPOUND
1181.	AEROSOL
1182.	AGARBATTI PERFUMERY COMPOUND
1183.	BEES WAX MANUFACTURE
1184.	CAMPHOR
1185.	CARDANOL FROM CASHEW NUT SHELL LIQUID
1186.	CASTOR OIL
1187.	CASTOR OIL DERIVATIVE OLEORESINS
1188.	CHILLI OIL
1189.	CITRONELLA OILS
1190.	CLOVE OIL
1191.	CONCENTRATE OF ROSE JASMINE & LILY ETC.
1192.	COLOURED FLAME CANDLE

Price Rs. 3675/- for each "Detailed Project Report" Payable in advance through Draft/Cash/M.O. in favour of "ENGINEERS INDIA RESEARCH INSTITUTE". 4449, Nai Sarak (D), Main Road Delhi - 110 006 OR Ask by V.P.P. ● Ph : 3918117, 391 6431, 392 0361, 396 0797
●Fax : 91-11- 391 6431 ●E-Mail : eirisidi@bol.net.in ● WebSite : www.startindustry.com

1193.	CANDLES (SEMI-AUTOMATIC)
1194.	CORN OIL (MAIZE OIL)
1195.	DEHYDRATED CASTOR OIL
1196.	EUGENOL FROM CINNAMON LEAF OIL
1197.	EXTRACTION OF ESSENTIAL OIL (CARDAMON, JEERA, AJOWAN, GINGER OILS ETC. & PACKAGING OF GROUND SPICES)
1198.	EXTRACTION OF JASMINE ESSENCE
1199.	EXTRACTION OF ESSENTIAL OILS BY SUPER CRITICAL FLUID METHOD FROM FLOWERS, HERBS & SPICES
1200.	EUCALYPTUS OIL
1201.	EXTRACTION OF OIL FROM OIL SEED EXPANDEREXTRUSION TECHNOLOGY)
1202.	FAT LIQUOR SULPHATED OIL
1203.	FLAVOURS FOR FOOD
1204.	GARLIC OIL & POWDER
1205.	GINGER OIL, SANDALWOOD OIL AND NAGARMOTHA OIL
1206.	GINGER OIL
1207.	GINGER OIL & GINGER DUST
1208.	INTEGERATED WAX COMPLEX
1209.	IONONE FROM LEMON GRASS OIL
1210.	JASMINE & LILLY FLOWER OIL
1211.	LEMON GRASS OIL
1212.	LIQUID PARAFFIN
1213.	LUBE OIL & GREASE
1214.	LUBRICATING OIL
1215.	MENTHOL CRYSTALS
1216.	MENTHOL OIL & CRYSTAL
1217.	MICRO CRYSTALLINE WAX
1218.	MUSTARD OIL (EDIBLE OIL)
1219.	OIL FROM ARTEMISIA HERBS
1220.	PALM OIL CRUSHING UNIT
1221.	PAN MASALA
1222.	PARAFFIN WAX
1223.	PARAFFIN WAX FROM SLACK WAX
1224.	REFINED OIL-SUN FLOWER OIL, GROUNDNUT OIL, STAFF FLOWER OIL & COTTON SEED OIL
1225.	REFINED VEGETABLE OIL
1226.	RECLAMATION OF USED ENGINE OIL
1227.	RICE BRAN OIL (R.B.O)
1228.	ROSE OIL EXTRACTION
1229.	SMOKE LESS CANDLE
1230.	SPICE OIL & OLEORESINS
1231.	SOLVENT EXTRACTION PLANT (OIL CAKE BASED)
1232.	SYNTHETIC ALMOND OIL
1233.	SYNTHETIC TALLOW
1234.	SYNTHETIC GHEE
1235.	VEGETABLE OIL EXTRACTION & REFINING
1236.	WADDING OIL (100%) FOR WADDING OF COTTON HOSIERY CLOTH IN DYEING PROCESS
1237.	WAX EMULSION FOR TEXTILE
1238.	WAX FLOOR POLISH

PAINT, ENAMEL, SOLVENTS, THINNERS, INKS & VARNISH

1239.	ACRYLIC EMULSION PAINTS
1240.	ALUMINIUM PAINT
1241.	AUTOMOBILE PAINTS
1242.	BALL POINT PEN REFILL INK
1243.	BITUMINIOUS ROAD EMULSION
1244.	BITUMEN
1245.	BITUMINIOUS FELTS FOR WATER & DAMP PROOFING
1246.	BITUMINIOUS ROAD EMULSION RAPID MEDIUM & SLOW SETTING
1247.	BUFFING & POLISHING
1248.	CEMENT PAINT FOR WHITE & GREY CEMENT
1249.	DISPERSANT
1250.	DRY DISTEMPER
1251.	DRY DISTEMPER & CEMENT PAINT
1252.	DUPLICATING INK BLACK FOR GESTNER DUPLICATOR
1255.	EMULSION PAINTS (WATER BASED)
1256.	HAMMERTONE PAINT
1257.	INSULATING VARNISH & WIRE ENAMEL
1258.	IRON OXIDE PIGMENTS
1259.	INSULATING VARNISH (POLY VINYL BUTYRAL BASED, FFC GRADE)
1260.	LIME COLOUR (CEMENT COLOUR)
1261.	SYNTHETIC RED OXIDE FOR FLOORINGS
1262.	SOLVENT & THINNERS
1263.	MARKING INKS (WATER PROOF)
1264.	METAL NAPHTHANATE (AS DRIER FOR PAINTS)
1265.	N.C. PUTTY
1266.	OFFSET PRINTING INK
1267.	OIL BOUND DISTEMPER PAINT
1268.	PAINT BRUSHES
1269.	PAINT REMOVERS
1270.	PAINT INDUSTRY
1271.	PAINT & VARNISH
1272.	PICTURE VARNISH
1273.	POWDER COATING PAINT
1274.	PRINTING INKS (OFFSET, FLEXO & ROTO GRAVURE)
1275.	PRIMER PAINT & ENAMEL PAINT
1276.	PUTTY & WATER PROOFING PAINT
1277.	PRINTING INKS (FLEXO-GRAPHIC INK)
1278.	PUTTY (METAL CASEMENT)
1279.	RED OXIDE PRIMER (ANTI CORROSIVE)
1280.	REFRECTORY PAINT (GRAPHITE BASED)
1281.	SCREEN PRINTING INKS
1282.	SILK SCREEN PRINTING INK FORMULATION FOR PLASTIC, PAPER, CLOTH
1283.	STAMP & PAD INK
1284.	STOVING PAINT
1285.	SPIRIT SOLUBLE MALEIC RESIN
1286.	TEXTURE PAINT
1287.	THINNERS AND ITS ALLIED PRODUCTS
1288.	TONER INK
1289.	VARNISH THINNER (SOLVENT)
1290.	VACUUM METALLIZING LACQUERS
1291.	WOOD PRIMER

PHARMACEUTICAL, DRUGS, AYURVEDIC/HERBAL COSMETICS & MEDICINES, HOMOEOPATHIC MEDICINES, DISPOSABLE SYRINGE, DENTAL COLLEGE & FINE CHEMICALS ETC.

1292.	AROMATIC PILLS
1293.	ASPIRIN
1294.	AYURVEDIC PAIN BALM OINTMENTS
1295.	AYURVEDIC CHURAN AND TABLETS
1296.	AYURVEDIC TABLETS (HAJMOLA TYPE)
1297.	AYURVEDIC/HERBAL PHARMACY
1298.	AYURVEDIC SHERBATS
1299.	AYURVEDIC PRODUCTS
1300.	BULK DRUGS (E.O.U)
1301.	BLOOD BAGS
1302.	CALCIUM GLUCONATE
1303.	CAPSULE, TABLET & INJECTION WITH MODERN INSTRUMENTS
1304.	CASHEW FENI
1305.	CHLOROQUINONE PHOSPHATE (BULK DRUGS)
1306.	CLINICAL THERMOMETER
1307.	DENTAL CLINIC

EIRI not only provides project reports but also provides turnkey services, liaisioning jobs, foreign collaborations & can also arrange loans.

Price Rs. 3675/- for each "Detailed Project Report" Payable in advance through Draft/Cash/M.O. in favour of "ENGINEERS INDIA RESEARCH INSTITUTE". 4449, Nai Sarak (D), Main Road Delhi - 110 006 OR Ask by V.P.P. ● Ph : 3918117, 391 6431, 392 0361, 396 0797
●Fax : 91-11- 391 6431 ●E-Mail : eirisidi@bol.net.in ● WebSite : www.startindustry.com

#	Item	#	Item	#	Item
1308.	DENTAL COLLEGE		PLASTIC BOTTLES)		PAPER WITH PRINTING
1309.	DENTAL GRADE EUGENOL	1351.	SORBITOL	1394.	LAMINATION & COATING ON PAPER
1310.	DEXTROSE MONOHYDRATE, LIQUID GLUCOSE	1352.	STARCH (MAIZE)	1395.	M.G. PAPER FROM WASTE PAPER
1311.	DEHYDRATED ONION & ONION POWDER	1353.	SURGICAL ADHESIVE PLASTER	1396.	MILL PAPER FROM WASTE PAPER
1312.	DEXTROSE POWDER (ANHYDROUS FROM STARCH)	1354.	SURGICAL BANDAGES	1397.	MILL BOARD FROM RICE & WHEAT STRAWS
1314.	DEXTROSE SALINE SOLUTION	1355.	SURGICAL GLOVES	1398.	MILL BOARD FROM WASTE PAPER
1315.	DISTILLERY (I.M.F.L)	1357.	SURGICAL COTTON		
1316.	DISPOSABLE NEEDLES FOR SYRINGES	1358.	SURGICAL COTTON AND BANDAGE	1399.	MINI PAPER PLANT FROM SISAL
1317.	DISPRIN	1359.	SYNTHETIC CAMPHOR POWDER	1400.	MINI PAPER PLANT
1318.	DISTILLED WATER	1360.	TABLETS & CAPSULES	1401.	MULTI WALL PAPER SACKS
1319.	EMPTY HARD GELATINE CAPSULES	1361.	TISSUE CULTURE	1402.	NEWS PAPER FOR CHILDREN
		1362.	TINCTURE FROM RECTIFIED SPIRIT	1403.	NEWS PRINT PAPER FROM RICE STRAW BAGASSE
1320.	FILLING & PACKING OF CAPSULES	1363.	TRIMETHOPIME	1404.	NEWS PAPER CHILDRENS
1321.	GLUCOSE - D - POWDER	1364.	VETERENARY MEDICINES (ONLY FORMULATIONS)	1405.	NEWS PRINT PAPER
1322.	GLYCERINE	1365.	VITAMIN 'C', SORBITOL' ANHYDROUS DEXTROSE, STARCH	1406.	OFFSET AND TREADLE TYPE PRINTING PRESS
1323.	HERBAL COSMETICS			1407.	MILL BOARD BASED ON RICE STRAW
1324.	HERBAL SHAMPOO				
1325.	HERBAL HAIR OILS (AYURVEDIC)		**PULP, PAPER, STRAW/GREY BOARD, KRAFT PAPER, PACKAGING, PAPER CARRY BAGE, PAPER FROM AGRO WASTE & STATIONERY ETC.**	1408.	PAPER AND BOARD FROM STRAW
1326.	HOMOE & BIO-MEDICINES WITH MOTHER TINCTURE			1409.	PAPER & PAPER PRODUCTS
1327.	HOMOEPATHIC MEDICINES			1410.	PAPER ENVELOPES
1328.	HYPODERMIC NEEDLES			1411.	PAPER CARRY BAGS
1329.	I.V. FLUIDS	1366.	AMMONIA PAPER	1412.	PAPER BOARD CARTON
1330.	IBUPROFEN	1367.	AUTOMATIC BOOK BINDING	1413.	PAPER CONES FOR LOUD SPEAKERS
1331.	INFUSION & TRANSFUSION SETS (I.V. SET)	1368.	ADHESIVE (FEVICOL TYPE)	1414.	PAPER FROM AKRA
1332.	INJECTABLE FOR PHARMACEUTICALS	1369.	ALL PIN & GEM CLIPS	1415.	PAPER FROM BAGASSE WITH CORRUGATED BOARD & BOXES
		1370.	CARBON PAPER		
1333.	INJECTION AMPOULES PACKAGING BOX	1371.	CARD BOARD		
		1372.	CARBON LESS PAPER	1416.	PAPER FROM BAMBOO
1334.	INTEGERATED SURGICAL COTTON	1373.	CELLPHANE PAPER	1417.	PAPER GLASSES FOR BEVERAGES
1335.	ICE MAKING PLANT	1374.	COMPUTER FORMS & SECURITY PRINTING PRESS		
1336.	ICE & COLD STORAGE			1418.	PAPER FROM RICE HUSK & WHEAT HUSK
1337.	LACTOSE & BY PRODUCTS PROCESSING FROM MILK	1375.	CORRUGATED BOARD & BOX (PRINTED & LAMINATED)	1419.	PAPER FROM TREE BARK, EUCALYPRUS WOOD
1338.	LICHEN (JATAMANSI CHARILA)	1376.	CORRUGATED BOARD AND BOXES FROM FROM CARD BOARDS	1420.	PAPER PRODUCTS
1339.	LIQUID GLUCOSE AND ITS BY-PRODUCTS			1421.	PAPER PLANT (WHITE WRITING & NEWS PAPER FOR PULP & WASTE PAPER)
1340.	L-LYSINE MONOHYDRO CHLORIDE	1377.	CORRUGATED CARTONS FROM PLAIN PAPERS		
1341.	LIQUID GLUCOSE FROM POTATOES	1378.	CORRUGATRED PACKING & MATERIAL (BULB & TUBES PACKING)	1422.	PAPER PLATES, PAPER GLASS
1342.	MEDICAL COLLEGE			1423.	PAPER CONES & TUBES
1343.	NICOTINE FROM TOBACCO WASTE	1379.	DESK TOP PUBLISHING	1425.	PAPER PLANT WITH DTP & PRINTING & PUBLISHING UNIT
		1380.	DEFOAMING AGENT FOR PAPER PLANT		
1344.	OINTMENT-AYURVEDIC (YELLOW & WHITE)	1381.	DRINKING STRAW PAPER	1426.	PAPER BASED PHENOLIC SHEET
		1382.	D.T.P CUM OFFSET PRESS		
1345.	PHARMACEUTICAL AND FOOD GRADE GELATINE	1383.	EGG TRAYS	1427.	PAPER CUP FOR ICE CREAM
		1384.	EXERCISE NOTE BOOK, REGISTER AND PAD	1428.	PAPER TUBES SPIRAL WINDING COMPOSIT CONTAINER
1346.	PHARMACEUTICAL INDUSTRY (TABLETS, CAPSULES, LIQUID, GEL, OINTMENT POWDER INJECTABLE)	1385.	FLEXOGRAPHIC INK		
		1386.	GREETING CARD BY OFFSET PRESS	1429.	PAPER LABLE FOR BEER BOTTLES
		1387.	HAND MADE PAPER FILTER PAPER	1430.	PARTICLE BOARD & BLACK BOARD WITH SANDING & LAMINATION OF PARTICLE BOARD
1347.	PHARMACEUTICAL UNIT (EOU) WITH FORMULA TIONS, INJECTABLES, ETC. PYRIDINE & DERIVATIVES	1388.	HARD BOARD		
		1389.	INJECTION AMPOULES PACKAGING BOXES	1431.	PARTICLE BOARD FROM RICE HUSK
1348.	SALT (IODIZED SALT)	1390.	INSULATIING PAPER		
1349.	SALINE & INJECTION WATER	1391.	KRAFT PAPER	1432.	POUCH FILLING & MAKING FOR TOMATO SAUCE
1350.	SALINE WATER & DEXTROSE SOLUTION (I.V. FLUID IN	1392.	KRAFT PAPER FROM BAGASSE		
		1393.	LAMINATED PACKAGING	1433.	POUCH MAKING &

Price Rs. 3675/- for each "Detailed Project Report" Payable in advance through Draft/Cash/M.O. in favour of *"ENGINEERS INDIA RESEARCH INSTITUTE"*. 4449, Nai Sarak (D), Main Road Delhi - 110 006 OR Ask by V.P.P. ● Ph : 3918117, 391 6431, 392 0361, 396 0797
●Fax : 91-11- 391 6431 ●E-Mail : eirisidi@bol.net.in ● WebSite : www.startindustry.com

1434.	GRAVURE PRINTING PROCESSING OF PAPER FOR FEEDING IN COMPUTER	
1435.	PULP FROM BAMBOO & WOOD	
1436.	PAPER FILES	
1437.	PLAYING CARDS	
1438.	ROSIN SIZING AGENT (FOR PAPER PLANT)	
1439.	SAND PAPER	
1440.	SANITRY NAPKINS	
1441.	SILICON COATED PAPER	
1442.	STENCIL PAPER	
1443.	STRAW BOARD AND GREY BOARD	
1444.	STRAW BOARD & MILL BOARD	
1445.	STRAW BOARD AND PAPER BOARD	
1446.	TISSUE PAPER FACIAL	
1447.	TISSUE MOIST TOILETERY CLEANSING TISSUE AND RELATED PRODUCTS	
1448.	TISSUE PAPER ROLLS	
1449.	TETRA PACK FOR MILK PACKAGING, GHEE & OTHER LIQUIDS	
1450.	TOILET PAPER ROLLS	
1451.	TOILET PAPER & NAPKINS	
1452.	WAX COATED PRINTED PAPER	
1453.	WET FACE FRESHNER TISSUE	
1454.	WHITE WRITING & PRINTING PAPER	
1455.	WRITING & PRINTING PAPER (PAPER MILLS)	

PLASTIC, B.O.P.P, ACRYLIC, DISPOSABLE PLASTIC PRODUCTS, PET PRODUCTS, P.V.C, H.D.P.E, P.P, L.D.P.E., P.U, A.B.S, THERMOFOARMING, MASTER BATCHES, & POLYMER AND RUBBER PRODUCTS, TYRE, TUBE, ADHESIVE, SHEET, COIR & MANY OTHERS

1456.	ABS GRANULES FROM ABS SCRAPS FROM OLD T.V. CABINETS, WHITE GOODS ETC.	
1457.	ACRYLIC BEADS	
1458.	ACRYLIC COPOLYMER EMULSION	
1459.	ACRYLIC LATEX	
1460.	ACRYLIC SHEET	
1461.	ACRYLIC SHEET & MOULDED PRODUCTS	
1462.	ACRYLIC TEETH	
1463.	AUTO TUBES	
1464.	AUTO FLAPS FOR TRUCKS & BUSES	
1465.	AUTO TYRES & TUBES	
1466.	BABY BOTTLES (PLASTIC) WITH WHITESILICON RUBBER NIPPLES	
1467.	B.O.P.P. FILM	
1468.	B.O.P.P. PRESSURE SENSITIVE SELF ADHESIVE TAPE	

1469.	BABY NIPPLE (SILICON)
1470.	BABY NIPPLE (BIG SIZE)
1471.	BALLOON PLASTIC ADVERTISING
1472.	BLISTER FILM PVC
1473.	BLISTER PACKAGING & POUCH PAKAGING
1474.	BLOW MOULDING PLASTIC CONTAINER
1475.	COATING ON METALIZED POLYESTER FILM/METALISED PAPER/ ALIMINIUM FOIL
1476.	COATING ON PLASTIC (ELECTROLYSIS) & GLASS
1477.	COIR FOAM (RUBBERISED)
1478.	COLOUR COATING ON PLASTICS
1479.	COLOUR MASTER BATCHES FOR VARIOUS PLASTICS
1480.	CYCLE TYRES AND TUBES
1481.	DISPOSABLE PLASTIC CUPS GLASSES, ETC.
1482.	DISPOSABLE PLASTIC SYRINGES & NEEDLES
1483.	DISPOSABLE PLASTIC SYRINGES
1484.	DOUGH MOULDING COMPOUND (D.M.C)
1485.	EPOXY RESIN
1486.	EXPANDED POLYESTRENE MOULDING (THERMOCOLE)
1487.	F.R.P SCOOTER ROOFS & CEILINGS
1488.	F.R.P PRODUCTS (HELMET, WASHBASIN SHEETS, ROOFING SHEETS)
1489.	FIBRE REINFORCED PLASTIC (HIGH PRESSURE MOULDING WITH SMC BMC AND DMC)
1490.	FIELD RUBBER CONVERTED TO THE 60% LATEX RUBBER
1491.	FLEXIBLE P.U. FOAM
1492.	FORMALDEHYDE CROCKERY & OTHER ITEMS
1493.	FORMALDEHYDE RESIN (UREA, PHENOL,MELEMINE)
1494.	GASKET SHEET
1495.	GUM BOTTLE (PVC)
1496.	GLASS BEADS
1497.	HDPE COATED PAPER SACK
1498.	H.D.P.E. BAGS
1499.	H.D.P.E. CONTAINERS (BLOW MOULDING)
1500.	H.D.P.E. CONTAINER, POLY JARS BY INJECTION MOULDING (FOOD GRADE)
1501.	H.D.P.E. JERRY CANS
1502.	HDPE MANUFACTURING FROM ETHYLALCOHOL
1503.	H.D.P.E PIPE AND FITTINGS
1504.	H.D.P.E. PIPES
1505.	H.D.P.E PRINTED BAGS
1506.	H.D.P.E TWINES AND ROPES
1507.	H.D.P.E. & L.D.P.E PIPES AND FITTINGS
1508.	H.D.P.E/PP BOX STRAPPING
1509.	H.D.P.E/PP WOVEN SACKS

	USING PLAIN LOOMS
1510.	HOLOGRAM STICKERS-3D
1511.	H.M BAG PLANT WITH PRINTING UNIT
1512.	HAWAI CHAPPALS (RUBBER)
1513.	I.V PLASTIC BOTTLE
1514.	ICE CREAM CUP (PLASTIC)
1515.	INJECTION MOULDED AUTO COMPONENTS
1516.	INJECTION & BLOW MOULDED PLASTIC PRODUCTS
1517.	INJECTION MOULDED PLASTIC PRODUCTS
1518.	INTEGRATED COMPLEX ESTER'S & ALLIED PRODUCTS (D.O.P,D.B.P, & ETHYL ACETATE, BUYTL ACETATE, WIRE ENAMELS, JELLY CABLE COMPOUND)
1519.	L.D.P.E. (LOW DENSITY POLY ETHYLENE) GRANULES FROM VIRGIN (L.D.P.E. RESIN)
1520.	INTEGRATED SURGICAL RUBBER GOODS INDUSTRY
1521.	INJECTION MOULDED PLASTIC BALLS
1522.	L.D.P.E FROM ETHYL ALCOHOL
1523.	LDPE MOULDED PRODUCTS
1524.	LAMINATION OF COEXTRUSION MULTILAYER FILM IN ROLL FORM
1525.	LATEX RUBBER
1526.	LATEX RUBBER CONDOM
1527.	MASTER BATCHES (COLOURED, P.V.C, L.D.P.E, H.D.P.E, ETC.)
1528.	MELAMINE FORMALHYDE RESIN
1529.	MOULDED LUGGAGE
1530.	MULTI-LAYER (3 LAYER BAGS)
1531.	MULTI-LAYER (3 LAYER) FILM WITH LAMINATION & PRINTING
1532.	OIL SEAL
1533.	PET BOTTLE/CONTAINERS
1534.	PET BOTTLES FROM PRE FORM
1535.	PET BOTTLE & MINERAL WATER
1536.	PET PRE-FORM FROM PET RESIN
1537.	PET PRE-FORM CUM PET BOTTLES
1538.	PET PRE-FORM PET BOTTLES CUM MINERAL WATERS
1539.	POLY CARBONATE RESIN
1540.	PTFE COMPONENTS
1541.	PU/PVC SOLE FOR SPORT SHOE BY IMPORTED M/C.
1542.	PVC BATTERY SEPARATOR
1543.	P.V.C COMPOUNDS (FRESH)
1544.	P.V.C COMPOUNDS (SCRAP)
1545.	P.V.C ELECTRICAL INSULATING TAPE
1546.	P.V.C. EXTRUSION PROFILES
1547.	P.V.C FITTINGS
1548.	P.V.C FLEXIBLE FUSIBLE POWDER HEAT FUSIBLE POWDER
1549.	P.V.C GRANULES (FOR

Price Rs. 3675/- for each "Detailed Project Report" Payable in advance through Draft/Cash/M.O. in favour of "ENGINEERS INDIA RESEARCH INSTITUTE". 4449, Nai Sarak (D), Main Road Delhi - 110 006 OR Ask by V.P.P. ● Ph : 3918117, 391 6431, 392 0361, 396 0797
●Fax : 91-11- 391 6431 ●E-Mail : eirisidi@bol.net.in ● WebSite : www.startindustry.com

	INSULATION & SHEETS GRADES)	1591.	TYPE RESIN COATED SAND REXINE	1631.	WALL PAPER VITON (FLUORO ELASTOMER)
1550.	P.V.C GRANULES FROM PVC SCRAPS (WITH POLLUTION CONTROL)	1592. 1593.	REXINE CLOTH & ALLIED PRODUCTS RUBBER ADHESIVE		**SOAP, COSMETICS & PERFUMS**
1551.	P.V.C HOSES	1594.	RUBBER AUTO PARTS	1632.	ACID SLURRY, SYNTHETIC
1552.	P.V.C LEATHER CLOTH	1595.	RUBBER BELTING		DETERGENT POWDER
1553.	P.V.C FLEXIBLE PIPES	1596.	RUBBER MOULDING UNIT	1632.	ACID SLURRY
1554.	P.V.C PIPES AND FITTINGS		INCLUDING LINING RUBBER	1633.	AGARBATTI SYNTHETIC,
1555.	POLYTHENE BAGS (PRINTED)		SHEETING		PERFUMERY COMPOUND
1556.	PVC PLASTICS FILM SHEET SOFT/RIGID	1597. 1598.	RUBBER RECLAIMING RUBBER ROLLERS FOR	1634. 1635.	AFTER SHAVE LOTION ANTISEPTIC CREAM
1557.	PVC RESIN AND COMPOUND		TEXTILE MILLS & PAPER	1636.	BETA IONONE
1558.	PVC RULAR		INDUSTRIES	1637.	BLEACHING POWDER
1559.	PVC STABLIZERS (SINGLE PACK SYSTEM)	1599.	RUBBER & PLASTIC SHEETS, MATS & FLAPS	1638.	BLUE DETERGENT POWDER
1560.	PVC WIRE AND CABLES	1600.	RUBBER SHEET AND ALLIED	1639.	CLEANING POWDER (VIM TYPE)
1561.	PAPER BASED PHENOLIC SHEET FOR ELECTRICAL	1601.	HOSPITAL RUBBER GOODS RUBBERIZED PVC GASKET	1640. 1641.	COLD CREAM COLOURED FLAME &
1562.	PHENOL FORMALDEHYDE RESIN	1602. 1603.	RUBBERISED COIR RUBBER COMPOUND FOR		PERFUMED CANDLES (RED, BLUE, GREEN FLAME)
1563.	PHENOLIC RESIN		AUTOMOBILES	1642.	COSMETIC INDUSTRY
1564.	PLASTIC BEADS FROM	1604.	SAFETY BELTS		(MODERN)
	PLASTIC SCRAPS	1605.	SILVER AND GOLD PLATING	1643.	COSMETIC INDUSTRY
1565.	PLASTIC BUTTONS		ON PVC AND NYLON-6		(SHAMPOO, SPRAY
1566.	PLASTIC CANS	1606.	SILICONE RUBBER NIPPLES/		PERFUME, TALCUM
1567.	PLASTIC COLLAPSIBLE TUBE		TEATS		POWDER
1568.	PLASTIC CORRUGATED SHEET & BOXES	1607.	SPECTACLE FRAMES (PLASTIC)	1644.	DETERGENT POWDER (ARIEL TYPE)
1569.	PLASTIC FILM AND SHEETS WITH PRINTING FLEXO & ROTO/LDPE/HDPE/PP/HM/PVC	1608. 1609.	SPUNGE RUBBER SURGICAL EXAMINATION GLOVES	1645.	DETERGENT POWDER (NIRMA TYPE) FULLY AUTOMATIC PLANT
1570.	PLASTIC FILTER MASTER BATCH & OTHER MASTER BATCHES FOR VARIOUS	1610. 1611.	SYNTHETIC PEARL COATING ON POLYSTYRENE BEADS SYNTHETIC RUBBER	1646. 1647.	DETERGENT WASHING POWDER FISH OIL SOAP
	PLASTICS		ADHESIVE	1648.	GLYCERINE TRANSPARENT
1571.	PLASTIC JERRY CANS	1612.	TEFLON MANUFACTURING		SOAP
1572.	PLASTIC GRANULES OR POWDER FROM PLASTIC	1613. 1614.	TEFLON TAPE TEFLON TAPES & CABLES	1649. 1650.	HAIR REMOVING CREAM HERBAL COSMETICS
	SCRAP	1615.	THERMOCOLE SHEET AND	1651.	HERBAL SHAMPO & CREAM
1573.	PLASTIC INJECTION MOULDED T.V. CABINETS		MOULDED PRODUCTS EXPANDED POLYESTERENE	1652.	HERBAL/AYURVEDIC COSMETICS
1574.	PLASTIC ITEMS MANUFAC TURE FROM POWDER MELAMINE	1616.	EXTRUSION PROFILES THERMOFORMED PACKAGING (BLISTER	1653. 1654.	INCENSE POWDER, INCENSE STICKS & INCENSE CAKE OPTICAL WHITENERS
1575.	PLASTIC GOODS		PACKAGING &	1655.	ROSE OIL EXTRACTION
1576.	PLASTIC PIPES & TARPAULINES		POUCH PACKAGING)	1656.	SHAMPOOS (COCONUT OIL
1577.	PLASTIC SHEET FROM SCRAP	1617.	THERMOPLASTIC		BASED COLD PROCESS)
1578.	PLASTIC PLANT (BLOW MOULDING & INJECTION MOULDING)	1618.	POLYURETHANE THERMOFORMED CUPS, PLATES & GLASS WITH HIPS	1657. 1658. 1659.	SHAVING CREAM SINDUR (KUMKUM) SOAP COATED PAPER
1579.	PLASTIC PRODUCTS (GOLD, SILVER, NICKEL)	1619.	SHEET THERMOCOLE	1660.	SPRAY DRIED DETERGENT POWDER
1580.	PLASTIC TOYS	1620.	THERMOCOLE BASED	1661.	STAIN REMOVER
1581.	POLYESTER BEADING		DISPOSABLE GLASS, CUPS &	1662.	TALCUM POWDER (FACE &
1582.	POLYESTER FILM		PLATES		TOILET POWDER)
1583.	POLYTHENE BAGS & AUTOMATIC PRINTING	1621. 1622.	TOOTH BRUSHES TOY BALLOON, DECORATIVE	1663. 1664.	TOILET AND HERBAL SOAP TOOTH PASTE & POWDER
1584.	POLYTHENE PRINTED BAGS		& INDUSTRIAL BALLOONS	1665.	WASHING DETERGENT
1585.	POLYURETHANE FOAM AND ITS PRODUCTS	1623. 1624.	TREAD RUBBER TYRE RETREADING (HOT)		POWDER AND WASHING SOAP
1586.	PROPYLENE FILM (PRINTED) & BAG MANUFACTURING	1625.	TYRE RETREADING BY COLD PROCESS	1666.	WASHING POWDER LIQUID DETERGENTS, LOTION &
1587.	PLASTIC MATS	1626.	TYRE TUBES & FLAPS		SHAMPOO
1588.	RAINBOW COLOUR ON PVC FILM & SHEET	1627. 1628.	TYRE & TUBES UNSATURATED POLYESTER		
1589.	RED MUD PVC PIPES AND FITTINGS	1629.	FOR REXINE V-BELT AND FAN BELT		
1590.	RE-RUBBERISED OF SOLID	1630.	VINYL ASBESTOS AND PVC		

Price Rs. 3675/- for each "Detailed Project Report" Payable in advance through Draft/Cash/ M.O. in favour of "ENGINEERS INDIA RESEARCH INSTITUTE". 4449, Nai Sarak (D), Main Road Delhi - 110 006 OR Ask by V.P.P. ● Ph : 3918117, 391 6431, 392 0361, 396 0797
●Fax : 91-11- 391 6431 ●E-Mail : eirisidi@bol.net.in ● WebSite : www.sfartindustry.com

TEXTILE INDUSTRIES, READYMADE GARMENTS, COTTON, DYEING, BLEACHING, CLOTH, HOSIERY, POWER LOOM, HAND LOOM, WOOLLEN, SILK, SOCKS, SURGICAL COTTON & MANY OTHERS

1667. ANGORA RABBIT WOOL
1668. BUCKRAM
1669. CANVAS SHOES, JUNGLE BOOT, BOOT RUBBER KNEES & BOOT COMBAT
1670. CARPET FROM COTTON WASTE
1671. CERAMIC THREAD GUIDE
1672. COTTON BUDS/SWABS
1673. COTTON FROM WASTE YARN
1674. COTTON ROLLS
1675. COTTON SPIDERS FOR LOUD SPEAKERS
1676. DENIM CLOTH
1677. DENIM CLOTH (INTEGERATED UNIT WITH BLEACHING, DYEING AND PRINTING)
1678. DISPERSENT FOR TEXTILE
1679. DYEING & BLEACHING
1680. DYEING OF HANK YARN
1681. EMULSIFIER FOR WOOL BATCHING OIL
1682. EMBROIDERY ON FABRICS
1683. GARMENT DYEING, WASHING & STITCHING (JEANS, JACKETS, SKIRTS & SHIRTS)
1684. GOVES KNITTING
1685. GUNNY BAGS
1687. HDPE WOVEN SACKS
1688. HDPE TARPAULINS USING PLAIN LOOM WITH LAMINATION
1689. HDPE/PP WOVEN SACKS USING CIRCULAR LOOMS
1690. HOSIERY CLOTH (COTTON) PROCESSING (BLEACHING, DYEING, FINISHING OF CLOTH)
1691. HOSIERY INDUSTRY
1692. HOSIERY MERCERISING
1693. HOSIERY PRODUCTS LIKE VEST, BRIEF, T-SHIRTS & SOCKS
1694. JACQUARD FABRICS
1695. JUTE COIR, GRASS ROPE/ SUTLI MAKING
1696. JUTE FELT
1697. JUTE TWINES
1698. KNITTED FABRICS
1699. LAMINATED JUTE BAGS
1700. LAMINATION OF HDPE WOVEN CLOTH (JUTE, COTTON, PAPER)
1701. NYLON YARN CRIMPING, DOUBLING AND 3LEACHING
1702. PIGMENT BINDER FOR TEXTILE PRINTING
1704. POLYESTER RESIN FOR WIRE ENAMEL
1705. POLYESTER RESIN
1706. POLYESTER YARN FROM WASTE POLYESTER ZIP FASTENERS
1707. POWER LOOM
1708. READYMADE GARMENTS & HOSIERY
1709. READYMADE GARMENTS MERCHANDISE
1710. READYMADE GARMENTS & COVERS
1711. READYMADE GARMENTS & EMBROIDERY OF GOWNS, SHIRTS, BLOUSES, T-SHIRTS ETC. (ONLY LADIES)
1712. READYMADE SALWAR SUIT
1713. RECOVERY OF NYLON FROM NYLON WASTE
1714. ROTARY PRINTING AND DYEING ON COTTON, SYNTHETIC TEXTILE
1715. SANITARY NAPKINS
1716. SCREEN PRINTING ON COTTON CLOTH
1717. SEWING THREAD REELS & BALLS MAKING INDUSTRIES
1718. SCREEN PRINTING ON COTTON, POLYESTER & ACRYLIC
1719. SHAWLS (WOOLLEN)
1720. SHOE LACES
1721. SILK FABRICS ON HANDLOOM
1722. SOCKS KNITTING
1723. SPINNING, DOUBLING DYEING MERCERISING & BLEACHING OF COTTON YARN
1724. SPINNING & CARDING OF WOOL INTO YARNS
1725. STARCH BOOK BINDING CLOTH
1726. SURAT JARI
1727. SURGICAL COTTON & BANDAGE
1728. SYNTHETIC TEXTILE INDUSTRY (SUITING, SHIRTING, SAREES) TERRY CLOTH
1729. T-SHIRTS
1730. TOWELS, BED SHEET COVERS
1731. TERRY TOWEL
1732. TERRY FABRICS WEAVING UNIT
1733. TEXTILE AUXILLIARIES & CHEMICALS
1734. TEXTILE BLEACHING, DYEING & FINISHING & PRINTING OF COTTON FABRICS
1735. TEXTILE (HOSIERY)
1736. TEXTILE MILL
1737. TEXTILE DYEING & PRINTING
1738. TEXTILE PRINTING (JOB WORK)
1739. TEXTILE PIGMENT PRINTING BINDER
1740. TOWEL (TERRY)
1741. VELVET CLOTH BY FLOCKING PROCESS
1742. VISCOSE STAPLE FIBRE
1743. WADDING OIL (100%) FOR WADDING OF COTTON HOSIERY CLOTH IN THE DYEING PROCESS
1744. WEAVING OF DASUTI CLOTH WITH PRINTING, DYEING, EMBROIDERY & FINISHING
1745. WASHING OF JEANS & OTHER GARMENTS
1746. WORSTED WOOLLEN YARN CLOTH
1747. ZARI GLITTER SALMA SITARA OF PLASTIC FILM

INFOTECH/IT, HOSPITALITY, HOSPITAL, COLLEGE, SCHOOL, MEDICAL, ENTERTAINMENT CLUB, WARE HOUSING & REAL ESTATE, PROJECTS

1748. AMUSEMENT PARK
1749. AMUSEMENT PARK CUM WATER PARK
1750. BANQUET HALL
1751. CALL CENTER (DOMESTIC)
1752. CALL CENTER (INTERNATIONAL)
1753. CHILDREN RECREATION CENTRE
1754. COLD STORAGE
1755. COMMUNITY HALL
1756. COMPUTER EDUCATION INSTITUTE
1757. COMPUTER SOFTWARE
1758. COLLEGE
1759. CYBER CAFE
1760. DENTAL CLINIC
1761. DENTAL COLLEGE
1762. DIAGONOSTIC CENTRE
1763. E-COMMERCE/BUSINESS
1764. E-SCHOOL (Rs. 5000/-)
1765. ENGINEERING COLLEGE
1766. ENTERTAINMENT CLUB
1767. ENTERTAINMENT CLUB, HOLIDAY RESORT, 4 STAR HOTEL, AMUSEMENT PARK CUM WATER PARK, MUSHROOM & ITS PRODUCTS, FISH FARMING, LAKE FOR BOATING, DEER PARK
1768. FASHION TECHNOLOGY INSTITUTE
1769. FAST FOOD PARLOUR
1770. FIVE STAR HOTEL
1771. FOOD PARLOUR
1772. FRANCHISE TRAINING PROGRAMME FOR IIT & ENGINEERING ENTRANCE EXAMS.
1773. GOLF COURSE
1774. HEALTH CLUB, BEAUTY PARLOUR
1775. HEALTH CLUB AND FITNESS CENTER
1776. HEALTH RESORTS
1777. HOLIDAY RESORTS
1778. HOLIDAY RESORT CUM

**Price Rs. 3675/- for each "Detailed Project Report" Payable in advance through Draft/Cash/ M.O. in favour of *"ENGINEERS INDIA RESEARCH INSTITUTE"*. 4449, Nai Sarak (D), Main Road Delhi - 110 006 OR Ask by V.P.P. ● Ph : 3918117, 391 6431, 392 0361, 396 0797
●Fax : 91-11- 391 6431 ●E-Mail : eirisidi@bol.net.in ● WebSite : www.startindustry.com**

1779. ENTERTAINMENT CLUB WITH 4 STAR HOTEL
1780. HOSPITALS
1781. ICE CREAM PARLOUR
1782. INTERNET SERVICE PROVIDER (I.S.P.)
1782. MEDICAL COLLEGE
1783. MEDICAL COLLEGE, HOSPITAL & RESEARCH INSTITUTE
1784. MEDICAL TRANSCRIPTION CENTRE
1785. MENTAL RETARDATION HOSPITAL & CEREBRAL PALSY
1786. MOTEL/SMALL HOTEL
1787. MULTISTOREY COMMERCIAL COMPLEX
1788. MULTISTOREY RESIDENTIAL COMPLEX
1789. NURSERY SCHOOL
1790. NATURE CARE CENTRE
1791. NURSING HOME
1792. ONLINE SHOPPING MALL (RS. 5000/- REPORT)
1793. PORTAL
1794. REHABILITATION CENTRE FOR AGED & NEEDY PERSONS
1795. RESIDENTIAL CUM COMMERCIAL COMPLEX
1796. RESTAURANT
1797. RESTAURANT WITH PUB
1798. SCHOOL (PRIMARY)
1799. SCHOOL (HIGHER SECONDARY)
1800. THREE STAR HOTEL
1801. TOURIST CLUB
1802. TRAINING INSTITUTE FOR MEDICAL TRANSCRIPTION
1803. VIDEO FILM STUDIO
1804. WARE HOUSE
1805. WEBSITE DESIGN & E-MAIL REGISTERING

AGRO BASED INDUSTRIES

1806. COAL BRIQUETTES FROM AGROWASTE
1807. FURFURAL FROM RICEHULL
1808. MUSHROOM CULTIVATION & PROCESSING (BUTTON)
1809. MUSHROOM GROWING & PROCESSING WITH AIR CONDITIONING
1810. MUSHROOM CULTIVATION & PROCESSING UNIT DEHYDRATION & PACKAGING OF OYSTER & PADDY STRAW MUSHROOMS
1811. ORGANIC MANURE
1812. PAPAYA CULTIVATION
1813. PAPAYA & TOMATO CULTIVATION
1814. PROCESSING & UTILISATION OF COCONUT
1815. PROCESSING OF SHEEP HAIR TO PRODUCE WOOL

BAKERY, CONFECTIONERY & FOOD PRODUCTS

1816. AGROLACTOR SOYA MILK
1817. APPLE FRUIT JUICE WITH CANNING BOTTLING
1818. AYURVEDIC SHARBAT
1819. BAKERY UNIT (PASTRIES, BREAD, BUNS, CAKE, TOFFEE ETC.)
1820. BAKING POWDER
1821. BANANA & ITS BY PRODUCTS
1822. BANANA POWDER
1823. BANANA WAFERS
1824. BANANA CULTIVATION
1825. BEER INDUSTRY
1826. DEHULLING OF JAUN FOR BEER
1827. BEER & WINE
1828. BEER, ALCOHOL, IMFL
1829. BESEN PLANT
1830. BISCUIT PLANT
1831. BREAD & BISCUIT PLANT
1832. BOTTLING PLANT COUNTRY LIQUOR FROM RECTIFIED SPIRIT
1833. BRANDY
1834. BREAD RUSKS
1835. CANNED FRUITS & VEGETABLES
1836. CANNING & PRESERVATION OF MEAT
1837. CANNING & PRESERVATION OF VEGETABLES
1838. CANNING OF MANGO PULP & MANGO SLICES
1839. CARBONATED BEVERAGS
1840. CASHEW FENI
1841. CASHEW NUT (DRIED & FRIED)
1842. CATTLE BREEDING
1843. CATTLE BREEDING & DAIRY FARM TO PRODUCE MILK
1844. CATTLE FEED FROM TAPIOCA
1845. CHEWING GINGER & AMLOKI
1846. CHEWING GUM
1847. CHILLI SAUCE
1848. CHILLI POWDER
1849. CHOCOLATE
1850. CIDER PLANT
1851. COCOA POWDER
1852. COCOA BUTTER & COCOA POWDER
1853. COCONUT SHELL POWDER
1854. COCONUT WATER
1855. COCONUT SWEET (WATERY)
1856. COCONUT MILK POWDER (DEHYDRATED)
1857. COCONUT PRODUCTS & BY PRODUCTS (INTEGRATED PLANT)
1858. COLD DRINK
1859. CURRY POWDER
1860. DAIRY FOR MILK PROCESSING (GHEE, BUTTER & PANEER)
1861. DAIRY PRODUCTS
1862. DAIRY PRODUCTS MILK PACKAGING IN POUCH (GHEE, BUTTER, ETC.
1863. DAIRY FARM TO PRODUCE MILK WITH PACKAGING (COW)
1864. DAIRY FARM TO PRDUCE MILK WITH PACKAGING (BUFALLOE)
1865. DAIRY FARM & MILK PRODUCTS
1866. DAL MOTH, CHANACHUR & BHUJIYA
1867. DEHYDRATION OF FRUITS & VEGETABLE
1868. DESICCATED COCONUT POWDER FROM COCONUTS
1869. DEHYDRATION & CANNING OF FRUITS & VEGETABLES
1870. DRY FRUIT ROASTING & PACKAGING
1871. DRYING OF RED CHILLIES, HALDI, DHANIYA, PEAS & GROUND NUT
1872. EGG POWDER
1873. FISH CANNING IN TIN & POUCHES
1874. FISH DEHYRATION (DRYING OF FISH)
1875. FISH MEAL
1876. FISH PROCESSING (BEAST FREEZING PROCESSES)
1877. FLAVOURS FOR FOOD INDUSTRIES
1878. FLOUR MILL (ROLLER)
1879. FROZEN MEAT
1880. FOOD DEHYDRATION (FRUITS & VEGETABLES)
1881. FRIED & ROASTED GROUND NUT, GRAMS, PEAR ETC.
1882. FRUIT JUICE MAKING & PACKAGING IN PLASTIC CONTAINER
1883. FRUIT JUICE IN TETRA PACK (DRINKS)
1884. FRUIT JUICE, SQUASHES, SAUCE & KETCHUP, JAM, JELLY, VINEGAR ETC.
1885. GARLIC FLAKES
1886. GARLIC POWDER
1887. GHEE & BUTTER
1888. GINGER (PULVERISED)
1889. GINGER GLAZING & PRESERVATION
1890. GINGER STORAGE
1891. GINGER PROCESSING
1892. GINGER OIL & GINGER DUST
1893. GINGER POWDER (DRY) & OLEORESIN
1894. GRAPE DEHYDRATION
1895. GRAPE CULTIVATION
1896. GRAPE JUICE
1897. HONEY PROCESSING & PACKAGING
1898. ICE CREAM & ICE CANDY
1899. ICE CUBE
1900. INVERT SUGAR
1901. IDLI MIX, DOSA MIX SAMBHAR MIX, VADA MIX, GULAB JAMUN MIX
1902. INSTANT COFFEE & INSTANT TEA

Price Rs. 3675/- for each "Detailed Project Report" Payable in advance through Draft/Cash/ M.O. in favour of *"ENGINEERS INDIA RESEARCH INSTITUTE"*. 4449, Nai Sarak (D), Main Road Delhi - 110 006 OR Ask by V.P.P. ● Ph : 3918117, 391 6431, 392 0361, 396 0797
●Fax : 91-11- 391 6431 ●E-Mail : eirisidi@bol.net.in ● WebSite : www.startindustry.com

#	Item	#	Item	#	Item
1903.	INSTANT NOODLES	1923.	MILK PRESERVATION & MARKETING TO WHOLE SELLERS	1942.	POTATO & ONION FLAKES
1904.	INSTANT SOUPS			1943.	POTATO CHIPS
1905.	IODIZED SALT FROM CRUDE SALT			1944.	POTATO GRANULES
1906.	JAM CHUTNEY PICKLES & SQUASHES	1924.	MILK PRESERVATION & MARKETING TO WHOLE SELLERS (IN POUCHES)	1945.	POUCH FILLING FOR SAUNF SUPARI ILAICHI ETC.
1907.	KATHA MANUFACTURING			1946.	PRESERVATION OF RAWS MANGO JUICE
1908.	LECITHIN (SOYA BASED)	1925.	MILK TOFFEE MANUFACTURES	1947.	PROCESSED CHEESE & MARINE PDTS.
1909.	LEMON & ITS PRODUCTS	1926.	MINERAL WATER	1948.	PULP FROM TARMARIND
1910.	MACARONI MANUFACTURING	1927.	MINERAL WATER IN POUCHES	1949.	READYMATE PROCESSED FOOD
1911.	MACARONI, SPAGHETTI, VERMICELLI & NOODLES	1928.	MINI FLOUR MILL ATTA MAIDA, SUJI & WHEAT BRAN	1950.	RICE & CORN FLAKES
1912.	MAIZE & ITS BY PRODUCTS MALTING PLANT			1951.	RICE BASMATI (TRADING)
1913.	MANGO PAPPAD (AAM PAPPAD)	1929.	MITHAI/HALWAI (SWEET & NAMKEEN)	1952.	RICE POLISHING & PACKAGING IN POUCH
1914.	MANGO POWDER RIPE	1930.	MUTTON PROCESSING	1953.	ROASTED/SALTED/MASALA/ CASHEW NUTS ALMONDS & PEA NUT
1915.	MANGO POWDER	1931.	PAN MASALA (MEETHA, SADA, ZARDA) MAKING & PACKING		
1916.	MANGO PROCESSING & CANNING (MANGO PULP)	1932.	PAN MASALA AND POUCH MAKING	1954.	ROLLER FLOUR MILL
1917.	MEAT PROCESSING (CHICKEN MUTTON)	1933.	PANEER (CHEESE)		**INFOTECH/IT PROJECTS**
		1934.	PAPAD & BARIYAN	1955.	MEDICAL TRANSCRIPTION
1918.	MEAT PROCESSING (BUFFALO)	1935.	PAPAD PLANT	1956.	E-COMMERCE
		1936.	PEPSICOLA IN POLYTUBES	1957.	CYBERCAFE
1919.	MENTHOL BOLD FROM MENTHOL FLAKES	1937.	PETHA PACKAGING	1958.	INTERNET SERVICE PROVIDER (ISP)
		1938.	PICKLES		
1020.	MILK POWDER	1939.	PIGGERY/MEAT/CHICKEN PROCESSING	1959.	COMPUTER EDUCATION CENTRE
1921.	MILK POWDER & GHEE				
1922.	MILK POWDER, GHEE & SPICES	1940.	PINE APPLE JUICE CANNING	1960.	PORTAL (WEBSITE DESIGN)
		1941.	POTATO & ONION POWDER	1961.	CALL CENTRE

TERMS AND CONDITIONS

FOR INDIA

1. Price Rs. 3,675/- (Rs. Three Thousand Six Hundred Seventy Five Only) for Each *Market Survey Cum Detailed Techno Economic Feasibility Report.* Payable in advance through Draft/M.O./Cash in favour of 'ENGINEERS INDIA RESEARCH INSTITUTE', Delhi. Delivery by Regd.post within 2 Days. (Postage Free)

2. Reputed Firms/Companies may place their orders by V.P.P. for full amount in India Only.

FOR OVERSEAS

1. Price US$ 250/- (US Dollars Two Hundred Fifty Only) for Each *Market Survey Cum Detailed Techno Economic Feasibility Report.*

2. Payable fully in advance through Draft in favour of 'ENGINEERS INDIA RESEARCH INSTITUTE', Delhi (Payable in India) Delivery by Regd. Air Mail Post within 2 Days.

ENGINEERS INDIA RESEARCH INSTITUTE

4449, Nai Sarak (D), Main Road, Delhi - 110 006 (India)
Ph:. 91-11-3918117, 3916431, 3920361, 3960797
Fax: 91-11- 3916431 E-Mail : eirisidi@bol.net.in
Website:www.startindustry.com
Also at : 4/27, Roop Nagar, Near Roop Nagar No. 1 School,
Delhi - 110 007 (India) Ph:. 396 0797, 392 0361

New Detailed Project Reports available on FOOD & ALLIED INDUSTRIES @ Rs. 3675/-

LIST OF READILY AVAILABLE DETAILED PROJECT REPORTS

- ACTIVATED CARBON FROM COCONUT SHELL & RICE HUSK
- AGRICULTURE IMPLIMENTS
- AMALA PLANTATION & PROCESSING (E.O.U)
- AYURVEDIC MADICINES
- BAKERY (BREAD/BISCUIT)
- BEER PLANT (EOU)
- BANANA POWDER (EOU)
- BONE CRUSHING PLANT
- BEE KEEPING
- BIO-FERTILIZER
- BREWERY & DISTILLERY
- CASHEW NUT SHELL LIQUID & KERNEL
- CATTLE & POULTRY FEED
- COCONUT PRODUCT & BY PRODUCTS
- CURRY PASTE
- CONFECTIONERY
- CUSTARD POWDER
- COLD STORAGE & ICE
- DALL MILL
- DAIRY FARM & PRODUCTS
- DAIRY FARM (MILK)
- DEHYDRATION OF FRUITS & VEGETABLE BY FREEZE DRYING METHOD
- EGG POWDER (E.O.U)
- FISH FARMING
- FLORICULTURE (CUT FLOWER)
- FLOUR MILL
- FOOD PROCESSING UNIT
- FOOD DEHYDRATION
- FROZEN MEAT
- HERBS CULTIVATION
- HERBS DRYING
- GINGER PROCESSING
- GOAT & SHEEP FARMING
- GOAT FARMING
- GUAR GUM
- GRANULATED MIXED FERTILIZER
- HONEY PROCESSING
- HYBRID SEEDS
- ICE CREAM (FOR ALL TYPE)
- INSECTICIDES FROM NEEM SEEDS, NEEM OIL & LEAVE
- INSTANT FOOD
- INSTANT NOODLES
- INVERT SUGAR
- IODIZED SALT
- KATTHA & CUTCH
- MANGO JUICE BOTTLING
- MANGO PRODUCTS
- MANGO PULP
- MAIZE & ITS BY PRODUCTS
- MENTHOL FLAKES & BOLD
- MUSHROOM
- MINERAL WATER
- OLEORESINS FROM CHILLI
- PAPAYA
- PEANUT BUTTER
- PIGGERY FARM
- PORK FARMING
- POTATO CHIPS
- ONION FLAKES
- POPLAR TREE
- RICE MILL
- SOYA BEAN OIL
- SOFT DRINK
- SPICES
- STARCH FROM MAIZE
- STRAWBERRY CULTIVATION
- TEA & COFFEE
- TEAK PLANT

Each 'EIRI' *Market Survey Cum Detailed Techno Economic Feasibility Report (Detailed Project Report)* covers Introduction, Properties, Market Survey, Process of Manufacture, Cost Economics with Profitability Analysis, Suppliers of Plant & Machineries and Raw Materials, Cash Flow Statement, Repayment Schedule, Depreciation Chart, Projected Balance Sheet etc.

Price **Rs. 3675/-** (Rs. Three Thousand Six Hundred Seventy Five Only) for Each. Send Draft/M.O. in favour of **"ENGINEERS INDIA RESEARCH INSTITUTE", DELHI**.

ENGINEERS INDIA RESEARCH INSTITUTE
4449, Nai Sarak (D), Main Road, Delhi - 110 006 (India)
Ph:. 3918117, 3916431, 3920361, 3960797 Fax: 91-11- 3916431
E-Mail : eirisidi@bol.net.in Website:www.startindustry.com

New Detailed Project Reports available on SPICES, FOOD ETC. INDUSTRIES @ Rs. 3675/- each

LIST OF READILY AVAILABLE DETAILED PROJECT REPORTS

- ASAFOETIDA (HING)
- ASAFOETIDA (SYNTHETIC)
- AJOWAN EXTRACTION FROM AJOWAN
- AMLA PLANTATION & PROCESSING (E.O.U)
- AMCHUR
- BLACK PEPPER
- BEE KEEPING
- BIO-FERTILIZER
- BREWERY & DISTILLERY
- CASHEW NUT SHELL LIQUID & KERNEL
- CHILLI OIL
- CORE OIL FROM CASHEW NUT OIL
- COCONUT PRODUCT & BY PRODUCTS
- CHILLI POWDER
- CARDANEL FROM CNSL
- CLOVE OIL
- COLD STORAGE & ICE
- DRYING OF RED CHILLI, HALDI, DHANIIA, PEAS ETC.
- DAIRY FARM & PRODUCTS
- DRY GINGER POWDER & OLEORESIN
- DRY GIBGER FROM GREEN
- GINGER
- EXTRACTION OF LARGE CARDAMOM
- FISH FARMING
- FLORICULTURE (CUT FLOWER)
- HERBS CULTIVATION
- HERBS DRYING
- GINGER PROCESSING
- GOAT & SHEEP FARMING
- GOAT FARMING
- GUAR GUM
- GARLIC OIL
- GARLIC POWDER
- GARLIC ACID
- GARLIC FLAKE & POWDER DEHYDRATION
- GINGER OIL
- GINGER OIL & GINGER DUST
- GINGER STORAGE
- MAIZE & ITS BY PRODUCTS
- MUSHROOM
- MINERAL WATER
- MUSTARD POWDE.
- PAPAYA
- OLEORESIN FROM CHILLI & GINGER
- OLEORESIN FROM CHILLI
- ONION FLAKES
- SPICES WITH PACKAGING & FORMULAES
- STARCH
- STRAWBERRY CULTIVATION
- THYMOL FROM AJOWAN OIL
- TOMATO, CHILLI & SOYABEAN SAUCE
- TARMARIND JUICE CONCENTRATE
- TARMARIND SEED
- TURMERIC POWDER
- TURMERIC PLANTATION
- TURMERIC OIL OLEORESIN
- WATER COCONUT SWEET

*Each 'EIRI' **Market Survey Cum Detailed Techno Economic Feasibility Report (Detailed Project Report)** covers Introduction, Properties, Market Survey, Process of Manufacture, Cost Economics with Profitability Analysis, Suppliers of Plant & Machineries and Raw Materials, Cash Flow Statement, Repayment Schedule, Depreciation Chart, Projected Balance Sheet etc.

*Price **Rs. 3675/-** (Rs. Three Thousand Six Hundred Seventy Five Only) for Each Report. Send Draft/M.O./Cash in favour of **"ENGINEERS INDIA RESEARCH INSTITUTE"**, DELHI. (Payable In India) (Delivery within Two Days)

ENGINEERS INDIA RESEARCH INSTITUTE
4449, Nai Sarak (D), Main Road, Delhi - 110 006 (India)
Ph:. 3918117, 3916431, 3920361, 3960797 Fax: 91-11- 3916431
E-Mail : eirisidi@bol.net.in * Website:www.startindustry.com

Useful Books on Cosmetics, Perfumes, Essential

HAND BOOK OF SYNTHETIC & HERBAL COSMETICS

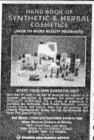

The Book covers Production Problems & Recommendations, Cosmetic and Drugs, Face Powder, Variations of Face Powder, Toilet Powder, Creams, Vanishing Creams, Foundation Creams, Hand Lotions, After Shaving Lotions, Deodorants, Mascara-eyebrow Pencils-Eye Shadows, Lipsticks, Shampoos, Depilatories, Shaving Cream, Cosmetics for Nails, Tooth Powder, Tooth Paste, Mouth Washes, Facial Masks, Cosmetics for Eyes, Cosmetic for Babies, Herbal Cosmetic for the Skin, Hair Shampoos, Anti Dandruff Preparations, Hair Straighteners, Hair Dyes, Bleaches, Colourings and Dye Removers, Oral Herbal Preparations, Govt. Regulations & Acts on Drugs & Cosmetics, Bath Preparations, Baby Preparations, Home Made Cosmetics, Herbal Preparations for Body, Skin Cleansing, Herbal Preparations for Feet & Hands, Herbal Shampoo and Setting, How to Layout a Cosmetic Factory, Project Profiles on Various Cosmetics with Herbal etc.

HAND BOOK OF PERFUMES & FLAVOURS

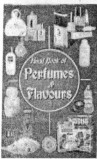

(With Directory of Plant & Equipment, Raw Material & Manufacturer/ Exporters/Suppliers of Perfumes)

The book covers new formulaes of various kinds of perfumes & flavours. The major chapters of the book are Perfume, Formulary of Perfume, Formulary of Flavour, Chemicals Specifications for Perfume & Flavour Components, Natural Odours Simulated with Aromatic Chemicals, Simulated Flower Scents, Simulated Marine Scents (Algae), Plant & Equipment Suppliers, Suppliers of Raw Materials, Manufacturer/Exporters/Suppliers of Perfumes. At the end of the book the last but not the least chapter project profiles has also included for the benefits of the new entrepreneurs.

Books Available at :
ENGINEERS INDIA RESEARCH INSTITUTE
4449, Nai Sarak, Main Road, Delhi-6
Ph:. 3918117, 3916431, 3920361, 3960797
* Fax: 91-11- 3916431
*E-Mail : eirisidi@bol.net.in

HAND BOOK OF ESSENTIAL OILS MANUFACTURING & AROMATIC PLANTS

With Directory of Plant & Machinery Suppliers, International Importers & Exporters and Manufacturers & Exporters of Essential Oils & Aromatic Chemicals

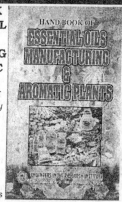

The book covers latest methods and formulaes to produce various type of Essential Oils and Aromatic Plants. The major chapters of the book are Trends in trade of essential oils, damask rose cultivation and processing, rose oil distillation method, chemistry of rose oil, cultivation of matricaria chamomilla, cultivation of davana for essential oil, cultivation and improvement of sweet marjoram, extraction of essential oils, essential chemical constituents profile in tree spice, folk medicinal uses of indigenous aromatic plants, essential oil bearing plants status, promising aromatic plants of industrial value, essential oil industry waste utilization, fractionation of essential oil in perfumery & turpentine industry, tagetes minuta, essential oil of hyptis suaveolens poit, super critical fluid extraction technology for spice extraction, citronella oil, clove oil, eucalyptus oil, ginger oil, jasmine rose & lily oil, jasmine flower oil etc.

ESSENTIAL OILS PROCESSES & FORMULATIONS HAND BOOK

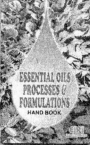

Essential Oils by Steam Distillation, Essential Oil Lemon Basil, Processing of Fresh Ginger (Zingiber Officinale Roscoe), Essential Oil from Cinnamomum glanduliferum (wal.) Nees, Kewda (Pandannus odoritissimus L.) flower distillation, Composition of essential oil from bottle brush (Callistemone lanceolatus) by capillary gas chromatography, Essentioal Oil of Ocimum basilicum L., Composition of essential oil from flowers of Keora (Pandanus odoratissimus Linn)., Manufacturers/Exporters/Importers & Traders of Essential oils and Aromatic Chemicals with Machinery Suppliers.

New Books Published from EIRI

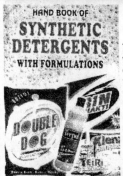

HAND BOOK OF SYNTHETIC DETERGENTS WITH FORMULATIONS

The unique and latest edition has just published. The book covers chapters viz. Group of Synthetic Detergents, Synthesis of Detergents, Manufacture of Finished Detergents, Formulations and Applications of Detergents, Perfuming of Soap and Detergents, Testing of Soaps and Detergents, Manufacturing of Herbal Synthetic Detergents, Detergents Bars, Herbal Liquid and Paste Detergents, Acid Slurry, Anionic Detergents, Detergent Washing Powder (Ariel Type- Enzyme Detergents), Synthetic Detergents (Blue Powder), Detergent Cake (Nirma Type), Cleaning Powder, Detergent Cake and Powder, Laundry and Dry Cleaners, Liquid Toilet Cleaner (Harpik Type), Acid Slurry (LAB), Nerol Laundry Soap, Liquid Detergents for Wool, Laundry for Clothes Washing, Nirma Type Detergent Powder, Non-Ionic Liquid Detergents, Detergent paste (Textile Grade), Spray Dried Detergent Powder, Washing & Laundry Soap, Zeolite -A Manufacturing (Detergent Grade), Detergent Washing Powder (Surf Excel Type), Detergent Powder Plants - Dry Mix Process, Laundry Soap Manufacturing Plant, Toilet (Bath) Soap Finishing Line, Detergent Cake Manufacturing Plants, Suppliers of Plant and Equipments and Raw materials etc.

HAND BOOK OF AGRO CHEMICAL INDUSTRIES (INSECTICIDES & PESTICIDES)

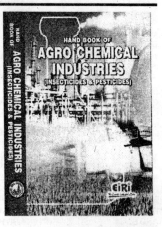

The Book covers Agro Chemical Industries with processes and Formulae including Organic Insecticides, BHC, Synthetic Insecticides, Fungicides, Nematicides, Rodenticides, Molluscicides, Fumigants, Acaricides, Herbicides, Plant Growth Regulators, Repellents, Attractants, Pheromones, Synergists, Synthetic Inhibitors & Proinsecticides, Toxicology and Safe Use of Pesticides, Insecticide Act, Pesticide Formulations, Pesticide Mixtures, Modern Equipments for a Pesticide Formulation Laboratory and Pilot Plant, Aerosol Formulations, Advances in Pesticides Formulations, Various different Project Profiles related with Insecticides and Pesticides including Neem Pesticides, Insecticides, Mosquito Agarbatti, Aerosol Insecticide Spray etc., Suppliers of Plant and Equipments and Raw Materials have also been provided for the new entrants in this line.

PAINT VARNISH SOLVENTS AND COATING TECHNOLOGY

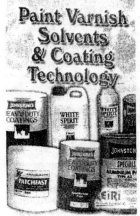

The Book 'Paint Varnish Solvents and Coating Technology' covers Introduction, General Pigments Physical Properties, Pigments Processing, Plasticizers and Solvents, Synthetic Resins, Cellulose Ester and Ether Products, Varnishes, Pigmentation, Paints (Decorative & Building), Coatings (Water Borne), Methods of Applications, Industrial Paints and Coatings, Industrial Finishes, Miscellaneous Coatings and Ancillary Materials, Testing and Evaluation, Miscellaneous Formulae, Project Profiles of Aluminium Paints, Cement Paints, Acrylic Emulsion Paints, Insulating Varnish, Powder Coating, Primer Paints and many others. Suppliers of Raw Materials, Suppliers of Plant and Machinery, Present Manufacturers, Packaging Material Addresses and many other details.

New Publications from EIRI

1. HAND BOOK OF EXPORT ORIENTED INDUSTRIES
2. HAND BOOK OF PLASTIC PROJECTS (HI-TECH PLASTIC PROJECTS)
3. AGRO BASED & FOOD PROCESSING WITH EXPORT ORIENTED INDUSTRIES
4. HAND BOOK OF PACKAGING INDUSTRIES
5. ALL CHEMICALS AND ALLIED INDUSTRIES
6. HAND BOOK OF HOSIERY READYMADE GARMENTS & TEXTILE PROJECTS
7. AGRO BASED INDUSTRIES HAND BOOK (PLANTATION & FARMING)
8. REAL ESTATE PLAZAS, HOTEL, MOTEL, HOSPITAL & COMMERCIAL COMPLEXES
9. WORLD IMPORTERS DIRECTORY OF AGRO BASED & FOOD PROCESSING
10. WORLD IMPORTERS YELLOW PAGES (ALL TRADE BUYERS DIRECTORY)
11. HAND BOOK OF PRINTING PROCESSES TECHNOLOGIES & INDUSTRIES
12. SMALL MEDIUM & LARGE SCALE CHEMICAL INDUSTRES
13. DAIRY FORMAULATIONS, PROCESSES & MILK PACKAGING INDUSTRIES
14. PLASTIC PROCESSING AND PACKAGING INDUSTRIES
15. STATIONERY, PAPER CONVERTING & PACKAGING INDUSTRIES
16. INDUSTRIAL DIRECTORY (ALL INDIA TRADE DIRECTORY)
17. FOOD PROCESSING AND AGRO BASED INDUSTRIES
18. AGRO BASED PLANTATION CULTIVATION AND FARMING HAND-BOOK
19. RUBBER CHEMICALS AND PROCESSING INDUSTRIES
20. PAINT PIGMENT VARNISH AND LACQUER MANUFACTURING
21. MODERN INKS FORMULAES AND MANUFACTURING INDUSTRIES
22. HAND BOOK OF BAKERY INDUSTRIES
23. INDUSTRIAL DIRECTORY OF DELHI AND SURROUNDING AREAS ON CD-ROM
24. START YOUR OWN COLD STORAGE UNIT
25. GARMENTS EXPORT DIRECTORY OF DELHI AND AROUND
26. MOULDS DESIGN AND PROCESSING HAND BOOK
27. PROFITABLE SMALL SCALE MANUFACTURE OF SOAPS & DETERGENTS
28. PET PRE-FORM AND ITS PRODUCTS (BOTTLES ETC.) MFG.
29. INDIAN INDUSTRIAL AND BUSINESS DIRECTORY
30. ESSENTIAL OILS MANUFACTURING & AROMATIC PLANTS
31. MODERN PACKAGING TECHNOLOGY FOR PROCESSED FOOD, BAKERY, SPICE & ALLIED FOOD
32. AGRO BASED HAND BOOK ON CULTIVATION, PLANTATION & FARMING
33. HAND BOOK OF PERFUMES & FLAVOURS
34. HAND BOOK OF SPICES & PACKAGING WITH FORMULAES
35. HAND BOOK OF HERBAL & SYNTHETIC COSMETICS
36. HAND BOOK OF ADHESIVES WITH THEIR FORMULAES
37. ELECTROPLATING ANODIZING & SURFACE TREATMENT TECHNOLOGY
38. HAND BOOK OF AYURVEDIC & HERBAL MEDICINES WITH FORMULAES
39. FRUITS & VEGETABLES PROCESSING HAND BOOK
40. HAND BOOK OF HERBS, MEDICINAL & AROMATIC PLANTS CULTIVATION
41. HAND BOOK OF CONFECTIONERY WITH & FORMULATIONS
42. MANUFACTURE OF SNACKS FOOD, NAMKEEN, PAPPAD & POTATO PRODUCTS
43. ESSENTIAL OIL PROCESSES AND FORMULATIONS HAND BOOK
44. SYNTHETIC RESINS TECHNOLOGY WITH FORMULATIONS
45. PAINT VARNISH SOLVENTS AND COATING TECHNOLOGY
46. COSMETICS PROCESSES AND FORMULATIONS HAND BOOK
47. HAND BOOK OF SYNTHETIC DETERGENTS WITH FORMULATIONS
48. AGRO CHEMICAL INDUSTRIES (INSECTICIDES AND PESTICIDES)
49. HERBAL COSMETICS AND BEAUTY PRODUCTS

Above all books available at :

ENGINEERS INDIA RESEARCH INSTITUTE

Regd. Off. :4449, Nai Sarak (B), Main Road, Delhi-110 006.(India)
Ph: 3916431, 3918117, 3920361, 3960797 * Fax: 91-11- 3916431
E-mail : eirisidi@bol.net.in, Website : www.startindustry.com

New Detailed Project Reports available on COSMETICS WITH HERBAL INDUSTRIES @ Rs. 3675/- each

LIST OF READILY AVAILABLE DETAILED PROJECT REPORTS

- AFTER SHAVE LOTION
- ANTISEPTIC CREAM
- ALLETHRIN MOSQUITO REPELLENT OIL
- AGARBATTI SYNTHETIC PERFUMERY COMPOUND
- BABY OIL
- BOROPLUS TYPE ANTISEPTIC CREAM
- AYURVEDIC MEDICINE
- BINDIYA
- BLACK TOOTH POWDER (MONKEY BRAND TYPE)
- BLACK HAIR DYE IN FORM OF HAIR OIL
- COLD CREAM
- COLD WAVE FOR HAIR CURLING
- COSMETIC UNIT (HERBAL AND SYNTHETIC)
- COSMETIC (MODERN)
- COSMETIC INDUSTRY, SHAMPOO, SPRAY PERFUME, TALCUM POWDER
- EGG SHAMPOO
- FACE MASK (LIQUID FORM)
- FISH OIL SOAP
- HAIR FIXER
- HAIR DYE POWDER
- HAIR DYE IN CREAM FORM
- HAIR REMOVING CREAM
- HAIR REMOVING WAX
- HAIR OILS
- HAIR FIXER & HAIR GEL
- HAIR STYLING GEL
- HENNA PASTE
- HERBAL COSMETICS
- HERBAL HAIR OIL
- HERBAL SHAMPOO & CREAM
- HERBAL TOOTH PASTE AND TOOTH POWDER
- HERBAL PRODUCTS COMPLEX
- KALI MEHANDI (HENNA)
- KAJAL
- KESH KALA TEL (HAIR DYE LOTION)
- LIQUID BINDI (KUMKUM TYPE)
- LIQUID BINDI AND SINDUR
- LIPSTICKS
- MEDICATED OIL
- MOSQUITO COIL & MATS
- NAIL POLISH & NAIL POLISH REMOVER
- NAIL ENAMEL
- NEUTRALIZER (FOR HAIR CURLING)
- SHAVING CREAM
- SINDUR
- TALCUM POWDER
- TOOTH PASTE AND POWDER
- TOILET AND HERBAL SOAP
- TOILET SOAP
- TOOTH PASTE (GEL TYPE)
- TOOTH PASTE FROM TOBACCO DUST
- WASHING AND LAUNDRY SOAP
- TOILET CLEANER (HARPIK TYPE)
- DOG SOAP

*Each 'EIRI' **Market Survey Cum Detailed Techno Economic Feasibility Report (Detailed Project Report)** covers Introduction, Properties, Market Survey, Process of Manufacture, Cost Economics with Profitability Analysis, Suppliers of Plant & Machineries and Raw Materials, Cash Flow Statement, Repayment Schedule, Depreciation Chart, Projected Balance Sheet etc.

*Price **Rs. 3675/-** (Rs. Three Thousand Six Hundred Seventy Five Only) for Each Report OR US$ 250/- for overseas clients. Just Send Draft/M.O./Cash in favour of **"ENGINEERS INDIA RESEARCH INSTITUTE", DELHI.** (Payable In India) (Delivery within Two Days)

ENGINEERS INDIA RESEARCH INSTITUTE
4449, Nai Sarak (D), Main Road, Delhi - 110 006 (India)
Ph:. 3918117, 3916431, 3920361, 3960797 Fax: 91-11- 3916431
E-Mail : eirisidi@bol.net.in * Website:www.startindustry.com